CANCER ETIOLOGY, DIAGNOSIS AND TREATMENTS

TAMOXIFEN CONCEPTS AND CANCER

NEW PARADIGMS

Cancer Etiology, Diagnosis and Treatments

Additional books in this series can be found on Nova's website under the Series tab.

Additional E-books in this series can be found on Nova's website under the E-book tab.

Pharmacology - Research, Safety Testing and Regulation

Additional books in this series can be found on Nova's website under the Series tab.

Additional E-books in this series can be found on Nova's website under the E-book tab.

CANCER ETIOLOGY, DIAGNOSIS AND TREATMENTS

TAMOXIFEN CONCEPTS AND CANCER

NEW PARADIGMS

RAMON ANDRADE DE MELLO
EDITOR

NOVA BIOMEDICAL

New York

For permission to use material from this book please contact us:
Telephone 631-231-7269; Fax 631-231-8175
Web Site: http://www.novapublishers.com

Library of Congress Cataloging-in-Publication Data

ISBN: 978-1-62081-520-5

Library of Congress Control Number: 2012947941

Published by Nova Science Publishers, Inc. † New York

Contents

Preface

Tamoxifen was first approved in 1977 and up to now remains a noteworthy therapeutic weapon to treat mainly breast cancer. However, further considerations exist regarding the tamoxifen profile. This book discusses recent research and future perspectives in the tamoxifen field. The topics discussed include tamoxifen pharmacokinetics, pharmacodynamics, adverse effects, clinical indications, therapeutic drug monitoring, autophagy mechanisms, tamoxifen topical formulation and breast cancer risk prevention, the use of tamoxifen in an estrogen-independent manner for various neoplasms (Hepatocellular carcinoma, renal cell carcinoma, high grade glioma), mechanisms of resistance, potential role of CYP2D6, tamoxifen and antidepressants interaction in a psychiatric view, obesity influence in tamoxifen treatment, electrical pulse-mediated tamoxifen delivery, and tamoxifen in melanoma treatment.

Chapter I - Currently, cancer is a disease highly prevalent worldwide. This is due to the new habits and lifestyle that increase overall risk in many populations regarding this disease. Furthermore, the constant increasing in life expectancy, mainly in developed countries, contributes to the emerging of several cancers. Breast cancer is the most prevalent type among women and many therapeutic weapons were developed toward the century in order to treat or reduce the risk of this entity. Tamoxifen was first approved in the cancer framework in the 1970s to the treatment of advanced breast cancer in post-menopausal women. Since 1977, tamoxifen was studied and applied in different treatment contexts, such as in adjuvant, or preventive setting. Moreover, the approach toward the hormonal receptors acquired a great benefit to the patients, due to the possibility of selecting those whom would have more clinical outcome. However, many researches in the field are still ongoing. Despite tamoxifen being a relatively old drug, its use is very important in the cancer setting and current studies may promise to bring novel issues in this regard. This chapter will briefly discuss and highlight introductory topics concerning tamoxifen approaches.

Chapter II - Tamoxifen is the most widely used anticancer drug in the world for the treatment of breast cancer. It is a selective estrogen receptor modulator (SERM) and exerts anti-estrogenic effect by binding to the estrogen receptor (ER) of breast cancer cells and thus inhibiting estrogen stimulated breast cancer growth. However, tamoxifen exhibits estrogenic activity in other tissues such as the uterus. Thus, the estrogen or anti-estrogen activity of tamoxifen depends on the target tissue. In tamoxifen treated breast cancer patients, tamoxifen has been detected in the uterus, liver, kidney, lung, pancreas, heart, and brain.

The metabolism of tamoxifen is complex, and shows considerable inter-individual variation. Genetic polymorphisms of tamoxifen-metabolizing enzymes and drug interactions have been shown to influence the metabolism of tamoxifen. Tamoxifen undergoes extensive hepatic metabolism by N-oxidation, hydroxylation, demethylation, sulfation, and glucuronidation. It has been regarded as a pro-drug that is hydroxylated to the clinically potent metabolite 4-hydroxytamoxifen (4OHtam). 4OHtam has a 30-100 fold higher anti-estrogenic activity compared to the parent drug. Another hydroxylated metabolite of tamoxifen, 4-hydroxy-N-desmethyltamoxifen (4OHNDtam, endoxifen) has been shown to be a potent anti-estrogen similar to 4OHtam. The efficacy of tamoxifen depends on the formation of these potent hydroxylated metabolites. N-desmethyltamoxifen (NDtam) is present in serum and tissues and at 30 times higher concentrations than that of the hydroxylated metabolites, and may contribute to both the anti-tumor effects and side effects of tamoxifen. The biological activity of NDtam appears to be similar to tamoxifen.

The most common side effects of tamoxifen are hot flashes and vaginal discharge and some patients also experience headaches, fatigue, nausea and/or vomiting, and vaginal dryness. Some serious side effects like thromboembolic disease and endometrial cancer are due to its estrogen agonistic effects. Despite its side effects, the benefits of tamoxifen treatment are considerably larger and are still without debate.

The tamoxifen dose used is based on the maximum tolerated dose rather than the optimal biological dose. In a short term clinical study we observed that a reduced dose from the conventional dose of 20 mg to 1 mg daily caused reduction or disappearance of the estrogen agonistic effects in blood parameters whereas the effects on the growth parameter Ki-67 was unchanged. In addition, studies suggest that a reduction in dose may decrease the side effects of tamoxifen. The high inter-subject variability in the measured serum levels of tamoxifen and its metabolites and the accepted criteria for therapeutic drug monitoring (TDM) that apply for tamoxifen suggests that TDM may be used to improve tamoxifen treatment.

Chapter III - Tamoxifen, a selective estrogen receptor modulator (SERM), is the most widely used antiestrogen monotherapy for the treatment of estrogen receptor positive (ER+) breast cancer. Although effective in reducing tumor growth and increasing overall patient survival, 20-30% of women treated with tamoxifen ultimately acquire resistance to the treatment. Resistance to tamoxifen has been attributed to both ER-dependent and ER-independent effects, but the underlying mechanisms are still not well understood. One of the many biological effects of tamoxifen is the induction of autophagy, a cellular process of "self-eating" that plays various roles in homeostasis, development, and stress adaptation. Autophagy has been implicated in the cellular response to numerous anticancer therapies, including tamoxifen. It is an evolutionarily conserved catabolic process that involves sequestration of long-lived proteins and organelles from the cytoplasm in a double membrane structure known as an autophagosome. The autophagosome fuses with a lysosome to form an autolysosome that enables the contents of the autophagosome to be degraded and released back into the cytoplasm for bioenergetic or biosynthetic processes. The roles of autophagy in breast cancer, as well as other cancer types, are still largely unknown. It was demonstrated that when breast cancer cell lines are treated with cytotoxic concentrations of tamoxifen, autophagy is increased. When tamoxifen treatment is combined with autophagy inhibition, breast cancer cell viability decreased. These observations indicate that autophagy has a primary survival or protective role in the context of the cellular response to tamoxifen. Further studies suggested that autophagy may play a critical role in the development of tamoxifen resistance. However, the molecular mechanisms that contribute to this outcome require further investigation. This chapter summarizes our current understanding of the interaction between tamoxifen and the autophagy pathway in breast cancer.

Chapter IV - Tamoxifen is widely used in the treatment of primary and recurrent breast cancer, and it can enter the aquatic environment in its native form or as transformed excretory products like other human pharmaceuticals. Therefore, the possible adverse effects of tamoxifen on aquatic animals, particularly on various species of fish, should be of concern. Moreover, against the pharmacology of a selective estrogen-receptor modulator (SERM), tamoxifen has become a powerful research tool in fish endocrinology and is recommended as a reference compound in fish testing to aid extrapolation across other SERMs. To date, the endocrine disruptions of tamoxifen in fish have been comprehensively assessed by biochemical endpoints, growth and morphological alternations and measurements of reproductive performance using several model fish. These results demonstrated that exposure to tamoxifen displayed the potential impacts on vitellogenin protein levels, gonad histology and reproductive capacity, although the exposure levels were considerably greater than the real environmental concentration. Recently, some works employing gene expression endpoints have provided more mechanistic understandings of the action of tamoxifen. Additionally, as an anti-estrogenic chemical, the modulatory influences of tamoxifen on the action of estrogens such as estradiol (E2) and ethinylestradiol (EE2) were evaluated, which showed that the presence of tamoxifen appeared to mask many signs of the impacts of environmental estrogens, but not neutralize the impaired reproductive capacity. Comparison of available toxicity data with environmental concentration indicates that tamoxifen may not induce adverse ecotoxicological effects in the aquatic system. However, considering the lack of information about the fate of tamoxifen and its possible interaction with other environmental pollutants, as well as the remained controversial results, more investigations are needed for accurate and comprehensive risk assessments of tamoxifen.

Chapter V - Tamoxifen has long been a mainstay of treatment of estrogen receptor (ER)-positive breast cancer in both the metastatic and adjuvant settings. In 1998, results from the large phase III Breast Cancer Prevention Trial (conducted by the National Surgical Adjuvant Breast and Bowel Project/NSABP) led to the Food and Drug Administration's approval of tamoxifen for reduction of breast cancer incidence in high-risk women. The toxicities associated with tamoxifen, particularly endometrial cancer and thromboembolic events, have hampered the drug's uptake by high-risk women who should benefit from its preventive effects. Among the strategies to overcome such obstacles to preventive tamoxifen use is the investigation of novel, and potentially safer, modes of delivery of this agent. Two novel approaches are discussed in this chapter. Low-dose tamoxifen, expected to confer fewer adverse events, is being examined by varying both dose and interval of administration. Low-dose tamoxifen is being investigated in in both clinical biomarker-based trials and observational studies. Modulation of systemic biomarkers, including lipid and IGF levels, and tissue biomarkers, including Ki-67, which are known to be favorably affected by conventional tamoxifen dosing, has been observed. These findings suggest possible beneficial clinical prevention effects from novel low-dose tamoxifen regimens. An alternative approach is administration of topical forms of tamoxifen directly to breast tissue in high-risk women. Avoidance of systemic administration is expected to limit the distribution of drug to tissues susceptible to tamoxifen-induced toxicity. While clinical trials of topical tamoxifen are still ongoing, laboratory data suggest that appropriate formulations of drug successfully penetrate the skin to reach breast tissue, where a preventive effect is expected.

Chapter VI - Tamoxifen has been shown to be an excellent treatment against neoplasms with increased expression of the estrogen receptor. In addition, tamoxifen and its metabolites have been shown to have antineoplastic activity through estrogen-independent inhibition of protein kinase C (PKC) pathways and MAP kinase cascades. This pathway has been used to treat a number of neoplasms including hepatocellular carcinoma, metastatic melanoma, prostate cancer and high-grade gliomas.

Early trials of the addition of tamoxifen to best available therapies for hepatocellular carcinoma and metastatic melanoma in small cohorts have shown improved survival. Additionally, studies of patients with recurrent high-grade gliomas demonstrated accumulation of tamoxifen in malignant cells by biopsy. Intracellular transport of tamoxifen in micromolar concentrations is sufficient to inhibit the PKC activity in glioma cell lines in vitro. These low doses are sufficient to induce apoptosis in these cell lines. Recent studies of the genomic and proteomic perturbations in high grade gliomas have shown an increased activity of protein kinase C (PKC) dependent pathways. Furthermore, tamoxifen and its metabolite, N-desmethyltamoxifen, have been shown to cross the blood-brain barrier and accumulate within tumors to therapeutic levels.

Through estrogen-independent modification of PKC, tamoxifen may present an additional treatment in the armamentarium against neoplastic diseases including high grade gliomas when used in conjunction with the standard of care. This chapter will review the pathways of tamoxifen induced apoptosis that are estrogen-independent as well as results from studies of the utility of tamoxifen in the treatment of various estrogen receptor negative cancers.

Chapter VII - Tamoxifen has become the drug of choice for the treatment of estrogen receptor positive (ER^{+ve}) early breast cancer; it has also gained recognition for its potential in the treatment of other disorders, including PCOS and bipolar mania. The duality of Tamoxifen action, acting as an antagonist in ER^{+ve} breast cancer and a partial agonist in other tissues, was originally unexpected as it was believed it would act as an antagonist throughout the body. This dual action has led to some highly beneficial effects, for example, prevention of osteoporosis, and some extreme side effects including increasing the risk for endometrial cancer. Tamoxifen has also found a role as a component of many complex treatments for various cancers and disorders, giving this drug new life and new expanded limitations. However, Tamoxifen faces stiff competition in the form of aromatase inhibitors that have been touted as being both more effective and having fewer side effects, although it has been proposed that some side effects, for example, memory impairment, may be even more severe for aromatase inhibitors. The undesired effects of aromatase inhibitors have been suggested to act through other mechanisms to produce some effects both intentional and undesired. Yet in the face of this competition and the unwanted side effects, Tamoxifen still holds the title of drug of choice.

The mechanisms of action, the side effects and the broad range of applications have led to Tamoxifen being intensively studied. While its target, the estrogen receptor (ER), explains many of the pathways Tamoxifen influences, its effects in other pathways are not so obvious. Recent studies have suggested that the number of signaling pathways affected by or affecting its action is very broad. The involvement of a wide range of signaling molecules has the potential to explain the effects, side effects and limitations of this drug. Furthermore, insight into these intracellular effects may unlock more surprises in the capabilities of this drug. The efficacy this drug demonstrates and its broad range of applications have been at the core of its success. This chapter seeks to examine the signaling pathways associated with Tamoxifen action and resistance and relate these to its effects on cancer and other disorders, as well as discussing the future implications for this drug.

Chapter VIII - Tamoxifen is the most widely used adjuvant endocrine therapy for breast cancer in pre- and postmenopausal women. Long-term studies have shown tamoxifen therapy to reduce the occurrence and reoccurrence of breast cancer and to prolong survival of patients with breast cancer and those predisposed to breast cancer. Early research with tamoxifen and other triphenylethylene compounds demonstrated their partial estrogenic activity but, perhaps more importantly, identified their antiestrogenic properties.

On the basis of this antiestrogenic activity, tamoxifen was approved in 1977 by the US Food and Drug Administration as adjuvant therapy in postmenopausal women with node positive breast cancer. Tamoxifen has also been approved to help reduce the risk for invasive breast cancer in women with ductal carcinoma *in situ* and to help reduce the incidence of breast cancer in women at high risk for such cancers. The demonstrated efficacy of tamoxifen in ER-positive breast cancers has led to the development and approval of aromatase inhibitor drugs, as well as to the conductance of large clinical trials comparing the two adjuvant hormonal therapies.

Clinical guidelines now recommend tamoxifen for premenopausal breast cancer patients and sequential aromatase inhibitor and tamoxifen therapies in postmenopausal patients especially those with high risk of recurrence. Long-term studies of tamoxifen have led to multiple discoveries: that to be optimally active tamoxifen must be metabolized to 4-hydroxytamoxifen and 4-hydroxy-N-desmethyltamoxifen (endoxifen) by cytochrome P450 systems, that CYP2D6 polymorphisms affect tamoxifen metabolism and may affect clinical outcomes, and that not all ER-positive breast cancer patients respond to tamoxifen.

Tamoxifen, as a selective estrogen receptor modulator, has direct estrogenic activities in that it preserves bone mineral density and has favorable effects on serum lipids. However, concerns with the drug include the invariable acquired resistance, a small but significant risk of developing uterine cancer, and in patients who took the drug for at least five years, the increased risk of developing ER-negative and perhaps more difficult to treat contralateral breast cancers.

Tamoxifen continues to be studied in preclinical and clinical settings and further genetic marker studies may identify populations that benefit most from adjuvant tamoxifen treatment.

Chapter IX - Tamoxifen is a well-established endocrine therapy used in the treatment of hormone-receptor positive breast cancer. In recent years, its role in adjuvant and advanced breast cancer settings has been superseded by aromatase inhibitors. The prodrug tamoxifen is metabolised in the liver into several primary and secondary metabolites via cytochrome P450 enzymes. The main active forms are endoxifen and 4-hydroxytamoxifen, with CYP2D6 being a key enzyme in the production of both.

There is evidence that tamoxifen-associated hot flushes are an indicator of clinical efficacy of tamoxifen. Co-prescription of CYP2D6 inhibitors, including selective serotonin re-uptake inhibitors (SSRIs) commonly used to treat hot flushes, may decrease the clinical efficacy of tamoxifen and should be used with caution. Moreover, there is evidence that patients with poor CYP2D6-mediated tamoxifen metaboliser phenotype have worse clinical outcomes, and fewer hot flushes, than those with other phenotypes.

Further research is necessary to clarify whether extensive metabolisers have the best clinical outcomes on tamoxifen.

Preliminary data suggest that in individuals of certain CYP2D6 phenotype, tamoxifen may have equivalent efficacy, and be considered as an alternative to aromatase inhibitors if there were concerns over the side effect profile and cost of the latter. Thus the role of tamoxifen may be redefined in a new era of personalised breast cancer treatment.

Chapter X - Breast cancer is the most commonly diagnosed cancer in women worldwide, and many patients experience clinically significant depression that require psychiatric intervention. Tamoxifen is a selective oestrogen receptor modulator that reduces the risk of recurrence in early-stage patients whose tumour cells express the oestrogen receptor. To be effective, it depends on metabolic activation via cytochrome P450 2D6 (CYP2D6). Many medications, including antidepressants used for hot flashes, pain or depression in breast cancer patients, may compromise CYP2D6 activity and interfere with plasma concentration of endoxifen (tamoxifen active metabolic), affecting survival in those patients. With so many treatment options, many questions arise about which antidepressant to choose in those patients. The data suggest that strong CYP2D6 inhibitors, such as fluoxetine and paroxetine, should probably be avoided, and weak inhibitors (venlafaxine, mirtazapine and citalopram) are safer choices, with less potential to decrease the clinical efficacy of tamoxifen. Studies with long follow-up periods and with greater power to look at individual antidepressants are necessary.

Chapter XI - *Background.* Breast cancer is the most frequent type of cancer in women. Epidemiological studies suggest that lifestyle factors including dietary patterns and physical activity play a significant role in the development and survival of breast cancer. In particular, there is convincing evidence that obesity is a potent risk factor for both cancer development and prognosis.

The pathophysiological link is not fully elucidated, but may include an increased estrogen production by adipose-tissue stromal cells, elevated levels of insulin and insulin-like growth factor (IGF)-1, increased adipose tissue-derived factors (adipokines), and possibly other mechanisms related to an expanded fat mass.

In addition, the pharmacological therapy in estrogen-positive breast cancer is a hormonal therapy focused in diminishing the estrogen levels, Tamoxifen. Thus, if high fat volume is associated with elevated levels of serum estrogen, an important question is whether obesity affects treatment efficacy, and if modifiable risk factors related to lifestyle and obesity could be an important and necessary part of the breast cancer treatment.

Conclusion. There is convincing evidence of the association between obesity and breast cancer risk and prognosis, consequently more studies of the effect of lifestyle factors such as diet patterns, physical activity and body mass index in breast cancer hormonal treatment as Tamoxifen are needed. Integral treatment including additional strategies that target other potential mediators of obesity-related prognostics effects are also necessary to improve prognosis in these patients.

Chapter XII - Tamoxifen is one of the most effective anti-hormonal agents for the treatment of estrogen receptor-positive breast cancer, for both pre- and post-menopausal patients. However, with its poor response rate of 21% to 41%, it is not benefitting all the estrogen receptor-positive (ER+) patients. This necessitates its delivery using other means, whose attributes include less-invasive, physical and lower dosages. Electrical pulse-mediated drug delivery is gaining momentum as a promising alternate technique. This involves the application of high intensity, short pulses that open up the normally impermeable cell plasma membranes allowing the external drug molecules in. This chapter presents the findings of the in vitro study of electrical pulse-mediated Tamoxifen delivery on MCF-7 breast cancer cells at low and high voltages and at various durations, from milli to micro to nanoseconds, and their efficacies. Our results indicate the proliferation control of breast cancer cells using as low as one to five μM dosages of Tamoxifen at an electric field strenth of 200V/cm and the potential of transferring this technique for clinical use for treating those patients who do not respond well to current Tamoxifen therapy.

Chapter XIII - Throughout the years, multiple studies showed the benefits of tamoxifen (Tam) for cancers, other than breast and ovarian cancers, such as advanced melanoma, mesothelioma tumors, glioblastomas, colon cancer, lung cancer and urological cancer. Although tamoxifen is widely used in conjunction with cytotoxic agents for advanced melanoma and may modify the disease response to such drugs in a positive manner, there is still some controversy as to whether strong evidence exists to support this practice. Moreover, debate continues on which is the main mechanism of action of Tam in melanoma, the most life threatening form of skin cancer. Melanoma is one of the most common forms of cancers in the U.S., with approximately 63,130 new cases of diagnosed in 2010, according to the figures from the National Cancer Institute.

Recent data indicate that the estrogen receptor (ER) blocker, tamoxifen, can induce cell death in malignant melanoma cells through a variety of mechanisms. It can even enhance the synergy with other drugs used in melanoma treatments such as cisplatin (DDP). The specific biochemical interaction through which tamoxifen produces its pharmacological effect in this cancer, has been shown to be through a calcium channel blocking property, delaying the resistance to DDP, and consequently, sensitizing melanoma cancer cells to chemotherapeutic agents. Tam also works by stimulating the immune system, increasing the level of natural killers, along with other important modifications, which in turn, helps constraining the growth control of the most deadly skin cancer of all. Moreover, it has been found that induction of apoptosis and inhibition of angiogenesis are alternative ways in which tamoxifen suppresses tumor cell growth. At the same time, it has the potential of acting through endocrine and paracrine mechanism inhibiting the anchorage- dependent growth of melanoma. Additionally, tamoxifen has been found to increase the secretion of the transforming growth factor- beta (TGF β), which inhibits the growth of several estrogen-receptor-negative cancers.

Even though the tamoxifen is still used in the therapy of advanced melanoma (Stages III-IV), debate continues among scientists on which is the explanation of its mechanism of action. This chapter presents the updated knowledge regarding the biochemical interactions, particularly on melanoma response and resistance, through which tamoxifen produces its pharmacological effect.

In: Tamoxifen Concepts and Cancer: New Paradigms
Editor: Ramon Andrade de Mello
ISBN: 978-1-62081-520-5

Chapter I

Introduction to Tamoxifen in Novel Approaches

Ramon Andrade de Mello[1,2,*]
[1]Department of Medicine, Faculty of Medicine,
University of Porto, Porto, Portugal
[2]Department of Medical Oncology,
Portuguese Oncology Institute, Porto, Portugal

Abstract

Currently, cancer is a disease highly prevalent worldwide. This is due to the new habits and lifestyle that increase overall risk in many populations regarding this disease. Furthermore, the constant increasing in life expectancy, mainly in developed countries, contributes to the emerging of several cancers. Breast cancer is the most prevalent type among women and many therapeutic weapons were developed toward the century in order to treat or reduce the risk of this entity. Tamoxifen was first approved in the cancer framework in the 1970s to the treatment of advanced breast cancer in post-menopausal women. Since 1977, tamoxifen was studied and applied in different treatment contexts, such as in adjuvant, or preventive setting. Moreover, the approach toward the hormonal receptors acquired a great benefit to the patients, due to the possibility of selecting those whom would have more clinical outcome. However, many researches in the field are still ongoing. Despite tamoxifen being a relatively old drug, its use is very important in the cancer setting and current studies may promise to bring novel issues in this regard. This chapter will briefly discuss and highlight introductory topics concerning tamoxifen approaches.

[*] E-mail: ramonmello@med.up.pt or ramondemello@gmail.com.

Introduction

Cancer is a highly prevalent disease worldwide. It is related with high mortality and morbidity. GLOBOCAM 2008 estimated about 12.7 million cancer cases and 7.6 million cancer-related deaths in 2008. Breast cancer is the most commom type among women and it is the leading cause of cancer-deaths among female in economically developing countries [1]. Research concerning its clinical management had been done throughout the centuries. Since 1977, tamoxifen was first approved by The Food and Drugs Administration (FDA) to the treatment of advanced breast cancer in postmenopausal women. This drug is an antiestrogenic selective agent, antineoplasic agent and selective estrogen receptor modulator. Many studies supported the role of tamoxifen in other therapeutic indications, such as adjuvant treatment or cancer prevention in the breast cancer setting. Therefore, taking into consideration all of those paramount features regarding tamoxifen, this chapter will highlight an introductory and brief discussion to the recent and future topics concerning tamoxifen approaches.

Metabolism and Pharmacogenomics Approaches

Tamoxifen acts mainly toward the interaction with estrogen receptors (ER) positive tumors. Some studies support that only a few number of ER positive cells in tumors are warranted to the patients who acquire benefits regarding hormonal therapy. Tamoxifen activity metabolites mainly are Alpha-hydroxy-, N-desmethyl- and N-didesmethyl-Tamoxifen. Recently, CYP3A4 and CYP2D6 seems to mediate tamoxifen metabolism and perhaps have influence in its activity [2]. Patients whom have reduced CYP2D6 activity, because of their genotype or either by the administration of drugs that inhibit CY2D6 function, produce less endoxifen than normal patients and thus have reduced therapeutic benefit from tamoxifen [3]. Then, this genetic polymorphism had been exhaustively studied in the pharmacogenomics field and perhaps may become a new weapon in the near future in order to improve patient's outcome. Also, it was previously demonstrated that tamoxifen acts through both ER α and ER β. However, the interaction between ER α seems to provide more clinical efficacy. Furthermore, tamoxifen‘s effects cannot be explained only by these estrogens receptors pathways. Further research supports the hypothesis that its drugs have also anti-apoptotic effects and influence in cell autophagy [4].

Safety Issues and Adverse Reactions

Normally, tamoxifen is a safe and very useful drug in the common oncology practice. However, medical oncologists should to be aware of the possible adverse reactions concerning this drug. Cardiovascular effects, such as vasodilatation, flushing, peripheral edema, and hypertension may occur in more than 10% of patients. Furthermore, the central nervous system's effects are frequently depression, mood changes and pain. In clinical practice, it is sometimes difficult to distinguish if the patients have depression due to use of tamoxifen, or due to the breast cancer itself. Other important side-effects commonly observed in the ambulatory are hot flashers, fluid retention, amenorrhea, vaginal discharge or bleeding, arthralgia, and weakness [5].

Warning and Precautions

Briefly, tamoxifen is a well-tolerated and safe drug. Nevertheless, patients and their physicians should to be aware somewhat to possible serious side-effects. First, bone marrow suppression may occur by the existence of thrombocytopenia and leucopenia. Second, some studies have reported hepatocellular carcinoma related to tamoxifen therapy [6], but the relationship in not entirely clear. Third, it is frequently reported that tamoxifen is associated with an increased risk of uterine and endometrial cancer in women at high risk to breast cancer or with ductal in situ carcinoma using this drug in order to breast cancer risk reduction [7]. Also, serious and life-threatening thromboembolic events, including stroke and pulmonary emboli have occurred at an incidence greater than placebo in women treated with tamoxifen [8].

Current Indications

Breast Cancer Adjuvant Treatment

In patients with estrogen receptor positive breast cancer, 5 years 20 mg/day of adjuvant tamoxifen can be indicated. Its approach reduces the 15 year relapse by approximately 40% and mortality 35% [9]. The treatment is recommended to begin after chemotherapy and radiotherapy. Further, adjustment with others drugs should be done considering its interactions, such as warfarin and anti-depressants.

Breast Cancer Metastatic

In the breast cancer metastatic setting, hormone-therapy has also a main role. Tamoxifen was established as a favorable toxicity and favorable response for metastatic estrogen positive breast cancer women. Postmenopausal women have an overall response rate of 30 to 60% and premenopausal women had lower response rate than those postmenopausal [10]. However, other hormone-therapy options, such as aromatase inhibitors and fulvestran, recently emerged as promising in the field.

Ductal Carcinoma in Situ

Ductal Carcinoma in Situ (DCIS) incidence has increased in the last decades mainly due to improvement of mammography screening technics. The key to successful treatment is to prevent the development of this invasive disease. Therapeutic options are surgery, radiotherapy and endocrine adjuvant therapy. The addition of tamoxifen to surgery and RT significantly showed reduced risk of ipsilateral invasive and contralateral in situ recurrence [11]. However, tamoxifen's benefit in this setting seems to be restricted to DCIS estrogen positive tumors [12].

Breast Cancer Prevention

Tamoxifen, as well as raloxifen, have anti-estrogenic activity that can also reduce epithelial cell proliferation. Thus, this property leads to many studies in the context of breast cancer prevention. Its related mechanism runs toward the reduction of transforming growth factor alfa, reduction of insulin like growth factor I, stimulation of transforming growth factor beta, binding to calmodulin and inhibition of protein kinase activity [13]. Nevertheless, many trials assessed the use of tamoxifen to reduce breast cancer risk in those women previous considered with high-risk of breast cancer. Those trials' results after assessment by meta-analysis showed a significant reduction of breast cancer risk after 5 years using tamoxifen. This effect remained at least 3 to 5 years after discontinuous therapy, but did not report effective in mortality [14]. Nowadays, novel studies [15-18] also suggest topical and transdermal applications of tamoxifen metabolites as promising approaches in order to prevent breast cancer in high-risk estrogen positive patients.

Off-Label Indications

Nowadays, off-label (unapproved) use of medications is a common practice and permitted in the United States and other territories worldwide. In 2010, an Israelite group conducted a study in order to assess the extent of off-label prescribing of tamoxifen and to ascertain what evidence is available to support the use of the drug for the off-label indications observed [5]. Here, there are somewhat off-labels indications reported in their study: ovarian cancer, Paget's disease of the breast, polycystic ovary syndrome (PCOS), precocious puberty and McCune-Albright syndrome (unlabeled use), and Metastatic melanoma. Of the 25 diagnosed categories of off-label indications, only 8 met criteria to be defined as "supported". Overall, tamoxifen was found to be off-label used in 5.8% of patients who received this drug in the study period and only 2.1% of all patients did receive tamoxifen for a diagnosis without efficacy supporting evidence. Thus, off-label use of tamoxifen seems not to be a health problem, but sometimes a rationale-based evidence option in difficult clinical situations.

Current and Future Directions

Nowadays, despite tamoxifen being an old drug, it still remains an important therapeutic option mainly to breast cancer prevention, in an adjuvant/metastatic setting and DCIS treatment. This drug may be considered one of the first target therapies in clinical practice, due to its property of interactions specific toward estrogen receptors. However, in the hormone-therapy class agents, aromatase inhibitors and fulvestran also emerged as good options in this framework. In the next chapters of this book, novel approaches and recent issues regarding this drug property, biological activities and health benefits will be discussed.

Acknowledgments

I would like to thank Ms. Cristina Rocha and Ms. Isabel Estrela, Department of Medical Oncology, Portuguese Oncology Institute, Porto, Portugal, for their technical support.

References

[1] Jemal, A., Bray, F., Center, M., Ferlay, J., Ward, E., D.F. Global cancer statistics. *CA Cancer J. Clin.* 2011;61(2):69-90.

[2] Li-Wan-Po, A., Girard, T., Farndon, P., Cooley, C., Lithgow, J. Pharmacogenetics of CYP2C19: functional and clinical implications of a new variant CYP2C19*17. *Br. J. Clin. Pharmacol.* 2010;69(3):222-30.

[3] Higgins, M., Rae, J., Flockhart, D., Hayes, D., Stearns, V. Pharmacogenetics of tamoxifen: who should undergo CYP2D6 genetic testing? *J. Natl. Compr. Canc. Netw.* 2009;7(2):203-13.

[4] Bursch, W., Ellinger, A., Kienzl, H., Török, L., Pandey, S., Sikorska, M., et al. Active cell death induced by the anti-estrogens tamoxifen and ICI 164 384 in human mammary carcinoma cells (MCF-7) in culture: the role of autophagy. *Carcinogenesis.* 1996 17(8):1595-607.

[5] Kahan, N., Waitman, D., Blackman, S., Vardy, D. Drug Use Evaluation of Tamoxifen Focusing on Off-Label Use in a Managed Care Population in Israel. *J. Manag. Care Pharm.* 2010;16(5):355-9.

[6] Moffat, D., Oien, K., Dickson, J., Habeshaw, T., McLellan, D. Hepatocellular carcinoma after long-term tamoxifen therapy. *Ann. Oncol.* 2000;11(9):1195-6.

[7] Karimi Zarchi, M., Behtash, N., Sekhavat, L., Dehghan, A. Effects of tamoxifen on the cervix and uterus in women with breast cancer: experience with Iranian patients and a literature review. *Asian Pac. J. Cancer Prev.* 2009;10(4):595-8.

[8] Noble, S., Pasi, J. Epidemiology and pathophysiology of cancer-associated thrombosis. *Br. J. Cancer.* 2010;102(Suppl 1):S2-9.

[9] Davies, C., Godwin, J., Gray, R., Clarke, M., Cutter, D., Darby, S., et al. Relevance of breast cancer hormone receptors and other factors to the efficacy of adjuvant tamoxifen: patient-level meta-analysis of randomized trials. *Lancet.* 2011 378(9793):771-84.

[10] Osborne, C. Tamoxifen in the treatment of breast cancer. *N. Engl. J. Med.* 1998;339(22): 1609-18.

[11] Petrelli, F., Barni, S. Tamoxifen added to radiotherapy and surgery for the treatment of ductal carcinoma in situ of the breast: a meta-analysis of 2 randomized trials. *Radiother. Oncol.* 2011;100(2):195-9.

[12] Eng-Wong, J., Costantino, J., Swain, S. The impact of systemic therapy following ductal carcinoma in situ. *J. Natl. Cancer Inst. Monogr.* 2010;2010(41):200-3.

[13] Friedman, Z. Recent advances in understanding the molecular mechanisms of tamoxifen action. *Cancer Invest.* 1998;16(6):391-6.

[14] Nelson, H., Fu, R., Griffin, J., Nygren, P., Smith, M., Humphrey, L. Systematic review: comparative effectiveness of medications to reduce risk for primary breast cancer. *Ann. Intern. Med.* 2009;151(10):703-15.

[15] Pujol, H., Girault, J., Rouanet, P., Fournier, S., Grenier, J., Simony, J., et al. Phase I study of percutaneous 4-hydroxy-tamoxifen with analyses of 4-hydroxy-tamoxifen concentrations in breast cancer and normal breast tissue. *Cancer Chemother. Pharmacol.* 1995;36(6):492-8.

[16] Rouanet, P., Linares-Cruz, G., Dravet, F., Poujol, S., Gourgou, S., Simony-Lafontaine, J., et al. Neoadjuvant percutaneous 4-hydroxytamoxifen decreases breast tumoral cell proliferation: a prospective controlled randomized study comparing three doses of 4-hydroxytamoxifen gel to oral tamoxifen. *J. Clin. Oncol.* 2005;23(13):2980-7.

[17] Chiesa, M., Passalacqua, R., Michiara, M., Franciosi, V., Di Costanzo, F., Bisagni, G., et al. Tamoxifen vs Tamoxifen plus 13-cis-retinoic acid vs Tamoxifen plus Interferon alpha-2a as first-line endocrine treatments in advanced breast cancer: updated results of a phase II, prospective, randomised multicentre trial. *Acta Biomed.* 2007;78(3):204-9.

[18] Lee, O., Ivancic, D., Chatterton, R., Rademaker, A., Khan, S. In vitro human skin permeation of endoxifen: potential for local transdermal therapy for primary prevention and carcinoma in situ of the breast. *Breast Cancer: Targets and Therapy.* 2011;3(1):61-70.

In: Tamoxifen Concepts and Cancer: New Paradigms
Editor: Ramon Andrade de Mello
ISBN: 978-1-62081-520-5

Chapter II

Tamoxifen Metabolism and Biological Activity

Jennifer Gjerde*[1,2,*]*, Line L. Haugan Moi*[1,3]*,
***Gunnar Mellgren*[1,2] *and Ernst A. Lien*[1,2]

[1]Institute of Medicine, University of Bergen, Bergen, Norway
[2]The Hormone Laboratory, Haukeland University Hospital, Bergen, Norway
[3]Department of Clinical Pathology,
The University Hospital of North Norway, Tromsø, Norway

Abstract

Tamoxifen is the most widely used anticancer drug in the world for the treatment of breast cancer. It is a selective estrogen receptor modulator (SERM) and exerts anti-estrogenic effect by binding to the estrogen receptor (ER) of breast cancer cells and thus inhibiting estrogen stimulated breast cancer growth. However, tamoxifen exhibits estrogenic activity in other tissues such as the uterus. Thus, the estrogen or anti-estrogen activity of tamoxifen depends on the target tissue. In tamoxifen treated breast cancer patients, tamoxifen has been detected in the uterus, liver, kidney, lung, pancreas, heart, and brain.

The metabolism of tamoxifen is complex, and shows considerable inter-individual variation. Genetic polymorphisms of tamoxifen-metabolizing enzymes and drug interactions have been shown to influence the metabolism of tamoxifen. Tamoxifen undergoes extensive hepatic metabolism by N-oxidation, hydroxylation, demethylation, sulfation, and glucuronidation. It has been regarded as a pro-drug that is hydroxylated to the clinically potent metabolite 4-hydroxytamoxifen (4OHtam). 4OHtam has a 30-100 fold higher anti-estrogenic activity compared to the parent drug. Another hydroxylated metabolite of tamoxifen, 4-hydroxy-N-desmethyltamoxifen (4OHNDtam, endoxifen) has been shown to be a potent anti-estrogen similar to 4OHtam. The efficacy of tamoxifen depends on the formation of these potent hydroxylated metabolites. N-desmethyltamoxifen (NDtam) is present in serum and tissues and at 30 times higher

* E-mail: Jennifer.Gjerde@med.uib.no.

concentrations than that of the hydroxylated metabolites, and may contribute to both the anti-tumor effects and side effects of tamoxifen. The biological activity of NDtam appears to be similar to tamoxifen.

The most common side effects of tamoxifen are hot flashes and vaginal discharge and some patients also experience headaches, fatigue, nausea and/or vomiting, and vaginal dryness. Some serious side effects like thromboembolic disease and endometrial cancer are due to its estrogen agonistic effects. Despite its side effects, the benefits of tamoxifen treatment are considerably larger and are still without debate.

The tamoxifen dose used is based on the maximum tolerated dose rather than the optimal biological dose. In a short term clinical study we observed that a reduced dose from the conventional dose of 20 mg to 1 mg daily caused reduction or disappearance of the estrogen agonistic effects in blood parameters whereas the effects on the growth parameter Ki-67 was unchanged. In addition, studies suggest that a reduction in dose may decrease the side effects of tamoxifen. The high inter-subject variability in the measured serum levels of tamoxifen and its metabolites and the accepted criteria for therapeutic drug monitoring (TDM) that apply for tamoxifen suggests that TDM may be used to improve tamoxifen treatment.

Introduction

Tamoxifen was patented by ICI Pharmaceuticals (AstraZeneca) as ICI46474 and is sold under the trade names Tamoxifen, Nolvadex, Tamofen, Isbutal, and Valodex. Tamoxifen is the trans-isomer of 1(p-β-dimethylaminoethoxy-phenyl)-1,2-dephenylbut-1-ene. It is a non-steroidal anti-estrogen and a selective estrogen receptor modulator (SERM) and exerts its effect by binding to the ER of breast cancer cells, thereby inhibiting estrogen stimulated breast cancer growth. Tamoxifen was introduced as an endocrine therapy in 1971 [1] and was approved by the US Food and Drug administration (FDA) as an adjuvant therapy with chemotherapy in 1986, as an adjuvant therapy alone in 1988, and has ever since been a front line drug in the treatment of breast cancer [2, 3]. Tamoxifen is the drug of choice in adjuvant endocrine treatment in premenopausal women and tamoxifen alone is still an option for postmenopausal patients [4, 5]. In 2011, tamoxifen is the most widely used anticancer drug for both treatment and prevention of breast cancer [5-7].

Breast Cancer Treatment

As a general priniciple, surgery with removal of the tumor and affected lymph nodes is the primary treatment of breast cancer, when possible. Adjuvant therapy including endocrine treatment (if hormone receptor positive cancer), trastuzumab (if human epidermal growth factor receptor 2/neu (HER-2/neu) positive cancer), chemotherapy and radiotherapy can be given in order to reduce the risk of recurrence due to microscopic spread of the disease or to stall disease progression. Chemotherapy, or less commonly endocrine therapy, can also be used in the neoadjuvant setting and is standard in locally advanced breast cancer.

Endocrine treatment is the first and oldest targeted therapy in breast cancer and considered a standard adjuvant therapy in all patients with endocrine-responsive tumors, i.e. immunohistochemical expression of estrogen receptor (ER) and progesterone receptor (PR).

It has been shown to improve long term relapse-free survival as well as overall survival in pre- as well as postmenopausal breast cancer patients. Tamoxifen treatment is the drug of choice in adjuvant endocrine treatment in premenopausal women. In postmenopausal patients aromatase inhibitors are recognized as the first line endocrine treatment in the adjuvant setting. However, selected patients could be treated with tamoxifen alone, or switched to tamoxifen if found to be intolerant or resistant to aromatase inhibitors. Tamoxifen is still widely used in the adjuvant setting also in male breast cancer. The antitumor effects of tamoxifen in advanced breast cancer have also been well documented for decades [8, 9]. In addition, it is the only drug approved for use in breast cancer chemoprevention.

Tamoxifen Metabolism

Tamoxifen is administered orally and undergoes extensive metabolism in the liver. The bioconversion of tamoxifen involves phase I and phase II metabolism [10]. Phase I metabolism occurs primarily in the liver and increases the water solubility of tamoxifen by introducing a hydroxyl group [11, 12]. The hydroxylated metabolites may undergo phase II metabolism by enzymes that catalyze glucuronidation or sulfation [10, 13-16]. The conjugated metabolites are hydrophilic and readily excreted from the body via bile and urine. Metabolic pathways of tamoxifen are depicted in Figure 1.

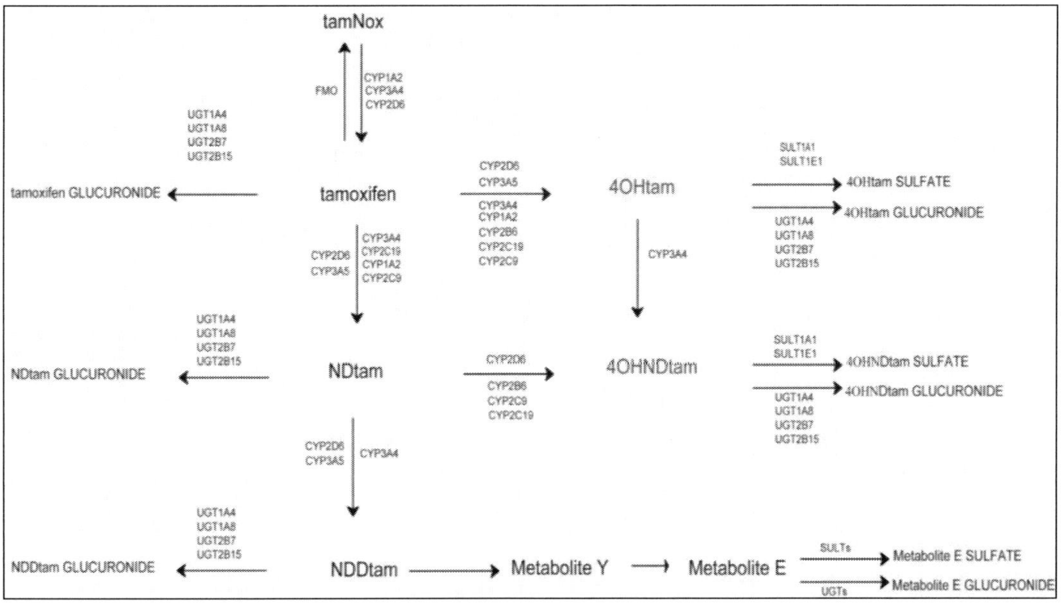

Figure 1. Schematic representation of tamoxifen metabolism and the enzymes involved. 4OHtam, 4-hydroxytamoxifen; 4OHNDtam, 4-hydroxy-*N*-desmethyltamoxifen; NDtam, *N*-desmethyltamoxifen; NDDtam, *N*-desdimethyltamoxifen; tamNox, tamoxifen-*N* -oxide; FMO, Flavin-Containing Monooxygenase; CYP,cytochrome P450; SULT, sulfotransferase; UGT, Uridine 5'-diphospho-glucuronosyltransferase; metabolite Y, the primary alcohol of tamoxifen, Metabolite E, tamoxifen without the aminoethoxide side chain.

Tamoxifen undergoes extensive hepatic metabolism by *N*-oxidation, hydroxylation, demethylation, sulfation, and glucuronidation [10-13, 15-25]. The metabolism of tamoxifen in the cytochrome P450 (CYP) system is complex, and shows considerable inter-individual variation [26, 27]. The major metabolite of tamoxifen is NDtam [28]. Tamoxifen undergoes *N*-demethylation of the tertiary amine to NDtam and further demethylation to *N*-desdimethyltamoxifen (NDDtam) [29]. This is catalyzed predominantly by CYP3A4 and CYP3A5 [12, 21, 22]. Studies have also shown that CYP2D6, CYP1A1, and CYP1A2 can *N*-demethylate tamoxifen [12, 24]. NDDtam is further metabolized by deamination to form the primary alcohol of tamoxifen (metabolite Y) [30] which is known to be a partial agonist with weak anti-estrogenic activity [31, 32]. Metabolite Y is possibly metabolized further by the removal of an ethoxy side chain forming metabolite E [33-35]. Metabolite E may be further conjugated by UDP-glucuronosyltransferase (UGT) and sulfotransferase (SULT). Therefore, it has been reported to be present in minute quantities of 0.9 – 2.0 ng/ ml in patient plasma [34]. The lack of the aminoethoxide side chain in Metabolite E may influence its activity. It has been reported to act as a pure estrogen agonist in both rat and mouse [36, 37].

CYP2D6 is the major contributor in the hydroxylation process of tamoxifen. Tamoxifen may be hydroxylated at the 4-position, generating 4OHtam from tamoxifen and 4OHNDtam from NDtam [13, 33, 38-40]. However, hydroxylation of tamoxifen and NDtam to the potent metabolites 4OHtam and 4OHNDtam also involves CYP2D6, CYP2B6, CYP2C9, and CYP2C19 [11, 12, 18, 23, 24, 41]. Furthermore tamoxifen *N*-oxidation is primarily catalyzed by flavin-containing monooxygenase (FMO) [17]. The tamoxifen-*N*-oxide (tamNox) produced can be reduced to tamoxifen by CYP enzymes such as CYP1A1, CYP1A2, CYP3A4, CYP2C9, CYP2C19, and CYP2D6 [18]. It may also be demethylated to NDtam [19, 20].

SULT1A1 plays a prominent role in the metabolism of a number of exogenous and endogenous compounds including estrogens [42, 43]. Tamoxifen is inactivated by SULT1A1 [14, 15, 44-46]. Furthermore, tamoxifen and its metabolites may be conjugated and inactivated by the polymorphic distributed UGT 1A4, 1A8, 2B7, and 2B15 [15, 46-48]. The genotypes of these enzymes may influence treatment outcome during tamoxifen therapy [49-54] some of which interact in the metabolism of estrogens. Accordingly we recently observed associations between estrogens and tamoxifen and its metabolites [55].

Tamoxifen Pharmacokinetics

Tamoxifen and its metabolites have a slow washout. They are extensively distributed into human tissues and have been observed to have a high distribution volume [31].The distribution volume of tamoxifen is 50-60 L/kg [40], with a distribution half-life of 7-14 hours [33]. The serum level of the major metabolite of tamoxifen, NDtam is about 2.5 times higher than the parent drug, tamoxifen [56], while the potent hydroxylated metabolites of tamoxifen, 4OHtam and 4OHNDtam are only 15% and 50% of tamoxifen, respectively. In 1973, Fromson *et al* first reported the presence of 4OHtam in human blood [33] while Lien *et al* identified 4OHNDtam in humans in 1988 [13, 31, 40]. 4OHtam, 4OHNDtam, and metabolite Y are known to contribute to the antitumor actions of tamoxifen. These metabolites inhibit the binding of 17-β-estradiol (E2) to the ER and exert antagonist activity [57].

In patients, the steady state concentrations of tamoxifen and NDtam are reached after 3-4 weeks and 8 weeks administration, respectively [58]. Upon stop of treatment, tamoxifen decline faster than NDtam with T ½ of 7 days for tamoxifen and 14 days for NDtam [59, 60]. Studies have shown that the traces of tamoxifen disappear after several months of drug withdrawal [31, 58, 61]. However, the serum levels of tamoxifen, 4OHtam, NDtam, metabolite E, and metabolite Y remain usually constant during 10 years of treatment [26].

The tamoxifen and metabolites are mainly excreted via feces, bile, and urine as conjugates. The unconjugated metabolite of tamoxifen, 4OHtam and 4OHNDtam are the predominating metabolites in feces [40, 62]. After deconjugation by intestinal microflora they may be partly reabsorbed resulting in a pronounced enterohepatic cycling [62, 63].

It has been suggested that the displayed marked inter-individual variation of tamoxifen metabolism is caused by differences in liver metabolism and absorption in the gastrointestinal tract [64]. However, studies have shown that this variation may also be caused by inter-individual differences in the activity of tamoxifen metabolizing enzymes due to inherited gene variants and concomitant medication with interacting drugs [41, 56, 65].

Drug Interaction

Several drugs interact with the metabolism of tamoxifen. In a clinical study we observed that 64% of breast cancer patients used additional drugs which may influence the pharmacokinetics of tamoxifen [27]. Some of these drugs may induce or inhibit the activity of CYP450 enzymes such as CYP2D6, CYP3A5 and CYP3A4 that metabolize tamoxifen to its active metabolites and may therefore influence the clinical efficiency and toxicity of tamoxifen.

Inhibition of warfarin metabolism upon combination with tamoxifen treatment has been observed [66]. Tamoxifen and warfarin are metabolized by CYP3A4. Tamoxifen increases the action of warfarin by competing with its metabolizing enzyme, CYP3A4 leading to potentially life-threatening bleeding. It has also been reported, increased digitoxin concentrations after administration of tamoxifen [66]. Thus, suggesting that digoxin is probably metabolized by the same enzyme system as tamoxifen and warfarin. Kivisto *et al* also showed that rifampin induces the activity of CYP3A4 resulting in reduced plasma concentrations of tamoxifen [67]. In addition, it was observed that one of the potent metabolites of tamoxifen, 4OHNDtam was not detectable in serum when patients were treated with tamoxifen and the enzyme inductor aminogluthethimide, a first generation aromatase inhibitor [68]. The observed reduction in serum concentrations of tamoxifen and its metabolites provides a potential explanation for the absence of beneficial effects of concomitant treatment with tamoxifen and aminoglutethimide over tamoxifen alone [69, 70]. Others have shown that the level of 4OHNDtam is dramatically reduced by co-medication with some anti-depressives [41]. Co-administration of tamoxifen and the selective serotonin reuptake inhibitor (SSRI) paroxetine or fluoxetine, which are inhibitors of CYP2D6, decreased the blood levels of 4OHNDtam [41].

These studies suggest that drug interactions should be considered in women using other drugs in addition to tamoxifen since these may influence the metabolism of the potent metabolites of tamoxifen, and hence influence its clinical efficiency, side-effects, and toxicity [41, 68].

Estrogen Receptor Binding and Biological Activities

The differences between the ER subtypes, ligand binding affinity and tissue distribution could contribute to the selective action of ER agonists and antagonists in different tissues [71]. Different estrogenic compounds have different binding affinities for ERα and ERβ. *In vitro* studies showed that tamoxifen is a mixed agonist-antagonist of ERα but is a pure antagonist of ERβ [72]. E2 binds 100% to ERα and ERβ. However, tamoxifen has 7% of the binding affinity of E2 [57] whereas NDtam has 1% the binding affinity of tamoxifen [73, 74]. The binding affinity for 4OHtam has been reported to be equal to E2 [73]. 4OHNDtam has identical properties to 4OHtam with regard to receptor affinity [75] and exists in higher concentration than 4OHtam [56]. The binding affinity of tamoxifen and its metabolites for the ER correlates with their growth inhibitory effect in MCF-7 breast cancer cells [74].

In vitro, the hydroxylated derivatives of tamoxifen were estrogen antagonist [57]. However, removal of the alkylaminoethoxy side chain from tamoxifen produced a full estrogen agonist with low potency. In contrast, removal of the side chain from 4OHtam produced a partial agonist indicating that this side chain is responsible for antagonistic effects. This suggests that altering the conformation of tamoxifen molecule may result in formation of different ER-complex with different activity.

ERα is a nuclear receptor that contains the common structural and functional features of a steroid/thyroid hormone receptor, and is a ligand-inducible transcription factor. The receptor contains activation function (AF)-1 and -2 domains. The autonomous AF-1 is located in the N-terminus and contributes to the constitutive estrogen-independent activation by the receptor. The ligand-binding domain (LBD) is composed of 12 helices and secures a ligand-binding pocket and the AF-2 and plays a critical role in the estrogen-dependent activation of ER. The DNA-binding domain (DBD) is responsible for specific binding of the ligand-receptor dimer complex to the estrogen responsive element (ERE) in the promoter of target genes [76] (Figure 2).

The binding of tamoxifen to the ER induces conformational changes in the LBD in the C-terminus of the receptor protein. 4OHtam, working as an ER antagonist, would upon binding to the ER induce a docking of helix 12 in the hydrophobic pocket formed by the LBD and part of the AF-2 domain of the ER [Beekman et al., 1993], thereby blocking the docking site for coactivators and instead recruiting corepressors such as NCOR and SMRT to the ERE [77-80].

Another factor that can affect the activity of tamoxifen is its recruitment of coregulators to the promoter and modulation of the cellular response to the ER-ligand complex [81-83]. In endometrium, binding of 4OHtam to ER leads to transcriptional activation through AF-1 by indirect binding to DNA via activator protein 1 (AP-1) and recruitment of the steroid receptor coactivator 1 (SRC-1) to the tamoxifen-ER complex. It is suggested that indirect binding of the tamoxifen-ER complex to DNA could induce conformational changes that favour binding of coactivators and transcriptional activation [Shang and Brown, 2002]. Thus, tamoxifen may function as an agonist by recruiting coactivators to E2-regulated genes and initiate transcription of the steroid responsive target genes [84] or as an antagonist, recruiting corepressors [85] and mediating inhibition of ER transactivation, Figure 3.

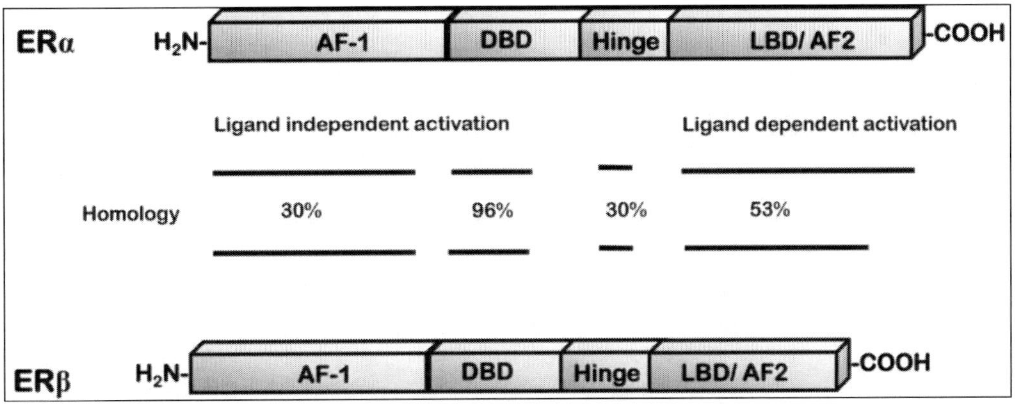

Figure 2. Schematic representation of the structural and functional domains of the estrogen receptor (ER). The activation function 1 (AF-1) is located in the N-terminus whereas the centrally-located DNA-binding domain (DBD) is responsible for specific binding of the ER to estrogen response elements (EREs) on its target genes.

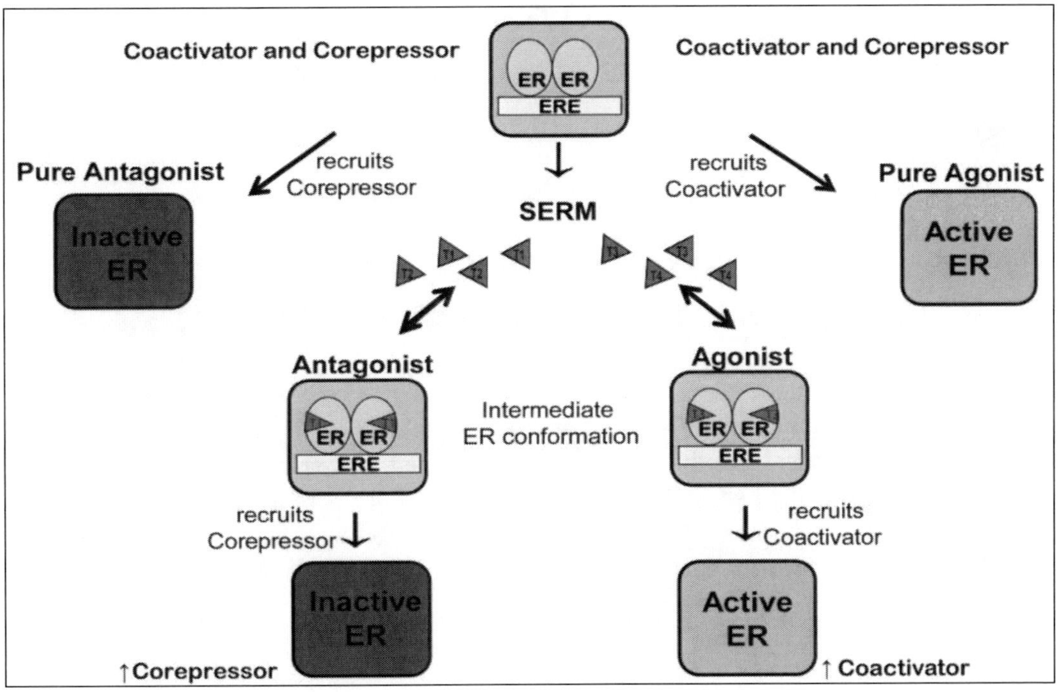

Figure 3. Proposed contributions of coactivators and corepressors to the tissue-specific agonist/antagonist activities of the selective estrogen receptor modulator (SERM), tamoxifen. ER, estrogen receptor; ERE, estrogen responsive elements; T1, 4OHtam; T2, 4OHNDtam; T3, metabolite E; T4, metabolite Y.

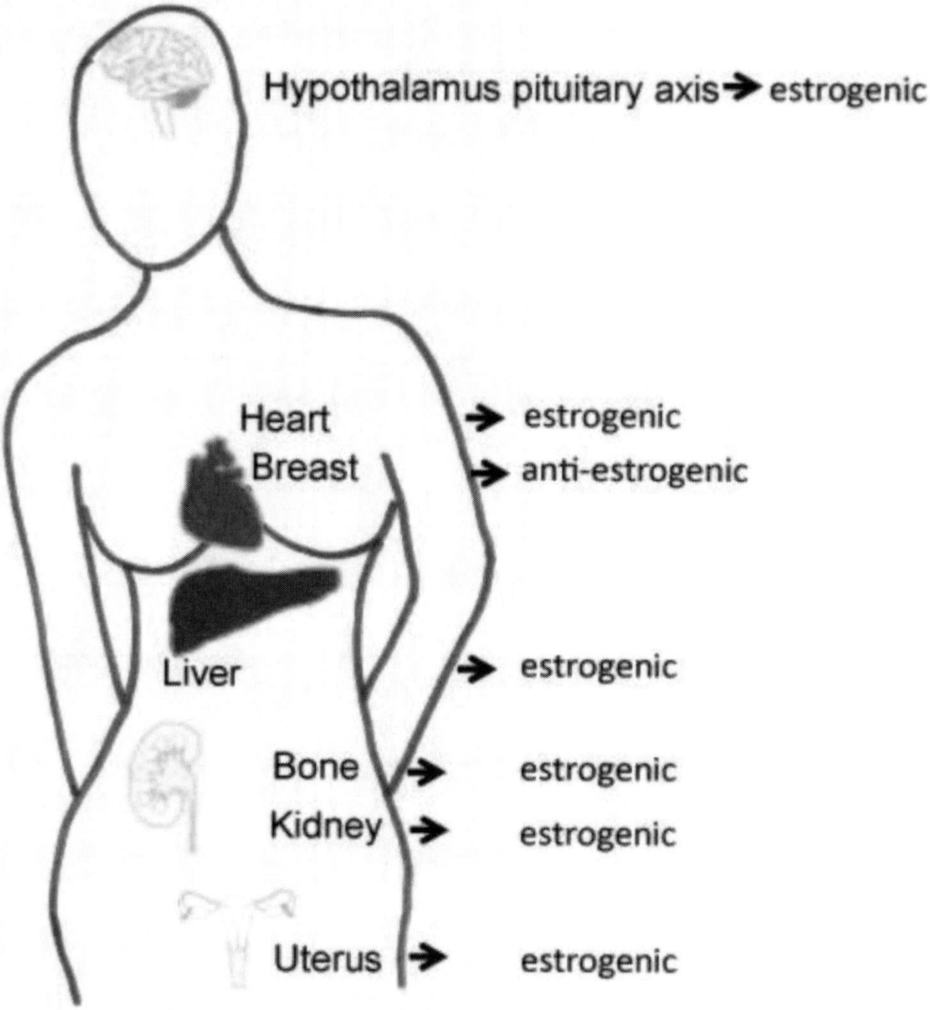

Figure 4. Schematic representation of the agonistic and antagonistic properties of tamoxifen in various target tissues.

Tamoxifen has distinct biological properties depending on the tissue environment. Tamoxifen's agonistic and antagonistic properties are related to its target tissue, figure 4. [86]. Besides breast tissue, tamoxifen has also been detected in the uterus, liver, kidney, lung, pancreas, heart, and brain [31, 33]. It has an anti-estrogenic activity in breast tissue and mediates competitive inhibition of estrogen binding to the ER. However metabolites that are hydroxylated in the 4-position have higher binding affinity for the ER than the parent drug [87]. 4OHtam has high affinity for the ER and may have anti-estrogenic activity during tamoxifen treatment, despite its relatively low concentration [56, 73]. 4OHNDtam is equipotent to 4OHtam in ER binding and has also been shown to have the same estrogen antagonist properties as 4OHtam determined by the suppression of estrogen stimulated breast cancer cell proliferation [41, 75]. Also NDtam has been shown to be as effective as tamoxifen and a higher effect is expected *in vivo* since the level of NDtam is much higher than 4OHtam [56, 73, 74].

Estrogenic actions of tamoxifen are observed in other tissues. Tamoxifen has tissue-specific and partially dose-dependent estrogenic effects in the hypothalamus-pituitary-axis [88], in the liver and in the vaginal epithelium of postmenopausal women [89]. In postmenopausal women with low levels of E2, tamoxifen treatment was shown to decrease the levels of follicle-stimulating hormone (FSH) and luteinizing hormone (LH) [90-92]. However, we observed that the concentration of 4OHNDtam was positively associated with FSH levels [56]. This observation suggests an anti-estrogenic effect only of this metabolite on the pituitary gland and strengthens the suggestions that this metabolite is the main anti-estrogenic tamoxifen compound [13, 75, 93].

Tamoxifens estrogenic effect on the liver is seen as a dose-dependent increase of sex hormone binding globulin (SHBG) [89]. SHBG levels are known to reflect tamoxifen estrogenicity in the liver as its level increases upon tamoxifen therapy [91, 92, 94]. Tamoxifen metabolism occurs in the liver and hepatic effects have been reported after tamoxifen administration [95, 96]. As for uterus, subjects taking tamoxifen have been shown to have a significant larger uterus and lower impedance to blood flow in uterine arteries [97]. In addition, 39% of women taking tamoxifen had histological evidence of an abnormal endometrium compared with 10% in the control group, suggesting an estrogenic effect of tamoxifen in the uterus. [98]. Tamoxifen has also an estrogenic effect on bone in postmenopausal [88, 99]. Patients treated with tamoxifen have a significant increase in bone mineral density when compared with control group, those receiving placebo [100, 101]. In addition, tamoxifen use has been associated with reduced osteoporotic fractures [102]. Tamoxifen also has an estrogenic effect on serum lipids [103] and this activity has been shown to be un-affected by reduction of tamoxifen dose [104]. Tamoxifen treatment results in decrease levels of low density lipoprotein (LDL) and cholesterol [105-109]. Thus, resulting in reduced cardiovascular risk in patients treated with tamoxifen [110].

Adverse Effects

Tamoxifen has been regarded as a pro-drug and the clinically potent metabolites; 4OHtam and 4OHNDtam have a higher affinity for the ER than tamoxifen itself [75, 111, 112]. NDtam is present in serum and tissues at about a 30 times higher concentration than 4OHtam [27, 31] and may also contribute to the anti-tumour effects of tamoxifen [113-115], as well as its side effects [116].

The most common side effects of tamoxifen are hot flashes and vaginal discharge and some patients experience headaches, fatigue, nausea and/or vomiting, and vaginal dryness. The cause of hot flashes is unclear. However, hormonal changes involving the elevation of serum concentrations of FSH and cessation of E2 levels during and after the menopause are related to the frequency of hot flashes [117, 118]. Notably, patients homozygous for the most common allele associated with the CYP2D6 poor metabolizer phenotype, CYP2D6*4, tend to have lower response rates to tamoxifen therapy and fewer hot flashes [52]. We propose that hot flashes, a major adverse effect of tamoxifen, may be due to the anti-estrogenic effects of 4OHNDtam on the pituitary gland based on the observation of an association between the serum level of FSH and 4OHNDtam [55]. This could also explain the association between hot flashes and disease outcome [119] and why patients most likely to benefit from tamoxifen may have the lowest compliance [120]. Patients who experience side effects are more likely to be noncompliant to tamoxifen treatment [121, 122]. Adverse effects of tamoxifen treatment that result in non-compliance may therefore increase the possibility of inadequate clinical response [123]. Non-compliance with tamoxifen is common, and may result in increased risk of local and distant disease recurrence [124].

Tamoxifen treatment has also some serious side effects such as an increased risk of thromboembolic disease and endometrial cancer, which are due to its estrogen agonistic effects. Studies have shown a significant correlation between long-term tamoxifen administration and endometrial proliferation [98]. An increased risk of endometrial cancer is associated with the duration of treatment and accumulated dose [6, 125]. The effect and side effects of tamoxifen may be attributed not only to concentrations of the parent drug but also to its biologically active metabolites and their accumulation in target tissues and side effects may be dose and concentration dependent, [126]

We have observed a higher level of NDtam in postmenopausal women compared to premenopausal women [127], and Peyrade *et al* showed that tamoxifen and metabolite concentrations significantly increase with age [116]. Notably, the levels of the demethylated tamoxifen metabolites have been reported to be increased in patients experiencing tamoxifen related side effects [116, 126]. A lower dose of tamoxifen could reduce the side-effects associated with treatment. Thus, tamoxifen treatment may be improved by administration of lower doses and therapeutic drug monitoring (TDM) [27, 55, 56, 104, 128].

Theraputic Drug Monitoring

There is more than a tenfold inter-individual difference in serum levels of tamoxifen and its metabolites and a positive correlation between serum and tissue levels of tamoxifen and its metabolites [27]. Differences in the activity of CYP2D6, CYP2C19, and SULT1A1 may partly explain the wide inter-individual variations in the serum levels of tamoxifen and its metabolites [55, 56].

Studies have shown that a steady state tamoxifen concentration in plasma does not predict treatment response [129, 130]. However in these studies the active hydroxylated metabolites of tamoxifen were not measured. It is suggested that TDM may be used to improve tamoxifen treatment by proper dosage, possibly lower than today's conventional dose [27, 55, 56, 128]. The conventional tamoxifen dosing regimen may be at the ceiling level of the dose response curve [131].

In distribution studies *in vivo*, it has been shown that kidney with low receptor content was fully saturated and the ligand more readily displaced [132]. Data also indicates that E2 binding to the ER is effectively blocked by tamoxifen and its metabolites using conventionally administered dose of 20 mg daily [74]. Thus, the use of lower dose of tamoxifen and TDM may improve its therapeutic utility and reduce its side effects. Moreover, doses lower than the conventional 20 mg/day may have a more favorable safety profile on serum biomarkers for cardiovascular disease [133]. In a short term clinical study we observed that a dose reduction from the conventional dose of 20 mg to 1 mg daily caused reduction or disappearance of the estrogen agonistic effects on blood parameters, whereas the effects on the growth parameter Ki-67 was unchanged [131].

The generally accepted criteria for TDM applies for tamoxifen, such as major individual variation of metabolism, possibility of interactions, difficult to clinically observe toxicity, compliance, and correlation between serum concentration and effect/side effects. Thus, adjustment of doses based on TDM may result in a lower dose with less side effects and better compliance. A 35.2% discontinuation rate of patients has been observed by the end of follow-up at 3.5 years [134]. TDM studies may also help clinicians to better select patients likely to benefit from adjuvant tamoxifen treatment. Hence, slow metabolizers with low levels of potent metabolites of tamoxifen experiencing side effects may not be candidates for tamoxifen treatment, and may benefit from other treatment strategies.

Conclusion

Tamoxifen has been the gold standard for treatment and prevention of breast cancer. Although tamoxifen is an "old drug" and the most used anti-cancer drug in the world, no proper dose findings studies of tamoxifen have been performed. New patented expensive drugs are often compared with the conventional tamoxifen regimens of 20 mg tamoxifen per day. However, it has not been discussed whether the tamoxifen regimen is optimal.

Since tamoxifen dose used is based on the maximum tolerated dose rather than the optimal biological dose and few dose finding studies of tamoxifen have been performed an optimal therapeutic serum concentrations has not been determined. Thus, examining associations between the serum concentrations of tamoxifen and its metabolites and clinical effects and adverse effects is warranted. This gives rise to important clinical-oncological questions and will bring personalized medicine a step forward.

References

[1] Cole, M.P., C.T. Jones, and I.D. Todd. A new anti-oestrogenic agent in late breast cancer. An early clinical appraisal of ICI46474. *Br. J. Cancer*. 1971; 25(2): 270-5.

[2] Legha, S.S. and S.K. Carter. Antiestrogens in the treatment of breast cancer. *Cancer Treat Rev*. 1976; 3(4): 205-16.

[3] Goldhirsch, A., W. Wood, R. Gelber, A. Coates, B. Thurlimann, H.J. Senn, and P. Members. Progress and promise: highlights of the international expert consensus on the primary therapy of early breast cancer 2007. *Ann. Oncol*. 2007; 18(7): 1133-44.

[4] Gnant, M., N. Harbeck, and C. Thomssen. St. Gallen 2011: Summary of the Consensus Discussion. *Breast care*. 2011; 6(2): 136-141.

[5] Goldhirsch, A., W.C. Wood, A.S. Coates, R.D. Gelber, B. Thurlimann, and H.J. Senn. Strategies for subtypes--dealing with the diversity of breast cancer: highlights of the St Gallen International Expert Consensus on the Primary Therapy of Early Breast Cancer 2011. *Annals of oncology: official journal of the European Society for Medical Oncology / ESMO*. 2011.

[6] Fisher, B., J.P. Costantino, D.L. Wickerham, C.K. Redmond, M. Kavanah, W.M. Cronin, V. Vogel, A. Robidoux, N. Dimitrov, J. Atkins, M. Daly, S. Wieand, E. Tan-Chiu, L. Ford, and N. Wolmark. Tamoxifen for prevention of breast cancer: report of the National Surgical Adjuvant Breast and Bowel Project P-1 Study. *J. Natl. Cancer Inst.* 1998; 90(18): 1371-1388.

[7] Cuzick, J., J. Forbes, R. Edwards, M. Baum, S. Cawthorn, A. Coates, A. Hamed, A. Howell, and T. Powles. First results from the International Breast Cancer Intervention Study (IBIS-I): a randomised prevention trial. *Lancet*. 2002; 360(9336): 817-824.

[8] Lonning, E. and E.A. Lien. Mechanisms of action of endocrine treatment in breast cancer. *Critical reviews in oncology/hematology*. 1995; 21(1-3): 158-93.

[9] Santen, R.J., A. Manni, H. Harvey, and C. Redmond. Endocrine treatment of breast cancer in women. *Endocr. Rev.* 1990; 11(2): 221-65.

[10] Poon, G.K., Y.C. Chui, R. McCague, P.E. Llnning, R. Feng, M.G. Rowlands, and M. Jarman. Analysis of phase I and phase II metabolites of tamoxifen in breast cancer patients. *Drug Metab. Dispos.* 1993; 21(6): 1119-1124.

[11] Crewe, H.K., S.W. Ellis, M.S. Lennard, and G.T. Tucker. Variable contribution of cytochromes P450 2D6, 2C9 and 3A4 to the 4-hydroxylation of tamoxifen by human liver microsomes. *Biochem. Pharmacol.* 1997; 53(2): 171-178.

[12] Desta, Z., B.A. Ward, N.V. Soukhova, and D.A. Flockhart. Comprehensive evaluation of tamoxifen sequential biotransformation by the human cytochrome P450 system in vitro: prominent roles for CYP3A and CYP2D6. *J. Pharmacol. Exp. Ther.* 2004; 310(3): 1062-1075.

[13] Lien, E.A., E. Solheim, S. Kvinnsland, and P.M. Ueland. Identification of 4-hydroxy-N-desmethyltamoxifen as a metabolite of tamoxifen in human bile. *Cancer Res.* 1988; 48(8): 2304-2308.

[14] Falany, C.N., J. Wheeler, T.S. Oh, and J.L. Falany. Steroid sulfation by expressed human cytosolic sulfotransferases. *J. Steroid Biochem. Mol. Biol.* 1994; 48(4): 369-375.

[15] Nishiyama, T., K. Ogura, H. Nakano, T. Ohnuma, T. Kaku, A. Hiratsuka, K. Muro, and T. Watabe. Reverse geometrical selectivity in glucuronidation and sulfation of cis- and trans-4-hydroxytamoxifens by human liver UDP-glucuronosyltransferases and sulfotransferases. *Biochem. Pharmacol.* 2002; 63(10): 1817-1830.

[16] Seth, P., K.L. Lunetta, D.W. Bell, H. Gray, S.M. Nasser, E. Rhei, C.M. Kaelin, D.J. Iglehart, J.R. Marks, J.E. Garber, D.A. Haber, and K. Polyak. Phenol sulfotransferases: hormonal regulation, polymorphism, and age of onset of breast cancer. *Cancer Res.* 2000; 60(24): 6859-6863.

[17] Mani, C., E. Hodgson, and D. Kupfer. Metabolism of the antimammary cancer antiestrogenic agent tamoxifen. II. Flavin-containing monooxygenase-mediated N-oxidation. *Drug Metab. Dispos.* 1993; 21(4): 657-661.

[18] Parte, P. and D. Kupfer. Oxidation of tamoxifen by human flavin-containing monooxygenase (FMO) 1 and FMO3 to tamoxifen-N-oxide and its novel reduction back to tamoxifen by human cytochromes P450 and hemoglobin. *Drug Metab. Dispos.* 2005; 33(10): 1446-52.

[19] Smuckler, E.A., E. Arrhenius, and T. Hultin. Alterations in microsomal electron transport, oxidative N-demethylation and azo-dye cleavage in carbon tetrachloride and dimethylnitrosamine-induced liver injury. *Biochem. J.* 1967; 103(1): 55-64.

[20] Jordan, V.C. New insights into the metabolism of tamoxifen and its role in the treatment and prevention of breast cancer. *Steroids*. 2007; 72(13): 829-42.

[21] Jacolot, F., I. Simon, Y. Dreano, P. Beaune, C. Riche, and F. Berthou. Identification of the cytochrome P450 IIIA family as the enzymes involved in the N-demethylation of tamoxifen in human liver microsomes. *Biochem. Pharmacol*. 1991; 41(12): 1911-1919.

[22] Coller, J.K., N. Krebsfaenger, K. Klein, R. Wolbold, A. Nussler, P. Neuhaus, U.M. Zanger, M. Eichelbaum, and T.E. Murdter. Large interindividual variability in the in vitro formation of tamoxifen metabolites related to the development of genotoxicity. *Br. J. Clin. Pharmacol*. 2004; 57(1): 105-111.

[23] Coller, J.K. Oxidative metabolism of tamoxifen to Z-4-hydroxy-tamoxifen by cytochrome P450 isoforms: an appraisal of in vitro studies. *Clin. Exp. Pharmacol. Physiol*. 2003; 30(11): 845-848.

[24] Crewe, H.K., L.M. Notley, R.M. Wunsch, M.S. Lennard, and E.M. Gillam. Metabolism of tamoxifen by recombinant human cytochrome P450 enzymes: formation of the 4-hydroxy, 4'-hydroxy and N-desmethyl metabolites and isomerization of trans-4-hydroxytamoxifen. *Drug Metab. Dispos*. 2002; 30(8): 869-874.

[25] Zhao, X.J., D.R. Jones, Y.H. Wang, S.W. Grimm, and S.D. Hall. Reversible and irreversible inhibition of CYP3A enzymes by tamoxifen and metabolites. *Xenobiotica*. 2002; 32(10): 863-878.

[26] Langan-Fahey, S.M., D.C. Tormey, and V.C. Jordan. Tamoxifen metabolites in patients on long-term adjuvant therapy for breast cancer. *Eur. J. Cancer*. 1990; 26(8): 883-888.

[27] Kisanga, E.R., J. Gjerde, A. Guerrieri-Gonzaga, F. Pigatto, A. Pesci-Feltri, C. Robertson, D. Serrano, G. Pelosi, A. Decensi, and E.A. Lien. Tamoxifen and metabolite concentrations in serum and breast cancer tissue during three dose regimens in a randomized preoperative trial. *Clin. Cancer Res*. 2004; 10(7): 2336-43.

[28] Adam, H.K., E.J. Douglas, and J.V. Kemp. The metabolism of tamoxifen in human. *Biochemical pharmacology*. 1979; 28(1): 145-7.

[29] Kemp, J.V., H.K. Adam, A.E. Wakeling, and R. Slater. Identification and biological activity of tamoxifen metabolites in human serum. *Biochemical pharmacology*. 1983; 32(13): 2045-52.

[30] Bain, R.R. and V.C. Jordan. Identification of a new metabolite of tamoxifen in patient serum during breast cancer therapy. *Biochemical pharmacology*. 1983; 32(2): 373-5.

[31] Lien, E.A., E. Solheim, and P.M. Ueland. Distribution of tamoxifen and its metabolites in rat and human tissues during steady-state treatment. *Cancer Res*. 1991; 51(18): 4837-4844.

[32] Jordan, V.C., R.R. Bain, R.R. Brown, B. Gosden, and M.A. Santos. Determination and pharmacology of a new hydroxylated metabolite of tamoxifen observed in patient sera during therapy for advanced breast cancer. *Cancer Res*. 1983; 43(3): 1446-50.

[33] Fromson, J.M., S. Pearson, and S. Bramah. The metabolism of tamoxifen (I.C.I. 46,474). II. In female patients. *Xenobiotica*. 1973; 3(11): 711-4.

[34] Murphy, C., T. Fotsis, P. Pantzar, H. Adlercreutz, and F. Martin. Analysis of tamoxifen and its metabolites in human plasma by gas chromatography-mass spectrometry (GC-MS) using selected ion monitoring (SIM). *J. Steroid Biochem*. 1987; 26(5): 547-555.

[35] Wiebe, V.J., C.K. Osborne, W.L. McGuire, and M.W. DeGregorio. Identification of estrogenic tamoxifen metabolite(s) in tamoxifen-resistant human breast tumors. *Journal of clinical oncology : official journal of the American Society of Clinical Oncology*. 1992; 10(6): 990-4.

[36] Lyman, S.D. and V.C. Jordan. Metabolism of nonsteroidal antiestrogens. *Estrogen/Antiestrogen Action and Breast Cancer Therapy*. 1986: 191-219.

[37] Swain, S.M. and M.E. Lippman. Endocrine therapies of cancer. in Cancer Chemotherapy: Principles and Practice. B.A. Chabner and J.M. Collins, Editors. 1990, J.B. Lippincott Company, Philadelphia: Grand Rapids. p. 59-109.

[38] Daniel, C.P., S.J. Gaskell, H. Bishop, and R.I. Nicholson. Determination of tamoxifen and an hydroxylated metabolite in plasma from patients with advanced breast cancer using gas chromatography-mass spectrometry. *The Journal of endocrinology*. 1979; 83(3): 401-8.

[39] Robinson, S.P., S.M. Langan-Fahey, and V.C. Jordan. Implications of tamoxifen metabolism in the athymic mouse for the study of antitumor effects upon human breast cancer xenografts. *European journal of cancer and clinical oncology*. 1989; 25(12): 1769-76.

[40] Lien, E.A., E. Solheim, O.A. Lea, S. Lundgren, S. Kvinnsland, and P.M. Ueland. Distribution of 4-hydroxy-N-desmethyltamoxifen and other tamoxifen metabolites in human biological fluids during tamoxifen treatment. *Cancer Res*. 1989; 49(8): 2175-83.

[41] Stearns, V., M.D. Johnson, J.M. Rae, A. Morocho, A. Novielli, P. Bhargava, D.F. Hayes, Z. Desta, and D.A. Flockhart. Active tamoxifen metabolite plasma concentrations after coadministration of tamoxifen and the selective serotonin reuptake inhibitor paroxetine. *J. Natl. Cancer Inst*. 2003; 95(23): 1758-1764.

[42] Harris, R.M., R.H. Waring, C.J. Kirk, and P.J. Hughes. Sulfation of "estrogenic" alkylphenols and 17beta-estradiol by human platelet phenol sulfotransferases. *J. Biol. Chem*. 2000; 275(1): 159-166.

[43] Adjei, A.A. and R.M. Weinshilboum. Catecholestrogen sulfation: possible role in carcinogenesis. *Biochem. Biophys. Res. Commun*. 2002; 292(2): 402-8.

[44] Raftogianis, R.B., T.C. Wood, D.M. Otterness, J.A. Van Loon, and R.M. Weinshilboum. Phenol sulfotransferase pharmacogenetics in humans: association of common SULT1A1 alleles with TS PST phenotype. *Biochem. Biophys. Res. Commun*. 1997; 239(1): 298-304.

[45] Nowell, S., C.B. Ambrosone, S. Ozawa, S.L. MacLeod, G. Mrackova, S. Williams, J. Plaxco, F.F. Kadlubar, and N.P. Lang. Relationship of phenol sulfotransferase activity (SULT1A1) genotype to sulfotransferase phenotype in platelet cytosol. *Pharmacogenetics*. 2000; 10(9): 789-797.

[46] Nowell, S.A., J. Ahn, J.M. Rae, J.O. Scheys, A. Trovato, C. Sweeney, S.L. MacLeod, F.F. Kadlubar, and C.B. Ambrosone. Association of genetic variation in tamoxifen-metabolizing enzymes with overall survival and recurrence of disease in breast cancer patients. *Breast Cancer Res. Treat*. 2005; 91(3): 249-258.

[47] Blevins-Primeau, A.S., D. Sun, G. Chen, A.K. Sharma, C.J. Gallagher, S. Amin, and P. Lazarus. Functional significance of UDP-glucuronosyltransferase variants in the metabolism of active tamoxifen metabolites. *Cancer Res*. 2009; 69(5): 1892-900.

[48] Levesque, E., M. Beaulieu, M.D. Green, T.R. Tephly, A. Belanger, and D.W. Hum. Isolation and characterization of UGT2B15(Y85): a UDP-glucuronosyltransferase encoded by a polymorphic gene. *Pharmacogenetics*. 1997; 7(4): 317-325.

[49] Schroth, W., L. Antoniadou, P. Fritz, M. Schwab, T. Muerdter, U.M. Zanger, W. Simon, M. Eichelbaum, and H. Brauch. Breast cancer treatment outcome with adjuvant tamoxifen relative to patient CYP2D6 and CYP2C19 genotypes. *J. Clin. Oncol.* 2007; 25(33): 5187-93.

[50] Nowell, S., C. Sweeney, M. Winters, A. Stone, N.P. Lang, L.F. Hutchins, F.F. Kadlubar, and C.B. Ambrosone. Association between sulfotransferase 1A1 genotype and survival of breast cancer patients receiving tamoxifen therapy. *J. Natl. Cancer Inst.* 2002; 94(21): 1635-1640.

[51] Wegman, P., L. Vainikka, and O. Stål. Genotype of metabolic enzymes and the benefit of tamoxifen in postmenopausal breast cancer patients. *Breast Cancer Res.* 2005; 7(3): 284-290.

[52] Goetz, M.P., J.M. Rae, V.J. Suman, S.L. Safgren, M.M. Ames, D.W. Visscher, C. Reynolds, F.J. Couch, W.L. Lingle, D.A. Flockhart, Z. Desta, E.A. Perez, and J.N. Ingle. Pharmacogenetics of tamoxifen biotransformation is associated with clinical outcomes of efficacy and hot flashes. *J. Clin. Oncol.* 2005; 23(36): 9312-9318.

[53] Goetz, M.P., S.K. Knox, V.J. Suman, J.M. Rae, S.L. Safgren, M.M. Ames, D.W. Visscher, C. Reynolds, F.J. Couch, W.L. Lingle, R.M. Weinshilboum, E.G. Fritcher, A.M. Nibbe, Z. Desta, A. Nguyen, D.A. Flockhart, E.A. Perez, and J.N. Ingle. The impact of cytochrome P450 2D6 metabolism in women receiving adjuvant tamoxifen. *Breast Cancer Res. Treat.* 2007; 101(1): 113-121.

[54] Wegman, P., S. Elingarami, J. Carstensen, O. Stal, B. Nordenskjold, and S. Wingren. Genetic variants of CYP3A5, CYP2D6, SULT1A1, UGT2B15 and tamoxifen response in postmenopausal breast cancer patients. *Breast Cancer Res.* 2007; 9(1): R7.

[55] Gjerde, J., J. Geisler, S. Lundgren, D. Ekse, J.E. Varhaug, G. Mellgren, V.M. Steen, and E.A. Lien. Associations between tamoxifen, estrogens, and FSH serum levels during steady state tamoxifen treatment of postmenopausal women with breast cancer. *BMC Cancer*. 2010; 10: 313.

[56] Gjerde, J., M. Hauglid, H. Breilid, S. Lundgren, J.E. Varhaug, E.R. Kisanga, G. Mellgren, V.M. Steen, and E.A. Lien. Effects of CYP2D6 and SULT1A1 genotypes including SULT1A1 gene copy number on tamoxifen metabolism. *Ann. Oncol.* 2008; 19(1): 56-61.

[57] Jordan, V.C., M.E. Lieberman, E. Cormier, R. Koch, J.R. Bagley, and P.C. Ruenitz. Structural requirements for the pharmacological activity of nonsteroidal antiestrogens in vitro. *Molecular pharmacology*. 1984; 26(2): 272-8.

[58] Adam, H.K., J.S. Patterson, and J.V. Kemp. Studies on the metabolism and pharmacokinetics of tamoxifen in normal volunteers. *Cancer Treat Rep.* 1980; 64(6-7): 761-764.

[59] Camaggi, C.M., E. Strocchi, N. Canova, B. Costanti, and F. Pannuti. Medroxyprogesterone acetate (MAP) and tamoxifen (TMX) plasma levels after simultaneous treatment with 'low' TMX and 'high' MAP doses. *Cancer chemotherapy and pharmacology*. 1985; 14(3): 229-31.

[60] Wilson, A.J., M. Baum, D.M. Brinkley, J.A. Dossett, K. McPherson, J.S. Patterson, R.D. Rubens, F.G. Smiddy, B.A. Stoll, D. Richards, and et al. Six-year results of a controlled trial of tamoxifen as single adjuvant agent in management of early breast cancer. *World journal of surgery*. 1985; 9(5): 756-64.

[61] Buckley, M.M. and K.L. Goa. Tamoxifen. A reappraisal of its pharmacodynamic and pharmacokinetic properties, and therapeutic use. *Drugs*. 1989; 37(4): 451-90.

[62] Kisanga, E.R., G. Mellgren, and E.A. Lien. Excretion of hydroxylated metabolites of tamoxifen in human bile and urine. *Anticancer Res.* 2005; 25(6C): 4487-4492.

[63] Adlercreutz, H., F. Martin, P. Jarvenpaa, and T. Fotsis. Steroid absorption and enterohepatic recycling. *Contraception*. 1979; 20(3): 201-23.

[64] McVie, J.G., G.P. Simonetti, D. Stevenson, R.J. Briggs, P.J. Guelen, and D. de Vos. The bioavailability of Tamoplex (tamoxifen). Part 1. A pilot study. *Methods Find Exp. Clin. Pharmacol*. 1986; 8(8): 505-12.

[65] Jin, Y., Z. Desta, V. Stearns, B. Ward, H. Ho, K.H. Lee, T. Skaar, A.M. Storniolo, L. Li, A. Araba, R. Blanchard, A. Nguyen, L. Ullmer, J. Hayden, S. Lemler, R.M. Weinshilboum, J.M. Rae, D.F. Hayes, and D.A. Flockhart. CYP2D6 genotype, antidepressant use, and tamoxifen metabolism during adjuvant breast cancer treatment. *J. Natl. Cancer Inst.* 2005; 97(1): 30-39.

[66] Lodwick, R., B. McConkey, and A.M. Brown. Life threatening interaction between tamoxifen and warfarin. *British medical journal*. 1987; 295(6606): 1141.

[67] Kivisto, K.T., K. Villikka, L. Nyman, M. Anttila, and P.J. Neuvonen. Tamoxifen and toremifene concentrations in plasma are greatly decreased by rifampin. *Clin. Pharmacol. Ther*. 1998; 64(6): 648-654.

[68] Lien, E.A., G. Anker, P.E. Lonning, E. Solheim, and P.M. Ueland. Decreased serum concentrations of tamoxifen and its metabolites induced by aminoglutethimide. *Cancer Res*. 1990; 50(18): 5851-7.

[69] Ingle, J.N., S.J. Green, D.L. Ahmann, H.J. Long, J.H. Edmonson, J. Rubin, M.N. Chang, and E.T. Creagan. Randomized trial of tamoxifen alone or combined with aminoglutethimide and hydrocortisone in women with metastatic breast cancer. *J. Clin. Oncol*. 1986; 4(6): 958-64.

[70] Rose, C., C. Kamby, H.T. Mouridsen, L. Bastholt, H. Brincker, H. Skovgaard-Poulsen, A.P. Andersen, H. Loft, P. Dombernowsky, and K.W. Andersen. Combined endocrine treatment of postmenopausal patients with advanced breast cancer. A randomized trial of tamoxifen vs. tamoxifen plus aminoglutethimide and hydrocortisone. *Breast Cancer Res. Treat*. 1986; 7 Suppl: S45-50.

[71] Kuiper, G.G., B. Carlsson, K. Grandien, E. Enmark, J. Haggblad, S. Nilsson, and J.A. Gustafsson. Comparison of the ligand binding specificity and transcript tissue distribution of estrogen receptors alpha and beta. *Endocrinology*. 1997; 138(3): 863-70.

[72] Barkhem, T., B. Carlsson, Y. Nilsson, E. Enmark, J. Gustafsson, and S. Nilsson. Differential response of estrogen receptor alpha and estrogen receptor beta to partial estrogen agonists/antagonists. *Mol. Pharmacol*. 1998; 54(1): 105-12.

[73] Fabian, C., L. Tilzer, and L. Sternson. Comparative binding affinities of tamoxifen, 4-hydroxytamoxifen, and desmethyltamoxifen for estrogen receptors isolated from human breast carcinoma: correlation with blood levels in patients with metastatic breast cancer. *Biopharm. Drug Dispos*. 1981; 2(4): 381-390.

[74] Coezy, E., J.L. Borgna, and H. Rochefort. Tamoxifen and metabolites in MCF7 cells: correlation between binding to estrogen receptor and inhibition of cell growth. *Cancer Res.* 1982; 42(1): 317-323.

[75] Johnson, M.D., H. Zuo, K.H. Lee, J.P. Trebley, J.M. Rae, R.V. Weatherman, Z. Desta, D.A. Flockhart, and T.C. Skaar. Pharmacological characterization of 4-hydroxy- N - desmethyl tamoxifen, a novel active metabolite of tamoxifen. *Breast Cancer Res. Treat.* 2004; 85(2): 151-159.

[76] Kumar, V., S. Green, G. Stack, M. Berry, J.R. Jin, and P. Chambon. Functional domains of the human estrogen receptor. *Cell.* 1987; 51(6): 941-51.

[77] Heinzel, T., R.M. Lavinsky, T.M. Mullen, M. Soderstrom, C.D. Laherty, J. Torchia, W.M. Yang, G. Brard, S.D. Ngo, J.R. Davie, E. Seto, R.N. Eisenman, D.W. Rose, C.K. Glass, and M.G. Rosenfeld. A complex containing N-CoR, mSin3 and histone deacetylase mediates transcriptional repression. *Nature.* 1997; 387(6628): 43-8.

[78] Shang, Y., X. Hu, J. DiRenzo, M.A. Lazar, and M. Brown. Cofactor dynamics and sufficiency in estrogen receptor-regulated transcription. *Cell.* 2000; 103(6): 843-52.

[79] Huang, H.J., J.D. Norris, and D.P. McDonnell. Identification of a negative regulatory surface within estrogen receptor alpha provides evidence in support of a role for corepressors in regulating cellular responses to agonists and antagonists. *Molecular endocrinology.* 2002; 16(8): 1778-92.

[80] Fleming, F.J., A.D. Hill, E.W. McDermott, N.J. O'Higgins, and L.S. Young. Differential recruitment of coregulator proteins steroid receptor coactivator-1 and silencing mediator for retinoid and thyroid receptors to the estrogen receptor-estrogen response element by beta-estradiol and 4-hydroxytamoxifen in human breast cancer. *J. Clin. Endocrinol. Metab.* 2004; 89(1): 375-83.

[81] Dutertre, M. and C.L. Smith. Molecular mechanisms of selective estrogen receptor modulator (SERM) action. *J. Pharmacol. Exp. Ther.* 2000; 295(2): 431-437.

[82] Edwards, D.P. The role of coactivators and corepressors in the biology and mechanism of action of steroid hormone receptors. *J. Mammary Gland Biol. Neoplasia.* 2000; 5(3): 307-24.

[83] Deroo, B.J. and K.S. Korach. Estrogen receptors and human disease. *J. Clin. Invest.* 2006; 116(3): 561-70.

[84] Shou, J., S. Massarweh, C.K. Osborne, A.E. Wakeling, S. Ali, H. Weiss, and R. Schiff. Mechanisms of tamoxifen resistance: increased estrogen receptor-HER2/neu cross-talk in ER/HER2-positive breast cancer. *J. Natl. Cancer Inst.* 2004; 96(12): 926-35.

[85] Shang, Y. and M. Brown. Molecular determinants for the tissue specificity of SERMs. *Science.* 2002; 295(5564): 2465-8.

[86] Lien, E.A. and P.E. Lonning. Selective oestrogen receptor modifiers (SERMs) and breast cancer therapy. *Cancer Treat. Rev.* 2000; 26(3): 205-227.

[87] Jordan, V.C., M.M. Collins, L. Rowsby, and G. Prestwich. A monohydroxylated metabolite of tamoxifen with potent antioestrogenic activity. *J. Endocrinol.* 1977; 75(2): 305-316.

[88] Fornander, T., L.E. Rutqvist, N. Wilking, K. Carlstrom, and B. von Schoultz. Oestrogenic effects of adjuvant tamoxifen in postmenopausal breast cancer. *Eur. J. Cancer.* 1993; 29A(4): 497-500.

[89] Ellmen, J., P. Hakulinen, A. Partanen, and D.F. Hayes. Estrogenic effects of toremifene and tamoxifen in postmenopausal breast cancer patients. *Breast Cancer Res. Treat.* 2003; 82(2): 103-11.

[90] Manni, A., J.E. Trujillo, J.S. Marshall, J. Brodkey, and O.H. Pearson. Antihormone treatment of stage IV breast cancer. *Cancer*. 1979; 43(2): 444-50.

[91] Jordan, V.C., N.F. Fritz, and D.C. Tormey. Long-term adjuvant therapy with tamoxifen: effects on sex hormone binding globulin and antithrombin III. *Cancer research*. 1987; 47(16): 4517-9.

[92] Jordan, V.C., N.F. Fritz, and D.C. Tormey. Endocrine effects of adjuvant chemotherapy and long-term tamoxifen administration on node-positive patients with breast cancer. *Cancer research*. 1987; 47(2): 624-30.

[93] Lim, Y.C., Z. Desta, D.A. Flockhart, and T.C. Skaar. Endoxifen (4-hydroxy-N-desmethyl-tamoxifen) has anti-estrogenic effects in breast cancer cells with potency similar to 4-hydroxy-tamoxifen. *Cancer Chemother. Pharmacol.* 2005; 55(5): 471-478.

[94] Barkhem, T., C. Andersson-Ross, M. Hoglund, and S. Nilsson. Characterization of the "estrogenicity" of tamoxifen and raloxifene in HepG2 cells: regulation of gene expression from an ERE controlled reporter vector versus regulation of the endogenous SHBG and PS2 genes. *J. Steroid Biochem. Mol. Biol.* 1997; 62(1): 53-64.

[95] Blackburn, A.M., S.A. Amiel, R.R. Millis, and R.D. Rubens. Tamoxifen and liver damage. *British medical journal*. 1984; 289(6440): 288.

[96] DeGregorio, M.W., V.J. Wiebe, A.P. Venook, and W.M. Holleran. Elevated plasma tamoxifen levels in a patient with liver obstruction. *Cancer Chemother. Pharmacol.* 1989; 23(3): 194-5.

[97] Kedar, R.P., T.H. Bourne, T.J. Powles, W.P. Collins, S.E. Ashley, D.O. Cosgrove, and S. Campbell. Effects of tamoxifen on uterus and ovaries of postmenopausal women in a randomised breast cancer prevention trial. *Lancet*. 1994; 343(8909): 1318-21.

[98] Uziely, B., A. Lewin, G. Brufman, D. Dorembus, and S. Mor-Yosef. The effect of tamoxifen on the endometrium. *Breast cancer research and treatment*. 1993; 26(1): 101-5.

[99] Vehmanen, L., I. Elomaa, C. Blomqvist, and T. Saarto. Tamoxifen treatment after adjuvant chemotherapy has opposite effects on bone mineral density in premenopausal patients depending on menstrual status. *J. Clin. Oncol*. 2006; 24(4): 675-680.

[100] Love, R.R., R.B. Mazess, H.S. Barden, S. Epstein, P.A. Newcomb, V.C. Jordan, P.P. Carbone, and D.L. DeMets. Effects of tamoxifen on bone mineral density in postmenopausal women with breast cancer. *N. Engl. J. Med*. 1992; 326(13): 852-6.

[101] Love, R.R., H.S. Barden, R.B. Mazess, S. Epstein, and R.J. Chappell. Effect of tamoxifen on lumbar spine bone mineral density in postmenopausal women after 5 years. *Archives of internal medicine*. 1994; 154(22): 2585-8.

[102] Cooke, A.L., C. Metge, L. Lix, H.J. Prior, and W.D. Leslie. Tamoxifen use and osteoporotic fracture risk: a population-based analysis. *J. Clin. Oncol*. 2008; 26(32): 5227-32.

[103] Bilimoria, M.M., V.J. Assikis, and V.C. Jordan. Should adjuvant tamoxifen therapy be stopped at 5 years? *The cancer journal from Scientific American*. 1996; 2(3): 140-50.

[104] Decensi, A., S. Gandini, A. Guerrieri-Gonzaga, H. Johansson, L. Manetti, B. Bonanni, M.T. Sandri, A. Barreca, A. Costa, C. Robertson, and E.A. Lien. Effect of blood tamoxifen concentrations on surrogate biomarkers in a trial of dose reduction in healthy women. *J. Clin. Oncol.* 1999; 17(9): 2633-2638.

[105] Schapira, D.V., N.B. Kumar, and G.H. Lyman. Serum cholesterol reduction with tamoxifen. *Breast cancer research and treatment*. 1990; 17(1): 3-7.

[106] Love, R.R., D.A. Wiebe, P.A. Newcomb, L. Cameron, H. Leventhal, V.C. Jordan, J. Feyzi, and D.L. DeMets. Effects of tamoxifen on cardiovascular risk factors in postmenopausal women. *Annals of internal medicine*. 1991; 115(11): 860-4.

[107] Dnistrian, A.M., M.K. Schwartz, E.J. Greenberg, C.A. Smith, and D.C. Schwartz. Effect of tamoxifen on serum cholesterol and lipoproteins during chemohormonal therapy. *Clinica chimica acta; international journal of clinical chemistry*. 1993; 223(1-2): 43-52.

[108] Love, R.R., D.A. Wiebe, J.M. Feyzi, P.A. Newcomb, and R.J. Chappell. Effects of tamoxifen on cardiovascular risk factors in postmenopausal women after 5 years of treatment. *Journal of the National Cancer Institute*. 1994; 86(20): 1534-9.

[109] Saarto, T., C. Blomqvist, C. Ehnholm, M.R. Taskinen, and I. Elomaa. Antiatherogenic effects of adjuvant antiestrogens: a randomized trial comparing the effects of tamoxifen and toremifene on plasma lipid levels in postmenopausal women with node-positive breast cancer. *Journal of clinical oncology : official journal of the American Society of Clinical Oncology*. 1996; 14(2): 429-33.

[110] Rutqvist, L.E. Long-term toxicity of tamoxifen. *Recent results in cancer research. Fortschritte der Krebsforschung. Progres dans les recherches sur le cancer*. 1993; 127: 257-66.

[111] Pasqualini, J.R., C. Sumida, and N. Giambiagi. Pharmacodynamic and biological effects of anti-estrogens in different models. *J. Steroid Biochem.* 1988; 31(4B): 613-643.

[112] Robertson, D.W., J.A. Katzenellenbogen, D.J. Long, E.A. Rorke, and B.S. Katzenellenbogen. Tamoxifen antiestrogens. A comparison of the activity, pharmacokinetics, and metabolic activation of the cis and trans isomers of tamoxifen. *J. Steroid Biochem.* 1982; 16(1): 1-13.

[113] Reddel, R.R. and R.L. Sutherland. N-desmethyltamoxifen inhibits growth of MCF 7 human mammary carcinoma cells in vitro. *Eur. J. Cancer Clin. Oncol.* 1983; 19(8): 1179-1181.

[114] Etienne, M.C., G. Milano, J.L. Fischel, M. Frenay, E. Francois, J.L. Formento, J. Gioanni, and M. Namer. Tamoxifen metabolism: pharmacokinetic and in vitro study. *Br. J. Cancer*. 1989; 60(1): 30-35.

[115] Mandlekar, S., V. Hebbar, K. Christov, and A.N. Kong. Pharmacodynamics of tamoxifen and its 4-hydroxy and N-desmethyl metabolites: activation of caspases and induction of apoptosis in rat mammary tumors and in human breast cancer cell lines. *Cancer Res*. 2000; 60(23): 6601-6606.

[116] Peyrade, F., M. Frenay, M.C. Etienne, F. Ruch, C. Guillemare, E. Francois, M. Namer, J.M. Ferrero, and G. Milano. Age-related difference in tamoxifen disposition. *Clin. Pharmacol. Ther.* 1996; 59(4): 401-10.

[117] Berstein, L.M., J.P. Wang, H. Zheng, W. Yue, M. Conaway, and R.J. Santen. Long-term exposure to tamoxifen induces hypersensitivity to estradiol. *Clin. Cancer Res.* 2004; 10(4): 1530-4.

[118] Randolph, J.F., Jr., M. Sowers, I. Bondarenko, E.B. Gold, G.A. Greendale, J.T. Bromberger, S.E. Brockwell, and K.A. Matthews. The relationship of longitudinal change in reproductive hormones and vasomotor symptoms during the menopausal transition. *J. Clin. Endocrinol. Metab.* 2005; 90(11): 6106-12.

[119] Mortimer, J.E., S.W. Flatt, B.A. Parker, E.B. Gold, L. Wasserman, L. Natarajan, and J.P. Pierce. Tamoxifen, hot flashes and recurrence in breast cancer. *Breast Cancer Res. Treat.* 2008; 108(3): 421-426.

[120] Rae, J., M. Sikora, N. Henry, S. Kim, S. Oesterreich, T.C. Skaar, A. Nguyen, and Z. Desta. Cytochrome P450 2D6 activity predicts adherence to tamoxifen therapy. *Breast Cancer Res. Treat.* 2007; S106(S1): S21.

[121] Demissie, S., R.A. Silliman, and T.L. Lash. Adjuvant tamoxifen: predictors of use, side effects, and discontinuation in older women. *J. Clin. Oncol.* 2001; 19(2): 322-8.

[122] Grunfeld, E.A., M.S. Hunter, P. Sikka, and S. Mittal. Adherence beliefs among breast cancer patients taking tamoxifen. *Patient Educ. Couns.* 2005; 59(1): 97-102.

[123] Owusu, C., D.S. Buist, T.S. Field, T.L. Lash, S.S. Thwin, A.M. Geiger, V.P. Quinn, F. Frost, M. Prout, M.U. Yood, F. Wei, and R.A. Silliman. Predictors of tamoxifen discontinuation among older women with estrogen receptor-positive breast cancer. *J. Clin. Oncol.* 2008; 26(4): 549-55.

[124] Ma, A.M., J. Barone, A.E. Wallis, N.J. Wu, L.B. Garcia, A. Estabrook, S.M. Rosenbaum-Smith, and P.I. Tartter. Noncompliance with adjuvant radiation, chemotherapy, or hormonal therapy in breast cancer patients. *Am. J. Surg.* 2008; 196(4): 500-4.

[125] van Leeuwen, F.E., J. Benraadt, J.W. Coebergh, L.A. Kiemeney, C.H. Gimbrere, R. Otter, L.J. Schouten, R.A. Damhuis, M. Bontenbal, F.W. Diepenhorst, and et al. Risk of endometrial cancer after tamoxifen treatment of breast cancer. *Lancet.* 1994; 343(8895): 448-52.

[126] Gallicchio, L., G. Lord, K. Tkaczuk, M. Danton, L.M. Lewis, C.K. Lim, and J.A. Flaws. Association of tamoxifen (TAM) and TAM metabolite concentrations with self-reported side effects of TAM in women with breast cancer. *Breast Cancer Res. Treat.* 2004; 85(1): 89-97.

[127] Lien, E.A., G. Anker, and P.M. Ueland. Pharmacokinetics of tamoxifen in premenopausal and postmenopausal women with breast cancer. *J. Steroid Biochem. Mol. Biol.* 1995; 55(2): 229-31.

[128] de Lima, G.R., G. Facina, J.Y. Shida, M.B. Chein, P. Tanaka, R.C. Dardes, V.C. Jordan, and L.H. Gebrim. Effects of low dose tamoxifen on normal breast tissue from premenopausal women. *Eur. J. Cancer.* 2003; 39(7): 891-898.

[129] Bratherton, D.G., C.H. Brown, R. Buchanan, V. Hall, E.M. Kingsley Pillers, T.K. Wheeler, and C.J. Williams. A comparison of two doses of tamoxifen (Nolvadex) in postmenopausal women with advanced breast cancer: 10 mg bd versus 20 mg bd. *Br. J. Cancer.* 1984; 50(2): 199-205.

[130] Watkins, S.M. The value of high dose tamoxifen in postmenopausal breast cancer patients progressing on standard doses: a pilot study. *British journal of cancer.* 1988; 57(3): 320-1.

[131] Decensi, A., C. Robertson, G. Viale, F. Pigatto, H. Johansson, E.R. Kisanga, P. Veronesi, R. Torrisi, M. Cazzaniga, S. Mora, M.T. Sandri, G. Pelosi, A. Luini, A. Goldhirsch, E.A. Lien, and U. Veronesi. A randomized trial of low-dose tamoxifen on breast cancer proliferation and blood estrogenic biomarkers. *J. Natl. Cancer Inst.* 2003; 95(11): 779-790.
[132] Katzenellenbogen, J.A., C.J. Mathias, H.F. VanBrocklin, J.W. Brodack, and M.J. Welch. Titration of the in vivo uptake of 16 alpha-[18F]fluoroestradiol by target tissues in the rat: competition by tamoxifen, and implications for quantitating estrogen receptors in vivo and the use of animal models in receptor-binding radiopharmaceutical development. *Nucl. Med. Biol.* 1993; 20(6): 735-45.
[133] Bonanni, B., H. Johansson, S. Gandini, A. Guerrieri-Gonzaga, M.T. Sandri, F. Mariette, E.A. Lien, and A. Decensi. Effect of tamoxifen at low doses on ultrasensitive C-reactive protein in healthy women. *J. Thromb. Haemost.* 2003; 1(10): 2149-2152.
[134] Barron, T.I., R. Connolly, K. Bennett, J. Feely, and M.J. Kennedy. Early discontinuation of tamoxifen: a lesson for oncologists. *Cancer.* 2007; 109(5): 832-9.

In: Tamoxifen Concepts and Cancer: New Paradigms
Editor: Ramon Andrade de Mello
ISBN: 978-1-62081-520-5

Chapter III

Tamoxifen and Autophagy: To Cease and Resist?

L. Phan[1,2] ***and S. M. Gorski***[1,2,*]
[1]The Genome Sciences Centre, BC Cancer Agency, Vancouver, BC, Canada
[2]Department of Molecular Biology and Biochemistry, Simon Fraser University, Burnaby, BC, Canada

Abstract

Tamoxifen, a selective estrogen receptor modulator (SERM), is the most widely used antiestrogen monotherapy for the treatment of estrogen receptor positive (ER+) breast cancer. Although effective in reducing tumor growth and increasing overall patient survival, 20-30% of women treated with tamoxifen ultimately acquire resistance to the treatment. Resistance to tamoxifen has been attributed to both ER-dependent and ER-independent effects, but the underlying mechanisms are still not well understood. One of the many biological effects of tamoxifen is the induction of autophagy, a cellular process of "self-eating" that plays various roles in homeostasis, development, and stress adaptation. Autophagy has been implicated in the cellular response to numerous anticancer therapies, including tamoxifen. It is an evolutionarily conserved catabolic process that involves sequestration of long-lived proteins and organelles from the cytoplasm in a double membrane structure known as an autophagosome. The autophagosome fuses with a lysosome to form an autolysosome that enables the contents of the autophagosome to be degraded and released back into the cytoplasm for bioenergetic or biosynthetic processes. The roles of autophagy in breast cancer, as well as other cancer types, are still largely unknown. It was demonstrated that when breast cancer cell lines are treated with cytotoxic concentrations of tamoxifen, autophagy is increased. When tamoxifen treatment is combined with autophagy inhibition, breast cancer cell viability decreased. These observations indicate that autophagy has a primary survival or protective role in the context of the cellular response to tamoxifen. Further studies suggested that autophagy may play a critical role in the development of tamoxifen

[*] E-mail: sgorski@bcgsc.ca.

resistance. However, the molecular mechanisms that contribute to this outcome require further investigation. This chapter summarizes our current understanding of the interaction between tamoxifen and the autophagy pathway in breast cancer.

Breast Cancer

Breast cancer is the third most common type of cancer after prostate and lung cancer but the most common cancer amongst women [1]. Worldwide, more than one million breast cancer cases occur annually with the most recent global reports indicating that approximately 400,000 or 1.6% of all female deaths occur each year from this disease [2]. Mortality is primarily associated with late detection and recurrence, which is often aggressive and unresponsive to most available treatments.

Breast Cancer Classification

Breast cancer prognosis and treatment options are assessed based on a number of characteristics depending on the stage of the disease, molecular signature of the tumor, and individual patient characteristics, including general health and age. Generally, breast cancers show significant variability in morphology, invasiveness, pathology, histology, ploidy, proliferation, and receptor expression. Molecular characterization of receptor status in breast cancers has revealed various subtypes that allow patient stratification with respect to treatment options and prognosis [3,4,5]. Three main receptors are screened to help determine the intrinsic breast cancer subtype: human epidermal growth factor receptor 2 (HER2), progesterone receptor (PR) and estrogen receptor (ER). The characterization of gene expression profiles and receptor status of breast cancers has also led to the classification of breast carcinomas into five types: luminal A (ER+, PR+, Her2-), luminal B (ER+, PR+, Her2+), HER2-positve (ER-, PR-, HER2+), basal-like (ER-, PR-, HER2-) and normal-like carcinomas (ER+ and HER2 normal) [6,7]. In the clinical management of breast cancer, determining receptor expression through methods such as immunohistochemistry (IHC) is required; for instance, the identification of hormone receptor status ER+ is used to initiate endocrine therapy.

Estrogen Receptors and Endocrine Therapies

The breast cancer estrogen receptor positive (ER+) subtype is found in approximately 70% of newly diagnosed breast cancers. Although there have been many pharmacological advances in screening and treating this subtype, it is associated with 30-50% of patients that have no initial response to the antiestrogen therapy or resistance is acquired after treatment [8]. The estrogen receptor is often a constitutively activated nuclear receptor in breast cancer cells. There are two main isoforms of the estrogen receptor, encoded by genes located on separate chromosomes: the canonical ER-alpha (chromosome 6q25.1) and ER-beta (chromosome 14q22–25) [9]. These isoforms act similarly, in that they vary their activity as nuclear transcription factors in response to ligands (e.g. estrogen). In breast cancer cells, they have antagonistic functions where ER-alpha stimulates growth and proliferation, while ER-beta inhibits this activity [10]. Present in nearly two thirds of breast cancers, the ER-alpha isoform is thought to have a larger role in breast cancers than ER-beta. Studies have indicated that measuring ER-alpha alone is sufficient to predict antiestrogen response [11].

Endocrine therapies act by preventing estrogen synthesis or by blocking estrogen binding to its receptor, thereby preventing growth and proliferation of an estrogen-sensitive tumor. 17-beta-estradiol is the cognate ligand to ER-alpha, and is antagonized by various selective estrogen receptor modulators (SERMs) and selective estrogen receptor down regulators (SERDs) [12]. SERDs, (e.g. fulvestrant) downregulate and degrade the estrogen receptor [13], while SERMs (e.g. tamoxifen) bind to estrogen receptors (alpha and/or beta) and depending on tissue, cell and gene or signaling pathways response, act as agonists or antagonists. For example, a SERM may stimulate ER function in the bone but inhibit ER function in the breast [14, 15].

Tamoxifen

Since the 1970s, tamoxifen, the first FDA approved non-steroidal SERM, has been the most extensively used first-line treatment for ER+ breast cancer [9]. Used as a preventative, adjuvant or neoadjuvant treatment option for breast cancer patients, tamoxifen is estimated to have saved the lives of over 400,000 women since its inception. However, since tamoxifen resistance is a common problem, other SERMS, like raloxifene, are used as second-line therapies. Alternative therapeutics for breast cancer can be used in combination with or instead of tamoxifen and include aromatase inhibitors (anastrazole, letrozole and exemestane) [16]. These drugs effectively block estrogen synthesis by inhibiting aromatase, the enzyme that converts androgen and other steroid precursors to estrogen. Despite the growing number of treatment options for ER+ breast cancer, treatment efficacy is still limited due to endocrine resistance.

Endocrine Resistance: Insights from Tamoxifen

Antiestrogen resistance occurs as a result of the cell's ability to exploit alternate mechanisms to enable estrogen-dependent and –independent cell growth and proliferation to occur. There are two main types of resistance associated with endocrine therapies: intrinsic (or *de novo*) resistance and acquired resistance. The main feature of intrinsic resistance appears to be a lack of estrogen receptor alpha expression. Another intrinsic mechanism, associated with tamoxifen resistance, is the disruption of cytochrome P450 2D6 (CYP2D6), an enzyme that metabolizes tamoxifen into its active forms [17]. Acquired resistance can occur through different mechanisms, most of which have been elucidated through studies of tamoxifen given its relatively long history of use in the clinic.

ER-Dependent Resistance Mechanisms

Many cells acquire tamoxifen resistance from prolonged ER-dependent stimulation of growth/survival pathways (illustrated in Figure 1) that cause the loss of ER functionality, dysregulation of ER co-regulators, or alterations in the protein partners that the ER interacts with (eg. NFkB, NCOA3, PELP1 and AP1) [18-22]. Alteration in protein interactions also includes increased molecular alteration through the activity of EGFR, HER2 or IGF1R that can lead to tamoxifen resistance, along with modifications in signalling pathway components including PI3K, PTEN, Akt, and mTOR [21, 23-26] (Figure 1). Inhibitors targeting components of such signal transduction pathways (e.g. Trastuzumab targeting HER2; Gefitinib targeting EGFR) are currently being evaluated in combination with endocrine therapies in clinical trials but further research in this area is required to identify effective combinations and the patients who will benefit from them.

ER-Independent Resistance Mechanisms

ER-independent mechanisms of tamoxifen resistance also exist. The ability of breast cancer cells to sustain growth in an estrogen independent manner was first shown by Clarke et al. (1993) who developed estrogen-independent but estrogen-responsive MCF7/LCC1 human breast cancer cells. A variant of this line, called MCF7/LCC2 was selected for resistance against 4-hydroxytamoxifen (4-OH), an active tamoxifen metabolite [27, 28].

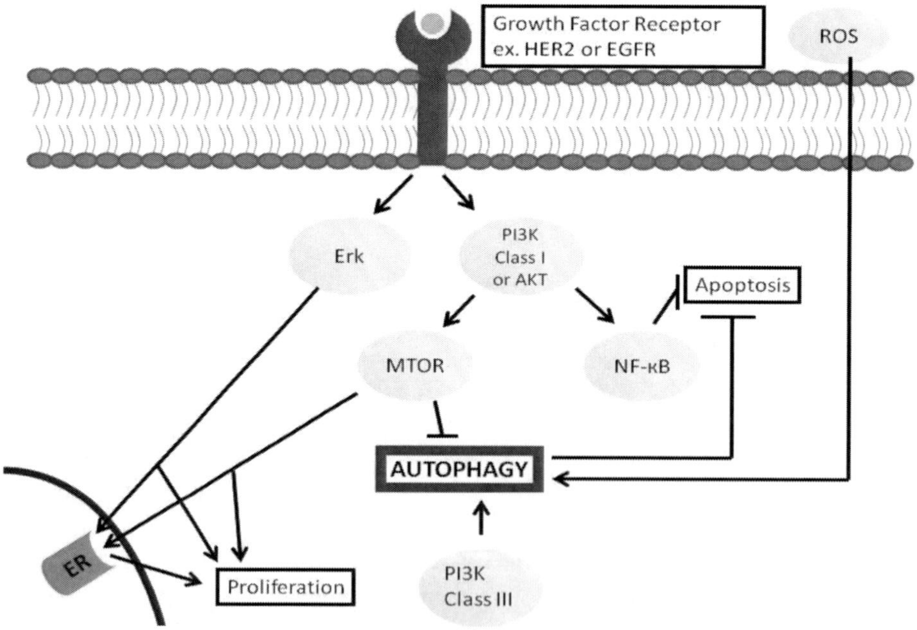

Figure 1. Mechanisms of endocrine resistance. Tamoxifen resistance often results from modulation of the estrogen receptor (ER) pathway or alterations in growth factor signal transduction pathways controlling apoptotic or anti-proliferative effects (illustrated with solid arrows). Autophagy's role in tamoxifen resistance has been linked to the inhibition of apoptosis and increased Beclin 1 expression, and may also be connected to alterations in the other denoted cellular signaling pathways.

These cells still expressed ER-alpha but could grow in the absence of estrogen and were resistant to tamoxifen *in vivo* and *in vitro* [9, 29], suggesting that even in the presence of a functional ER, the cells were resistant to the growth inhibitory effects of tamoxifen. Another ER-independent mechanism of resistance has since been shown to involve the induction of the oxidative stress response [30]. Other ER-independent effects or mechanisms of resistance include cellular membrane structure disruptions, inhibition of the Ca+ binding protein calmodulin, and changes in protein kinase C activation and subcellular localization [21]. These mechanisms were associated with relatively high (micromolar) concentrations of tamoxifen that normally result in apoptosis-associated cytotoxic effects in breast cancer cells (reviewed in 31). In addition to the above outlined mechanisms, a cellular process called autophagy has been implicated in antiestrogen therapy resistance. Like the ER signaling network, autophagy is also associated with several genetic, molecular, and signaling networks that make studying the mechanisms behind autophagy-mediated resistance complex (Figure 1).

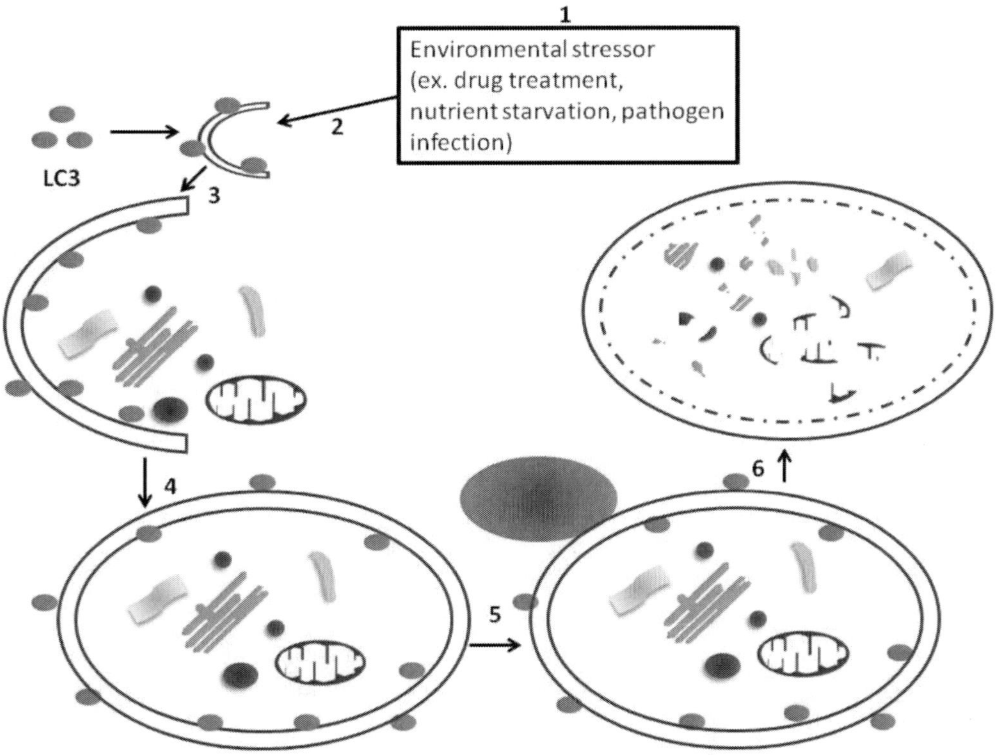

Figure 2. The cellular events of autophagy can be divided into specific steps: 1. Induction - environmental conditions such as drug treatment, nutrient starvation, and pathogen infection are stressors that can induce autophagy. 2. Vesicle nucleation – this is where the double-membrane bound structure/phagophore is initiated. 3. Vesicle elongation – the double membrane elongates, sequestering cytoplasmic proteins and organelles. 4. Vesicle completion – the ends of the double membrane fuse to form the circular autophagosome. 5. Docking and fusion – lysosomes dock and fuse with the autophagosome to form an autolysosome. 6. Degradation – the inner membrane and contents of the autophagosome are degraded by lysosomal hydrolases.

Autophagy

Autophagy, a term derived from the Greek words meaning "self" and "eating", is a degradative process conserved in all eukaryotes [32, 33]. It was first described in the 1960s by Christian de Duve [33] and has gathered increasing attention as the genes involved have been uncovered and methods of detection have evolved [34]. The model system used to uncover the molecular mechanisms of autophagy was the yeast, *Saccharmyces cervisiae.* Genetic screens using this model have identified at least 32 autophagy-related genes (*ATG*) with orthologues in many other species including *C. elegans, D. melanogaster,* and mammals [35-41]. The functions of the *ATG* gene products in yeasts are comparable to those of their mammalian counterparts. There are three main defined types of autophagy that each participate in the proteolytic degradation of cytosolic components by the lysosome: macroautophagy, micro-autophagy and chaperone-mediated autophagy [42]. This chapter focuses on macroautophagy (hereafter referred to as autophagy).

Autophagy is primarily a cell survival process, involved in energy homeostasis and mitigation of cellular damage, which provides nutrients and energy by recycling damaged or aggregated proteins and organelles. Autophagy functions at a basal rate under normal conditions, but is upregulated during cellular stress (e.g., nutrient deprivation, anticancer therapy). Autophagy's cytoprotective role is also associated with immune responses against foreign invaders detected by the cell [43, 44]. The importance of autophagy in organismal survival was underscored by studies showing that the autophagy-related genes (*ATG*), *ATG5* or *ATG7*, knocked out in mice result in neonatal lethality [47-49]. This indicates that *ATG* are important in cell and organismal survival. Conversely, prolonged autophagy can degrade necessary cellular constituents causing cellular degeneration, or may reach a point where apoptotic or non-apoptotic cell death occurs [50-52].

The Autophagy Pathway

The autophagic process can be described in 6 main steps: 1) induction 2) vesicle nucleation 3) membrane elongation 4) autophagosome completion 5) docking and fusion, and 6) vesicle breakdown and degradation (Figure 2) [53].

Autophagy *induction* occurs when external factors lead to the formation of the Atg1:Atg13:Atg17 complex in yeast and its mammalian counterpart, the ULK1:Atg13:FIP200 complex [54]. A key regulator that inhibits autophagy is the target of rapamycin (TOR). Under growth-promoting conditions, mTOR (i.e. mammalian TOR) acts to suppress autophagy by inhibiting ULK1 kinase activity. However following autophagy-initiating signals such as starvation, stress or rapamycin, mTOR becomes repressed and ULK1 catalytic activity is stimulated [55, 56].

Vesicle *nucleation* involves the initial assembly of the autophagosome through the class III phosphatidylinositol 3-kinase (PIK3C3; or its yeast ortholog vps34) and Beclin 1 (mammalian orthologue of essential yeast *ATG6/vps30* gene [57]. PIK3C3, p150 (mammalian orthologue of yeast vps15), Atg14L, and Ambra1 form a complex that is directed to the organizing center of autophagosome formation known as the phagophore (preautophagosomal structure [PAS] in yeast).

Elongation of the autophagosome membrane is then mediated by two ubiquitin-like pathways: i) Atg12 is covalently conjugated to Atg5 through the action of Atg7 and Atg10 and ii) Atg8 (mammalian MAP1LC3B or LC3) is lipidated by conjugation to phosphatidylethanolamine (PE) through enzymatic action of Atg7 and Atg3 [57]. The lipidation of LC3 is a critical step in the pathway that only occurs upon stimulation of autophagy and converts LC3-I (a cleaved form of LC3) to LC3-II; that is, from its soluble cytoplasmic form to the membrane-bound form, respectively [58, 59]. This lipidated form of LC3 can be found on the outer and inner membranes of the autophagosome (Figure 2).

Autophagosome membrane elongation and membrane-end fusion result in *autophagosome completion*; if it fuses with an endosome then it is termed an amphisome [59].

Mature autophagosomes or amphisomes undergo trafficking and subsequent *docking and fusion* with lysosomal compartments to form autolysosomes [61-63]. The proteins that regulate the intracellular transport include Rab GTPase, SNARE (Soluble *N*-ethylmaleimide-sensitive factor attachment protein receptors), LAMP2 (lysosomal-associated membrane protein 2) and ESCRT (endosomal sorting complex required for transport) [64]. These trafficking events are further regulated by Beclin 1 through its interaction with Rubicon and UVRAG either by upregulating (via Beclin 1:Vps34:p150:UVRAG:Bif-1complex) or downregulating (via Beclin 1:Vps34:p150:UVRAG:Rubicon complex) the maturation of autophagosomes and endocytic trafficking [65-67].

Finally, *vesicle breakdown and degradation* is mediated by the function of the acidic degradative compartments (autolysosomes) and controlled by proteins that include v-ATPase, LAMP proteins, lysosomal carriers, and lysosomal hydrolases.

Detection of Autophagy in Mammalian Cells

Microscopy and Staining

Detection of the double-membrane autophagosome and its fusion with the lysosome is used to assess autophagy status in cells. The first direct observation of the autophagosome occurred by transmission electron microscopy (TEM) and continues to be a widely used method of detection in conjunction with other approaches such as the imaging of acidic compartments by staining with the autofluorescent compound monodansylcadaverine (MDC) or LysoTracker stains (indicating possible accumulation of autolysosomes) [33, 68-71]. However, as MDC is not a specific marker for autophagy, complementary methods are necessary to detect autophagic structures and measure autophagic flux (i.e. degradative completion of autophagy).

MAP1LC3β

The autophagy protein microtubule-associated protein light chain 3β, MAP1LC3β (LC3B, or simply LC3, in mammals and Atg8 in yeast), is the most commonly used specific marker for autophagic structures. Unprocessed (pro)LC3 is a full-length cytosolic protein involved in autophagosome formation that is cleaved by Atg4B, a cysteine protease, to generate LC3-I. The LC3-I protein is transferred to Atg3 before it becomes conjugated to phosphatidyl-ethanolamine (PE) to generate processed LC3-II. LC3-II is then recruited and integrated into the growing autophagosome with the help of Atg5-Atg12 and is found on both external and internal membranes of the autophagosome [72]. Thus, LC3-II is a useful marker as it can be used to detect autophagosome membranes as well as autophagy induction. LC3 can also be fused to fluorescent proteins such as GFP so that it can be readily observed and quantified in GFP-LC3 transfected cells using fluorescence microscopy. GFP-LC3 appears diffuse in the cytoplasm under normal conditions, but appears as measurable punctate structures when inserted into the autophagosome membrane upon autophagy induction (Figure 3).

Another standard technique for autophagy detection is Western blot analysis to detect conversion of LC3-I to LC3-II. The cytosolic form of LC3-I becomes lipidated, forming LC3-II, and moves to the autophagosome membrane where it is eventually degraded following fusion with a lysosome. The addition of lysosomal inhibitors, such as bafilomycin A1 (baf A1) or chloroquine, are used to help measure LC3-II processing and determine whether a given treatment results in autophagic flux (i.e. the completion of the autophagic pathway) [68]. LC3-II protein levels on a Western blot that show an increased accumulation in the presence of a lysosomal inhibitor compared to a control with no inhibitor, indicate that the treatment under question normally induces autophagy flux. If no further increase in LC3-II is observed, this suggests that the treatment in question does not induce flux, but instead signifies impaired lysosomal proteolytic activity, delayed trafficking to the lysosomes, or reduced fusion between compartments [55, 73].

p62/SQSTM1

LC3-II is thought to act as a phagophore 'receptor' that facilitates selective uptake and degradation of autophagic targets expressing 'adaptor' molecules, such as p62/SQSTM1. p62/SQSTM1 promotes turnover of poly-ubiquinated protein aggregates [59, 74] and is degraded in autolysosomes along with the target protein. Therefore, degraded or decreased expression levels of p62 following autophagy induction indicate functional flux, while a block in flux is associated with an increased p62 level. The function of p62 in other cellular processes is not well known, so p62 levels should not be relied on as a sole indicator of autophagy flux. Together, p62 and LC3-II autophagy assays provide a more reliable evaluation of autophagic flux, but timing and inhibitor concentrations are key parameters that must be carefully monitored. In summary, the recommended method of autophagy detection is through a combination of assays to identify morphological structures as well as to determine autophagic flux.

The Role of Autophagy in Cancer and Cancer Therapy

Dysfunction of autophagy can lead to various pathologies such as neurodegenerative and cardiovascular disorders, infectious disease and cancer [56]. Autophagy has been shown to play dual roles facilitating either tumor suppression or tumor survival in cancer. In breast cancer cells, Liang et al. (1999) demonstrated the association between Beclin1 and tumorigenicity. They showed decreased levels of Beclin 1 in breast cancer cells compared to normal adjacent breast tissue. When a construct expressing Beclin 1 was reintroduced into MCF7 breast cancer cells, it induced autophagy and inhibited tumorigenesis, suggesting that autophagy plays a tumor suppressor role in breast cancer cells. Subsequent studies have led to a generally accepted model whereby autophagy functions as a tumor suppressor by clearing damaged materials within the cell that may otherwise lead to genomic damage, inflammation and an overall environment conducive to tumor growth [75-78]. Alternatively, autophagy may promote tumorigenesis by enabling the survival of cancer cells. For example, the central region of a tumor is often starved of nutrients and oxygen and may rely on autophagy for survival. To reconcile the dual roles it plays in cancer, autophagy can be considered to play a tumor suppressor role in normal or pre-cancerous cells, but may function to promote tumor progression by facilitating survival in established cancer cells.

Pathways Involved in Autophagy and Tumorigenesis

Many of the signaling pathways that regulate tumorigenesis are also linked to the regulation of autophagy. Aberrant mTOR signaling is a common feature of cancers [79] and, as described above, mTOR functions as a negative regulator of autophagy in response to a variety of stimuli. Several upstream inhibitors of mTOR, including the tumor suppressors PTEN, TSC1, and TSC2, enhance autophagy [80]. One of the most prolifically mutated tumor suppressors in human cancers, p53, also positively regulates autophagy[81, 82]. Additional positive regulators of autophagy involved in the response to cellular stress are JNK, PERK, and NFκB. Conversely, the oncogenes PI3-kinase and Akt function to inhibit autophagy in most cases [80]. Growth factor receptor signaling pathways such as IGFR, EGFR and HER2 also function to suppress autophagy, and blockage of these pathways by drugs or by crosstalk with other signaling molecules leads to autophagy upregulation (reviewed in 83; 56, 84). While many of these signaling molecules and pathways are also linked to tamoxifen resistance (Figure 1), it remains to be determined whether autophagy levels are a contributing factor to their tumor suppressor or oncogenic effects.

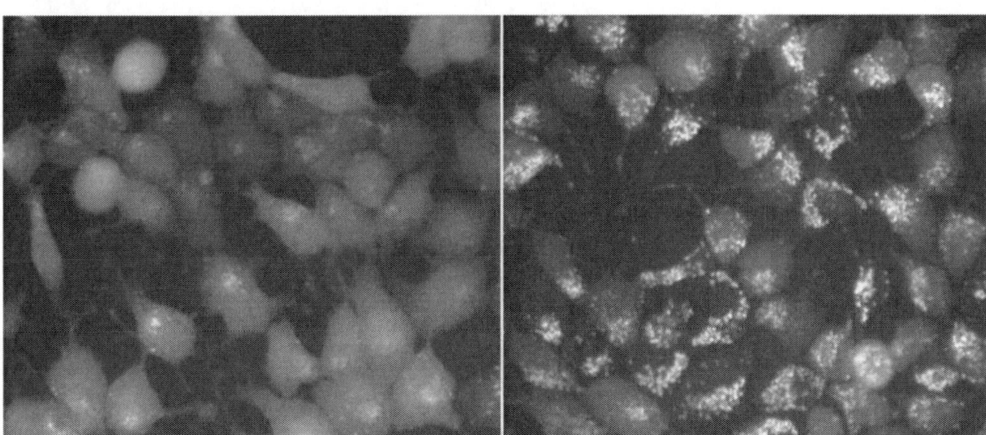

Figure 3. Autophagy detection by GFP-LC3. MCF7 cells stably transfected with GFP-LC3 were treated with vehicle control (left) or 5uM tamoxifen (right) for three days. Flourescence microscopy analysis revealed a dramatic increase in GFP-LC3 puncta in the tamoxifen treated MCF7 cells compared to the control MCF7 cells.

Autophagy Response to Anti-Cancer Therapeutics

In a number of cancer cell lines, including breast cancer cells, the induction of autophagy was demonstrated in response to stress conditions, including treatment with a variety of anti-cancer therapeutics [85-87]. Genetic or pharmacological inhibition of autophagy in combination with chemotherapies has revealed that, in this context, autophagy represents a cytoprotective response that enables cancer cells to cope with the stress induced by treatment [88]. Pharmacological (non-specific) inhibitors of autophagy include 3-methyladenine (3MA), chloroquine, bafilomycin A1 (BafA1) or hydroxychloroquine. Autophagy inhibition, using these drugs and/or *ATG* targeted siRNAs, in combination with radiation or chemotherapeutics resulted in increased sensitization and/or enhanced levels of apoptosis in a variety of breast and other cancer cell lines, as well as in mouse models [56; 89-95]. Together, these findings provide a strong rationale for pursuing autophagy inhibition in anticancer combination therapy. Notably, recent reports have indicated that inhibition of autophagy may also be an effective strategy for enhancing the efficacy of tamoxifen treatment [96, 97].

Tamoxifen and Autophagy

Tamoxifen Induces Autophagy in Association with Cell Death

The induction of autophagy by tamoxifen was first described in 1996 by Bursch et al. who used electron microscopy analysis to show that addition of the antiestrogens tamoxifen, 4-hydroxy-tamoxifen (4-OH) and ICI 164 384 to MCF7 breast carcinoma cells in culture led to the formation of autophagic vacuoles [98]. While treatment of MCF7 cells with 10uM tamoxifen led to extensive necrosis within 24hr, treatment with 1uM tamoxifen had primarily cytostatic effects followed by delayed cell death. The cells treated with 1uM tamoxifen contained numerous autophagic vacuoles and most had normal appearing nuclei, though 20-25% of the cells had nuclei with altered morphology that included pyknosis (nuclear condensation), crescent pieces of chromatin, or fragmentation. Upon addition of 3-methyladenine three or four days after tamoxifen treatment there was a modest reduction in nuclear alterations, with 1-5% of cells affected. These results were interpreted to mean that in response to tamoxifen, the cells were undergoing *autophagic cell death* – defined at that time on a morphological basis (i.e. the dying cells had morphological features of autophagy). A subsequent investigation found that tamoxifen also induced signs of autophagy in the FM3a murine breast tumor cell line, and cell death was similarly assumed to occur in part *via* autophagy [99]. Today, most evidence from studies exploring "autophagic cell death" suggests that *autophagy occurs in association with cell death* rather than contributing to it; instead, autophagy represents a failed attempt at cell survival [56, 100, 101]. However, these initial observations of tamoxifen-induced autophagy [98, 99] were instrumental in setting the stage for later studies that would directly test the function of autophagy in tamoxifen treated breast cancer cell lines (see below).

Mechanisms Underlying the Induction of Autophagy by Tamoxifen

How does tamoxifen lead to the stimulation of autophagy? The following are some of the suggested mechanisms:

Lipids

Multiple lipids have been implicated in the regulation of autophagy induction by tamoxifen. The sphingolipid ceramide has established roles in the response to cellular stress, and Scarlatti et al. (2004) showed that C2-ceramide stimulated an increase in mRNA and protein expression of Beclin 1 in MCF7 cells. Further, the addition of myriocin, an inhibitor of ceramide *de novo* synthesis, resulted in reduced Beclin 1 levels and a reduction in autophagic vacuole accumulation in response to tamoxifen [102]. In 2009, Medina et al investigated the cellular effects of the antiestrogen binding site (AEBS) ligands, tamoxifen and N-pyrrolidino-(phenylmethyphenoxy)-ethanamine, HCl (PBPE), a tamoxifen derivative, on breast cancer cells and they found that they induced autophagy in MCF7 cells. They showed that the induction of autophagy was dependent on sterol accumulation, and that the sterols stimulate the production of reactive oxygen species (ROS). These authors found that while accumulation of sterols was required for autophagy, the production of reactive oxygen species (ROS) was not required in this system. Interestingly, different AEBS ligands resulted in the accumulation of different sterol precursors that induced autophagy to different extents. These findings indicate that accumulation of sterols is one mechanism by which tamoxifen induces autophagy.

Zinc Ions and Reactive Oxygen Species

A recent study indicated that zinc (2+) ions may also contribute to the induction of autophagy by tamoxifen [103]. Labile Zn^{2+} ions were found to accumulate in most LC3-positive vacuoles in tamoxifen-treated MCF7 cells, and addition of a Zn^{2+} chelator, N,N,N',N'-tetrakis (2-pyridyl-methyl) ethylenediamine (TPEN), led to decreased LC3-II levels, a reduction in phosphorylated Erk, and reduced vacuole formation. These authors found that ROS levels did affect tamoxifen-induced autophagy since treatment with the antioxidant NAC resulted in reduced Zn^{2+} levels, reduced LC3-II conversion. Thus, this study attributed autophagy induction to the presence of both Zn^{2+} ions as well as ROS, the latter consistent with previous reports demonstrating the activation of autophagy by ROS [104, 105].

Autophagy Contributes to Cell Survival and Resistance to Tamoxifen

Multiple lines of evidence now support a survival role for autophagy in response to tamoxifen treatment. The function of autophagy in response to tamoxifen was first tested in two studies reported in 2008 [96, 97] Qadir et al (2008) used a siRNA-based approach to target three essential autophagy components (*ATG5*, *Beclin 1*, and *ATG7*) in MCF7 cells. Knockdown of any of these targets in combination with micromolar concentrations of tamoxifen resulted in decreased viability compared to tamoxifen alone, and was associated with an increase in mitochondrial-mediated apoptosis as measured by an increase in Annexin-V positive cells and a decrease in mitochondrial transmembrane potential. The effect of *ATG* gene silencing on tamoxifen sensitivity was also determined in two cell lines with increased resistance to tamoxifen, T47D and MCF7-HER2. Tamoxifen induced autophagy in both cell lines, and reduction in autophagy by *ATG*-siRNAs led to reduced viability, suggesting its role as a drug-induced survival mechanism. Interestingly, knockdown of *Beclin 1* had the greatest effect on viability in all three cell lines examined, and this may be due in part to autophagy-independent functions. Together, the results from Qadir et al (2008) suggested that autophagy inhibition can sensitize ER+ breast cancer cells, including tamoxifen-resistant breast cancer cells, to tamoxifen therapy. Additional support for a pro-survival function for autophagy in response to tamoxifen came from a study by Schoenlein and colleagues (2008, 2009) who showed that autophagy knockdown by *Beclin 1* siRNA or by 3-methyladenine (3-MA) resulted in increased MCF7 cell death in combination with micromolar concentrations of 4-hydroxytamoxifen (4OH). Cell death exhibited features of apoptosis, including activation of caspase-9 and caspase-6. Furthermore, MCF7 cells were subjected to a step-wise drug selection protocol using 4OH to derive tamoxifen-resistant cell lines. Detailed characterization of autophagy status in one of these lines showed that treatment resulted in relatively high levels of autophagy, and autophagy inhibition with 3-MA, bafilomycin A1 (bafA1) or *Beclin 1* siRNA induced a robust death response. In summary, these studies suggest that autophagy contributes to survival and is associated with tamoxifen-resistance in ER+ breast cancer cells.

Subsequent studies further supported a survival role for autophagy in response to tamoxifen treatment. In 2009, Medina et al showed that inhibition of autophagy with *Beclin 1* siRNA, 3-methyladenine, or (bafA1), sensitized cells to tamoxifen and AEBS ligands resulting in increased cell death as measured by Trypan blue exclusion [106]. Another study investigated the effects of combination treatment with tamoxifen and a histone deacetylase (HDAC) inhibitor in ER+ breast cancer cells [107]. The HDAC inhibitor was found to increase both apoptosis and autophagy in tamoxifen-treated cells, and the combination was associated with a decrease in Bcl-2 (a regulator of apoptosis and autophagy) and an increase in Beclin 1 protein. Despite enhanced apoptosis, a small population of cells remained resistant to the combination treatment and exhibited high levels of autophagy. Inhibition of autophagy in these remaining cells by either *Beclin1*-siRNA or chloroquine treatment led to apoptosis [107]. Together these results support a survival function for autophagy and also suggest that the triple combination of tamoxifen, an HDAC inhibitor and an autophagy inhibitor may be an effective treatment strategy for ER+ breast tumors.

Potential Mechanisms of Autophagy-Mediated Survival and Tamoxifen Resistance

This section discusses some of the mechanisms by which autophagy facilitates survival and resistance to tamoxifen:

Apoptosis Inhibition

The studies that have been discussed indicate that autophagy may contribute to survival of ER+ breast cancer cells, at least in part, by mitigating apoptosis (Figure 1). Consistent with these observations, it is well established that micromolar concentrations of tamoxifen and 4-hydroxytamoxifen (4OH) have cytotoxic effects in addition to cytostatic effects in breast cancer cells (reviewed in Mandlekar and Kong, 2001). The cytotoxic apoptosis-inducing effects of tamoxifen are considered to be predominantly ER-independent, and include involvement of caspases, mitochondria, ceramide, MAPK, JNK, PKC TGFb and c-myc (reviewed in 32). While many connections between apoptosis and autophagy regulation have been uncovered (reviewed in 53; 110, 111), the specific molecules involved in the context of tamoxifen treatment are just beginning to be identified. The studies described above implicate mitochondria, caspase, and Bcl-2 regulation as important factors [96, 97, 107], and several additional reports described below have provided further insights into the mechanisms related to autophagy's survival role in response to tamoxifen.

Modulation of ER-Alpha Function

Although it seems that tamoxifen-induced autophagy may be ER-independent (based on the cytotoxic concentrations of tamoxifen employed), some studies indicate that at least some effects may still be ER-mediated. A recent report suggested that tamoxifen induces *Beclin 1* expression via increased transcription mediated by the ER [107]. Interestingly, the Thomas laboratory suggested that Beclin 1 may function to sequester ER-alpha, resulting in reduced ER-alpha function [112], and they showed that Beclin 1 overexpression in MCF7 cells resulted in a decreased proliferative response to estrogen, the down-regulation of several estrogen-responsive genes, decreased Akt phosphorylation, and reduced sensitivity to the antiestrogens 4-hydroxytamoxifen and raloxifene. Co-immunoprecipitation of ER-alpha and Beclin 1 indicated that these proteins may interact directly in cells [112]. Thus, an increase in Beclin 1 protein (associated with induction of autophagy) could lead to reduced ER-alpha function and a corresponding decrease in tamoxifen sensitivity. In other words, a key autophagy protein, Beclin 1, may have an additional autophagy-independent role in the context of ER-alpha function and antiestrogen sensitivity.

Other Factors Identified by Large Scale Screening Approaches

Gene expression and function-based screening have provided new insights into possible mechanisms related to autophagy-mediated resistance in cancer cells. Gonzalez-Malerva et al. used high-throughput functional cell-based screening to identify more than 31 candidate kinases associated with resistance to tamoxifen. These kinases included previously described EGFR, HER2, and IGF1R, and also a newly identified kinase, HSPB8. They found that, like EGFR, HER2, and IGF1R, the overexpression of HSPB8 resulted in reduced autophagy, but the significance of this effect with respect to the observed resistance phenotype remains to be investigated [113]. Another study employing high throughput functional screening identified prolylcarboxypeptidase (PRCP) as a tamoxifen resistance factor associated with elevated autophagy. Knockdown of PRCP decreased proliferation, LC3-II, MDC-staining and BSA-proteolysis, and enhanced 4-hydroxytamoxifen-induced cytotoxicity [114]. Similarly, Namgoong et al found that high levels of the prolyl isomerase, Pin1, correlated with high levels of LC3 in tamoxifen-resistant breast cancer and that Pin1-siRNA resulted in robust induction of apoptosis in combination with 4-hydroxytamoxifen [115]. While further investigations are required, these results suggest that PRCP and/or Pin1 may confer tamoxifen resistance, at least in part, through upregulation of autophagy.

Conclusion

The induction of autophagy is one of the many cellular responses to the antiestrogen tamoxifen. However, this autophagy response still requires investigation in tumor models *in vivo* and in breast cancer patient specimens. Mounting evidence from *in vitro* studies supports a survival or protective role for autophagy in the response to tamoxifen treatment and suggests that autophagy may contribute to tamoxifen resistance. These observations suggest potential strategies to enhance responsiveness to tamoxifen, and perhaps other antiestrogens, by inhibiting autophagy. The non-specific inhibitors of autophagy, chloroquine and hydroxychloroquine, are already being investigated as combination therapy agents in numerous clinical trials in a variety of cancers (http://www.cancer.gov/clinicaltrials), and small molecule screens are underway to identify specific autophagy inhibitors [116]. The proteasome and autophagy inhibitor bortezomib [117] or agents targeting Beclin 1 or Pin1 may also provide effective treatment options for anti-estrogen resistant ER+ breast cancers. Additional biological targets will be realized as further studies reveal the molecular mechanisms involved in regulating autophagy and its roles in cell survival and tamoxifen resistance.

Acknowledgments

The authors thank Patricia Schoenlein, Adrienne Kyle, Svetlana Bortnik, Chandra Lebovitz, and Mario Jardon for helpful discussions and/or comments on the manuscript, and thank Amy Leung for providing the images for Figure 3. Research in the area of breast cancer and autophagy is conducted in SMG's laboratory with support from CIHR grants GPG102167 and MOP78882. SMG is supported in part by a CIHR New Investigator Award.

References

[1] N. Wadden and G.P. Doyle, *Association Of Radiologists Journal,* 56(5), 271-275 , (2005).

[2] D.M. Parkin, F. Bray, J. Ferlay, and P. Pisani, CA A Cancer Journal for Clinicians, 55(2), 74-108, (2005)

[3] D. J. Brennan, S. L. O'Brien, A. Fagan, A. C. Culhane, D. G. Higgins, M. J. Duffy, and W. M. Gallagher, *Expert Opinion on Biological Therapy, 5*(8), 1069-1083, (2005).

[4] L. Dunn and A. Demichele, *Molecular Diagnosis and Therapy, 13*(2), 73-90, (2009).

[5] V. Kaklamani, *Expert Review of Molecular Diagnostics, 6*(6), 803-809, (2006).

[6] L. A. Carey, *Clinical Breast Cancer, 10*(3), 188-195, (2010).

[7] F.A. Tavassoli, *International Journal Of Surgical Pathology, 18*(3 Suppl), 167S-169S, (2010).

[8] W.J. Gradishar, *Cancer Investigation, 28*(4), 433-442, (2010).

[9] R. Clarke, M.C. Liu, K.B. Bouker, Z. Gu, R.Y. Lee, Y. Zhu, T.C. Skaar et al., *Oncogene, 22*(47), 7316-7339, (2003).

[10] V.V. Tyulmenkov, S.C. Jernigan, and C.M. Klinge, *Molecular And Cellular Endocrinology*, *165*(1-2), 151-161, (2000).
[11] Y. Miyoshi, K. Murase, M. Saito, M. Imamura, and K. Oh, *Medical Molecular Morphology*, *43*(4), 193-196, (2011).
[12] S. Kocanova, M. Mazaheri, S. Caze-Subra, and K. Bystricky, *BMC Cell Biology*, 11, 98, (2010).
[13] Howell et al., Best Pract Res Clin Endocrinol Metab, 18(1), 47-66, (2004).
[14] V.C. Jordan, and B.W. O'Malley, *Journal of Clinical Oncology: Official Journal of the American Society of Clinical Oncology*, *25*(36), 5815-5824, (2007).
[15] Cummings et al., *JAMA*, 281(23), 2189-97, (1999).
[16] Geisler, *Breast Cancer*, 15(1), 17-26 (2008).
[17] Hoskins et al., *Nature Rev. Cancer*, 9(8), 576-86, (2009).
[18] Gururaj et al, *Clinical Cancer Research*, 12, 1001s-1007s, (2006).
[19] Johnston et al, *Clinical Cancer Research* 5(2), 251-6, (1999).
[20] Zhou et al, *BMC Cancer*, 7, 59, (2007).
[21] G. Arpino, C. De Angelis, M. Giuliano, A. Giordano, C. Falato, M. De Laurentiis, and De Placido, *Oncology*, 77, 23-37, (2009).
[22] S. Masri, S. Phung, X. Wang, and S. Chen, *The Journal Of Steroid Biochemistry And Molecular Biology*, 118(4-5), 277-282, (2010).
[23] G. Bunone et al, *EMBO J.*, 15, 2174-83 1996.
[24] Campbell et al, *J. Biol. Chem.*, 276, 9817, (2001).
[25] S. Kato et al, *Breast Cancer*, 8, 3, (1995).
[26] Musgrove and Sutherland, *Nat. Rev. Cancer*, 9, 631, (2009).
[27] M.F. Barginear, M. Jaremko, I. Peter, C. Yu, Y. Kasia, *Nature Clinical Pharmacology and Therapeutics*, 90, 605, (2011).
[28] M. Jaremko, Y. Kasai, M. Barginear, G. Raptis, R. Desnick, and C. Yu, *Analytical Chemistry*, 82(24), 10186-10193, (2010).
[29] Brunner et al., *Cancer Res.*, 53(14), 3229-32, (1993).
[30] G.E. Weitsman, W. Weebadda, K. Ung, and L.C. Murphy, *Breast Cancer Research And Treatment*, 118(2), 269-279, (2009).
[31] Mandlekar and Kong, *Apoptosis*, 6(6), 269-77, (2001).
[32] D. Glick, S. Barth, and K.F. Macleod, *The Journal of Pathology*, 221(1), 3-12, 2010.
[33] D. J. Klionsky, H. Abeliovich, P. Agostinis, D.K. Agrawal, G. Aliev, D.S. Askew, M. Baba, et al., *Autophagy*, 4(2), 151-175, (2008).
[34] Daniel J. Klionsky, *Nature Reviews. Molecular Cell Biology*, 8(11), 931-937, (2007).
[35] M. Baba et al., *J. Cell Biol.*, 124(6), 903-13, (1994).
[36] M. Tsukada et al., *FEBS*, 331, 169-74, (1993).
[37] T.M. Harding et al, *J. Biol. Chem.*, 271(30), 17621-4, (1996).
[38] C. He, and Daniel J. Klionsky, *Annual Review of Genetics*, 43(1), 67-93, (2009).
[39] A. Longatti and S.A. Tooze, *Cell Death Differ.*, 16(7), 956-965, (2009).
[40] H. Nakatogawa, K. Suzuki, Y. Kamada, and Yoshinori Ohsumi, *Nat. Rev. Mol. Cell Biol.*, 10(7), 458-467, (2009).
[41] M.H. Stipanuk, *Nutrition Reviews*, 67(12), 677-689, (2009).
[42] Y. Dong, V.V. Undyala, R.A. Gottlieb, R.M. Mentzer and K. Przyklenk, *Journal Of Cardiovascular Pharmacology And Therapeutics*, 15(3), 220-230, (2010).

[43] J. Nedjic, M. Aichinger, J. Emmerich, Noboru Mizushima and L. Klein *Nature*, 455(7211), 396-400,(2008).
[44] A. Orvedahl, and B. Levine, *Cell Death and Differentiation*, 16(1), 57-69, (2009).
[45] Qu et al., *J. Clin. Invest.*, 12(12), 1809-20, (2003).
[46] Zhenyu Yue, S. Jin, C. Yang, A.J. Levine and N. Heintz, *Proceedings of the National Academy of Sciences of the United States of America*, 100(25), 15077 -15082, (2003).
[47] V.M. Aita, X.H. Liang, V.V. Murty, D.L. Pincus, W.Yu, E. Cayanis, E., S. Kalachikov, et al., *Genomics*, 59(1), 59-65, (1999).
[48] A. Kuma, M. Hatano, M. Matsui, A. Yamamoto, H. Nakaya, Tamotsu Yoshimori, Yoshinori Ohsumi, et al., *Nature*, 432(7020), 1032-1036, (2004).
[49] Komatsu et al, *J. Cell Biol.*, 169(3), 425-34, (2005).
[50] M.B. Azad, Y. Chen, E.S. Henson, J. Cizeau, E. McMillan-Ward, S.J. Israels, and S.B. Gibson, *Autophagy*, 4(2), 195-204, (2008).
[51] T. Kanzawa, Y. Kondo, H. Ito, S. Kondo and I. Germano, *Cancer Research*, 63(9), 2103-2108, (2003).
[52] S. Shimizu, T. Kanaseki, Noboru Mizushima, T. Mizuta, S. Arakawa-Kobayashi, C.B. Thompson, and Y Tsujimoto, *Nature Cell Biology*, *6*(12), 1221-1228, (2004).
[53] M.C. Maiuri, E. Zalckvar, A. Kimchi and G. Kroemer, *Nature Reviews. Molecular Cell Biology*, *8*(9), 741-752, (2007).
[54] M. Mehrpour, A. Esclatine, I. Beau, I. and P. Codogno, *Cell Research*, (2010).
[55] N. Mizushima, *Genes and Development*, 21(22), 2861-2873, (2007).
[56] B. Levine, and G. Kroemer, *Cell*, 132(1), 27-42, (2008).
[57] M. Mehrpour, A. Esclatine, I. Beau, and P. Codogno, *American Journal Of Physiology. Cell Physiology*, 298(4), C776-C785, (2010).
[58] H. Nakatogawa, K. Suzuki, Y. Kamada, and Yoshinori Ohsumi, *Nat. Rev. Mol. Cell Biol.*, 10(7), 458-467, (2009).
[59] S. Pankiv et al, *J Biol Chem*, 282(33), 24131-45, (2007).
[60] P.E. Strømhaug, and P.O. Seglen, *The Biochemical Journal*, 291 (Pt 1*)*, 115-121, (1993).
[61] E-L. Eskelinen, *Autophagy*, 1(1), 1-11, (2004).
[62] C.M. Fader and M.I. Colombo, *Cell Death Differ.*, 16(1), 70-78, (2008).
[63] Z. Yang and Daniel J. Klionsky,*Current Topics In Microbiology And Immunology*, 335, 1-32, (2009).
[64] T.E. Rusten and H. Stenmark, *Journal of Cell Science*, 122(13), 2179 -2183, (2009).
[65] C. Liang, P. Feng, B. Ku, I. Botan, D. Canaani, B-H. Oh and J.U. Jung, J. U. , *Nat. Cell Biol.*, *8*(7), 688-698,(2006).
[66] Y. Zhong, Q.J. Wang, X. Li, Y. Yan, J.M. Backer, B.T. Chait, N. Heintz, N., et al. *Nat. Cell Biol.*, 11(4), 468-476, (2009).
[67] Yang and Klionsky, *Curr. Opin. Cell Biol.*, 22(2), 124-31, (2010).
[68] S. Barth, D. Glick, D., and K.F. Macleod, *The Journal of Pathology*, 221(2), 117-124, (2010).
[69] E.-L. Eskelinen, *Methods in Molecular Biology (Clifton, N.J.)*, 445, 11-28, (2008).
[70] C.L. Vázquez and Maria Isabel Colombo, *Methods In Enzymology*, 452, 85-95, (2009).
[71] Mizushima et al., *Cell*, 140(4), 313-26, (2010).
[72] N. Mizushima, T. Noda, T. Yoshimori, Y. Tanaka, T. Ishii, M.D. George, D.J. Klionsky, et al., *Nature*, 395(6700), 395-398, (1998).

[73] I. Tanida et al., *Autophagy*, 1(2), 84-91, (2005).
[74] G. Bjørkøy et al., *Methods Enzymol.*, 452, 181-97, (2009).
[75] K. Degenhardt et al., *Cancer Cell*, 10(1), 51-64, (2006).
[76] R. Mathew, S. Kongara, B. Beaudoin, C.M. Karp, K. Bray, K. Degenhardt, G. Chen, et al., *Genes and Development*, 21(11), 1367-1381, (2007).
[77] Maiuri et al., *Cell Death Differ.*, *16(1)*, 87-93, (2009).
[78] Y. Kondo, T. Kanzawa, R. Sawaya, and S. Kondo, *Nature Reviews. Cancer*, *5*(9), 726-734, (2005).
[79] Menon and Manning, *Oncogene*, Suppl 2:S43-51, (2008).
[80] Z. Yang, and Daniel J. Klionsky, *Current Topics In Microbiology And Immunology*, 335, 1-32, (2009).
[81] DW Meek, *Nat. Rev. Cancer*, 9(10), 714-23, (2009).
[82] J. Chung, *Curr. Drug Targets*, 11(6), 667-81, (2010).
[83] Ogier-Denis and Codogno, *Biochem. Biophys. Acta*, 1603(2), 113-28, (2003).
[84] Kroemer et al, *Mol. Cell*, 40(2), 280-93, (2010).
[85] Y. Kondo, T. Kanzawa, R. Sawaya, and S. Kondo, *Nature Reviews. Cancer*, 5(9), 726-734, (2005).
[86] V. Karantza-Wadsworth and E. White, *Autophagy*, 3(6), 601-3, (2007).
[87] P.V. Schoenlein, S. Periyasamy-Thandavan, Julia S. Samaddar, W.H. Jackson, and John T. Barrett, *Autophagy*, *5*(3), 400-403, (2009).
[88] Rubinsztein et al., *Nat. Rev. Drug Discov.*, 6(4), 304-12, (2007).
[89] A. Apel, I. Herr, H. Schwarz, H.P. Rodemann, and A. Mayer, *Cancer Research*, 68(5), 1485-1494, (2008).
[90] M.J. Abedin, D. Wang, M.A. McDonnell, U. Lehmann, A. Kelekar, *Cell Death and Differentiation*, 14(3), 500-10, (2007).
[91] Gupta et al., *Proc. Natl. Acad. Sci.*, 107(32), 14333-8, (2010).
[92] Lopez et al., *Cancer Res.*, 71(1), 185-96, (2011).
[93] R.K. Amaravadi, D. Yu, J.J. Lum, T. Bui, M.A. Christophorou, G.I. Evan, A. Thomas-Tikhonenko, et al. *The Journal of Clinical Investigation*, 117(2), 326-336, (2007).
[94] W.-L. Sun, Juan Chen, Y.-P. Wang and H. Zheng, *Autophagy*, *7*(10), (2011).
[95] A. Vazquez-Martin, C. Oliveras-Ferraros and J.A. Menendez, *PloS One*, 4(7), e6251, (2009).
[96] J. S. Samaddar, V. T. Gaddy, J. Duplantier, S. Periyasamy-Thandavan, M. Shah, M. J. Smith, D. Browning, et al., *Molecular Cancer Therapeutics*, 7(9), 2977-2987, (2008).
[97] M.A. Qadir, B. Kwok, W.H. Dragowska, K.H. To, D. Le, M.B. Bally, M. B., and S.M. Gorski, *Breast Cancer Research and Treatment*, 112(3), 389-403, (2008).
[98] Bursch et al, *Carcinogenesis*, 17(8), 1595-607, (1996).
[99] A. Bilir, M.A. Altinoz, M. Erkan, V. Ozmen and A. Aydiner *Pathobiology: Journal of Immunopathology, Molecular and Cellular Biology*, 69(3), 120-126, (2001).
[100] J. Debnath et al., *Autophagy*, 1(2), 66-74, (2005).
[101] C. Giusti. et al., *Autophagy*, 6(6), 823-4, (2010).
[102] F. Scarlatti et al, *J. Biol. Chem.*, 279(18), 18384-91, (2004).
[103] Hwang et al, *Biometals*, 23(6), 997-1013, (2010).
[104] R. Sherz-Shouval et al., *EMBO J.*, 26(7), 1749-6, (2007).
[105] R. Sherz-Shouval and Z. Elazar, *Trends Biochem. Sci.*, 36(1), 30-8, (2011).
[106] P. de Medina et al, *Autophagy*, 5(7), 1066-7, (2009).

[107] S. Thomas et al, *Breast Cancer Res. Treat.*, 130(2), 437-47, (2011).
[108] M. German and R.S. Slack, *Autophagy*, 7(5), 549-51, (2011).
[109] V. Betin V. and J.D. Lane, *J. Cell Sci.*, 122, 2554-66, (2009).
[110] M. Schwarten et al., *Autophagy*, 5(5), 690-8, (2009).
[111] R. Kang et al., *Autophagy*, 7(4), 442-4, (2011).
[112] John et al, *Cancer Res.*, 68(19), 7855-63, (2008).
[113] Gonzalez-Malerva et al, *Proc. Natl. Acad. Sci. USA*, 108(5), 2058-63, (2011).
[114] L. Duan, N. Motchoulski, B. Danzer, I. Davidovich, Z. Shariat-Madar and V.V. Levenson, *The Journal Of Biological Chemistry*, 286(4), 2864-2876, (2011).
[115] Namgoong et al, *J. Biol. Chem.*, 285(31), 23829-41, (2010).
[116] Shu et al, *J. Biomol. Screen*, 16(2), 174-82, (2011).
[117] Periyasamy-Thandavan et al, *Autophagy*, 6(1), 19-35, (2010).

Reviewed by Patricia Schoenlein, PhD, Developmental Therapeutics, Georgia Health Sciences University, USA.

In: Tamoxifen Concepts and Cancer: New Paradigms
Editor: Ramon Andrade de Mello ISBN: 978-1-62081-520-5

Chapter IV

Ecotoxicological Effects of Tamoxifen in the Aquatic Environment

Liwei Sun, Jian Chi, Xinhua Hu and Zhengwei Fu*
College of Biological and Environmental Engineering,
Zhejiang University of Technology, Hangzhou, PR China

Abstract

Tamoxifen is widely used in the treatment of primary and recurrent breast cancer, and it can enter the aquatic environment in its native form or as transformed excretory products like other human pharmaceuticals. Therefore, the possible adverse effects of tamoxifen on aquatic animals, particularly on various species of fish, should be of concern. Moreover, against the pharmacology of a selective estrogen-receptor modulator (SERM), tamoxifen has become a powerful research tool in fish endocrinology and is recommended as a reference compound in fish testing to aid extrapolation across other SERMs. To date, the endocrine disruptions of tamoxifen in fish have been comprehensively assessed by biochemical endpoints, growth and morphological alternations and measurements of reproductive performance using several model fish. These results demonstrated that exposure to tamoxifen displayed the potential impacts on vitellogenin protein levels, gonad histology and reproductive capacity, although the exposure levels were considerably greater than the real environmental concentration. Recently, some works employing gene expression endpoints have provided more mechanistic understandings of the action of tamoxifen. Additionally, as an anti-estrogenic chemical, the modulatory influences of tamoxifen on the action of estrogens such as estradiol (E2) and ethinylestradiol (EE2) were evaluated, which showed that the presence of tamoxifen appeared to mask many signs of the impacts of environmental estrogens, but not neutralize the impaired reproductive capacity. Comparison of available toxicity data with environmental concentration indicates that tamoxifen may not induce adverse

* E-mail: azwfu2003@yahoo.com.cn.

ecotoxicological effects in the aquatic system. However, considering the lack of information about the fate of tamoxifen and its possible interaction with other environmental pollutants, as well as the remained controversial results, more investigations are needed for accurate and comprehensive risk assessments of tamoxifen.

Introduction

Pharmaceuticals are a class of emerging environmental contaminants that have received growing attention in recent years [1-3]. In the European Union (EU), about 3000 different substances are used in human medicine [2]. Many human pharmaceutical compounds can enter the aquatic systems in the form of the non-metabolized parent compounds or as metabolites, following manufacture, use or ingestion/excretion [4]. As their continual introduction to waste-receiving water, certain pharmaceuticals exhibit pseudo-persistence even without high persistence rates [1]. In the last two decades, various pharmaceuticals have been detected in many countries in influents and effluents from sewage treatment plants, surface water, groundwater and even drinking waters [3-5]. Therefore, it compels the scientific community to be in agreement with the possibility that detrimental effects may arise from the presence of pharmaceuticals for human health as well as for aquatic organisms.

In general, pharmaceuticals are designed to target specific metabolic and molecular pathways in humans. When introduced into the aquatic environment, they may affect the same pathways in fish or other aquatic animals with identical or similar target organs, tissues, cells or biomolecules [2]. However, certain target receptors or biomolecules in lower vertebrates and invertebrates may be different or lacking. Additionally, the specific modes of action for many pharmaceuticals are not well known and, often not only just one but many different modes of actions may occur. It is also important to keep in mind that the routes of uptake of a drug in a mammal and a fish are quite different. Xenobiotic uptake in fish is across the gills, whereas in mammals, it will usually be across the lining of the alimentary canal [6]. Therefore, some pharmaceuticals may induce unexpected effects in lower organism than the primary therapeutic pharmacology observed in humans, due to biological differences in pharmacodynamics, pharmacokinetics and physiology [2].

Tamoxifen, a non-steroidal triphenylethylene derivative, is widely used in the treatment of primary and recurrent breast cancer [7]. Its pharmaceutical action is forming a relatively complex with the estrogen receptor (ER) and thereby reducing the number of receptors available for subsequent E2 binding [8]. Based on their mechanism of action derived from the studies using mammalian animal models, tamoxifen can be classified into direct-acting anti-estrogens belonging to the endocrine disrupting chemicals (EDCs) as it interferes with estrogen signaling directly [9]. Some studies show that tamoxifen also has estrogen agonistic properties, depending on the species and tissue. Owing to its multiple actions, tamoxifen is referred to as a selective estrogen-receptor modulator (SERM) [10]. However, many gaps, which concern the ecotoxicological effects of tamoxifen on the aquatic ecosystem, should be filled before more reliable environmental risk assessment with much lower uncertainty can be performed.

The object of our paper is to compile and review the present knowledge about the environmental occurrence and fate of tamoxifen in the aquatic environment, to describe the ecotoxicological effects on the aquatic organisms, particularly on fish, and to attempt to discuss the potential mechanisms of action based on the available studies.

Fate and Occurrence of Tamoxifen in Aquatic Environment

The fate and behavior of pharmaceuticals needs to be completely understood for environment risk assessment. Therefore, the knowledge of physical, biological, and chemical processes in the aquatic system is of great importance. However, as for tamoxifen, very limited information on these processes is available to date.

In general, pharmaceuticals can enter waters via a number of pathways, and the main pathway from humans should be ingestion followed by subsequent excretion. Based on the pharmacokinetics data of mammal, tamoxifen is extensively metabolized and produced to demethylated and hydroxylated derivatives [11]. The N-desmethyltamoxifen has estrogenic properties similar to tamoxifen. Another metabolite is 4-hydroxytamoxifen which shows much higher ER binding affinity (approximately a 100-fold) and anti-estrogenic activity, and can therefore be referred to as the hormonally active metabolite of tamoxifen [10, 11]. With regard to the transformation for tamoxifen, DellaGreca et al. [12] found that dispersion of tamoxifen in water exposed to prolonged sunlight (1 month) caused 50% conversion. Isomerization and cyclization are the main photoinduced reactions of tamoxifen under natural conditions [12]. Photooxygenation can also occur [12] which corresponding to the studies on antioxidant properties of the drug which have shown its capability of reacting with OH radicals [13]. Moreover, it found that the degradation rate increased at acidic pH which could be due to greater solubility of the protonated drug in water than the neutral form. While in the presence of nitrate and humic acid, tamoxifen remained stable [12].

To confirm pharmaceutical occurrences in the aquatic environment, it is essential for assessing their potential risks. However, as mentioned before, thousands of different human pharmaceutical substances are registered for use, and it is therefore necessary to rank substances on their relative risk, enabling those substances with the greatest potential to pose a risk to the aquatic environment to be identified. Using a combination of traditional risk assessment procedures, persistence, bioaccumulation, toxicity data, occurrence data from other countries, etc., tamoxifen was identified to be as one of about ten human pharmaceuticals for priority investigation based on a ranking procedure conducted by the UK Environment Agency [4, 14]. Hilton and Thomas [15] developed a suite of methods for the environmental analysis of tamoxifen, as well as other targeted pharmaceutical compounds and pharmaceutical metabolites, which using a generic solid-phase extraction (SPE) and preconcentration procedure, followed by liquid chromatography-electrospray tandem mass spectrometry (LC-ESI-MS/MS) analysis. Application of this method to samples collected from UK sewage treatment work (STW) effluents and surfacewaters showed that the concentration of tamoxifen was below the limit of detection (<10 ng/L). Using the same analysis method, the data based on another investigation of the STW and surface water demonstrated that tamoxifen was detected twice in STW effluent samples at concentration of 20 ng and 40 ng/L, but was not detected in surface water samples [4]. Also, Thomas and Hilton [16] determined the concentration of 14 pharmaceutical compounds and their metabolites, including tamoxifen, in UK estuarine surface. Four of the estuarine samples contained tamoxifen at concentration of between 13 and 71 ng/L, while no tamoxifen was detected in any of the river water samples analyzed. However, in a monitoring program studying the surface water of the lower river in the UK, tamoxifen was detected in 100% of all samples with concentrations ranging from 27 to 212 ng/L [17]. Moreover, it was surprising to observe an increase of tamoxifen in median concentration between the raw STW effluent and the final pre-ultra violet disinfected effluent, and the percentage changes of tamoxifen was 30% [17]. The authors believed that this increase in concentration was due to the suppression of MS/MS detector signal caused by the high concentration of organic matter in the raw wastewater effluent [17]. However, on the other hand, this increase may imply that the sufficiently persistent character of tamoxifen, and the STW process, even in tertiary treatment plant, is insufficient to remove this substance. In a more recent study, Zhou et al. [18] determined the concentrations of a range of pharmaceuticals including tamoxifen in the wastewater from a STW daily, and found that tamoxifen was detected in 100% waste, at 0.1–1.3 ng/L in influent and 0.1–0.5 ng/L in effluent samples with the overall removal efficiency varying from 32 to 45%. In a river close to the effluent discharge of this STW, the concentration of tamoxifen was, on average, below the limit of the detection. All of the mentioned monitoring studies demonstrated that the residues of tamoxifen in treated wastewater and surface water were very widespread and varied considerably on the concentration. However, to the best to our knowledge, no monitoring studies performed targeting the metabolites of tamoxifen.

Ecotoxicological Effects

General Toxicity

As mentioned above, the pharmaceuticals are designed to have a specific mode of action, and therefore, most of them are suggested to pose only a low risk for acute toxicity. When tested on non-target aquatic organisms (*Brachionus calyciflorus*, *Thamnocephalus platyurus*, and *Daphnia magna*), tamoxifen affects the exposed organisms, with 24h-L(E)C50 being 0.97 mg/L for the rotifer *B. calyciflorus*, 0.40 mg/L for the crustacean *T. platyurus* and 1.53 mg/L for *D. magna*. With regarding to its photoproducts, the L(E)C50s values ranging from 0.95 to 1.31mg/L for *B. calyciflorus* and 0.47 to 1.59 mg/L for *T. platyurus* [12]. As for fish, it was reported that the 96h-LC50 value was 230 and 410 μg/L in juvenile bluegill sunfish and rainbow trout, respectively [19].

Since many aquatic organisms are continuously exposed to waterborne pharmaceutical residues over long periods of time or even over their entire life, investigation of long-term (even multi-generation life-cycle) exposure will be more valuable for assessing the implications of pharmaceutical residues in aquatic systems. In the chronic bioassays based on the population growth inhibition in 7 d of exposure, *Ceriodaphnia dubia* was proved to be very sensitive with an EC50 value of 0.81 μg/L for tamoxifen and EC50 values ranging from 0.41 to 2.8 μg/L for its photoproducts, which being toxic three orders of magnitude higher than acute tests [12]. For chronic data to *Acartia tonsa*, EC50 was found to be 49 μg/L [20]. With regard to fish, using a partial life-cycle assay with zebrafish (*Danio rerio*), mortality was observed in larvae at 27000 nM (about 10 mg/L), while adult and juvenile fish exposed to 2700 nM (about 1 mg/L) or greater resulted in hemorrhages as well as disturbed locomotion and respiration [21]. Moreover, in the F1 generation, dysmorphogenesis associated with lethality in embryos and high mortality (88%) in hatched larvae observed at 270 nM (about 100 μg/L). Other pathological conditions included pancreatic inflammation with hyperemia, infiltration of mononuclear cells, and fibrosis. It was also observed that exposure to tamoxifen was associated with severe inflammation of the gills, skin pathology, and muscular necrosi [21]. However, the data from partial and full life-cycle studies (maximum exposure periods of 42 and 211 d, respectively) demonstrated that survival of fathead minnows (*Pimephales promelas*) was unaffected by tamoxifen (tamoxifen citrate) exposure over 42 d to 18 μg/L and over 211 days to 5.12 μg/L, respectively [19].

Endocrine Disruption Effects as a SERM

Against its pharmaceutical action, tamoxifen has become a powerful research tool in fish endocrinology and has its application in aquaculture and ecotoxicology [19]. Furthermore, in terms of understanding the potential impacts of SERMs in aquatic life, a 2003 Society of Environmental Toxicology and Chemistry (SETAC) Pellston workshop recommended that tamoxifen be used as a reference compound in fish testing, supplemented by mechanistic biomarkers to aid interspecies extrapolation [22]. Here, we briefly review the current literatures about the endocrine disruption effects of tamoxifen.

Initially, tamoxifen was primarily used as an antagonist to estrogen in revealing the estrogen signaling pathway. This anti-estrogenic activity was mostly reflected by the inhibition of tamoxifen to estrogen-response endpoints, such as vitellogenin (VTG). VTG is produced in the liver of oviparous species in response to simulation by endogenous estrogens or exogenous estrogenic chemicals, which has been successfully exploited as the most specific and accepted biomarker for exposure to estrogenic compounds [23]. Since the VTG induction can be measured not only *in vivo* but also in fish hepatocyte *in vitro*, the use of VTG induction in isolated fish liver cells has been suggested as an *in vitro* screen for identifying estrogenic-active substances. Pelissero et al. [24] assessed the estrogenic potency of several xenobiotic compounds, including phytoestrogens, by VTG induction based on cultured rainbow trout hepatocytes, and found that when the estrogenic-active substances were tested in the presence of tamoxifen, the production of VTG reduced significantly, demonstrating that the estrogenic action of all of these compounds was most likely mediated by the estrogen receptor. Latonnelle et al. [25] developed the cell culture technique with hepatocytes from sturgeon (*Acipenser baeri*) , and found that tamoxifen strongly inhibited the VTG synthesis induced by E2, while only partially reduced the estrogenic effects of phytoestrogen.

In the *in vivo* test, the SERM property of tamoxifen was clearly confirmed. Chikae et al. [26] investigated the effects of oral administration of tamoxifen on plasma VTG levels of adult Japanese medaka (*Oryzias latipes*). As expected, tamoxifen significantly increased the VTG levels in males, but inhibited the normal VTG inductions in females in the high concentration groups. Similarly, in our study [27], all concentrations of tamoxifen (1-625 μg/L) caused a significant and concentration-dependent increase in plasma VTG levels of male medaka. In contrast, the plasma VTG concentrations of females decreased significantly in the high exposure groups. It is suggested that tamoxifen binds to the ER and forms a receptor complex that is only partially active in initiating gene activation (may cause a single round of gene transcription [28]) and ultimately VTG synthesis. This mechanism may explain the weak estrogenic activity of tamoxifen observed in male fish. However, this weak potential was masked owing to the higher estradiol level in the females. The antagonistic action of tamoxifen at high concentration in females may be due to competing with endogenous estradiol for estrogen receptor, which is very comparable to the pharmacological action of tamoxifen. In a research into the combined effects of EDCs with different properties using Japanese medaka, we found that the plasma VTG concentrations induced by E2 were significantly reduced in both sexes, when combined with TAM exposure [29]. In contrast, Leanos-Castaneda et al. [30] reported that tamoxifen alone did not affect the vitellogenesis in Nile tilapia(*Oreochromis niloticus*), but it inhibited E2 or *o,p'*-DDT stimulated vitellogenesis. Such contrasting results were also been found between a partial and full life-cycle studies using fathead minnows. It was reported that exposure of adult fish in the 42-d study had no influence on plasma VTG levels; however, there was a significant (almost 50%) reduction in whole body VTG levels in F1 fish larvae at 28 dph. Conversely, during the fish full life-cycle study, there was a significant increase in plasma VTG in F0 males at 211 dph and in F1 males at 112 dph [19]. Also, in the partial life-cycle assay with zebrafish, both VTG immunostaining in the plasma and liver basophilia in males remained unchanged after exposure to tamoxifen. In females, however, the VTG immunostaining in the plasma decreased with increased concentration of tamoxifen; while in the liver, the immnumostaining was very intense in all females irrespective of tamoxifen treatment [21]. In the case of hatching alligators, tamoxifen acted as a pure antiestrogen which completely blocked the effects of estradiol-induced hepatic VTG secretion and oviductal hypertrophy [31].

Besides the vitellogenesis, the measurement of tissue steroid concentration can also be used as a useful endpoint in assessing the endocrine status of sexually mature fish [9]. In male tilapia, the lowered plasma T caused by E2 was potentiated by tamoxifen [30]. However, although neither tamoxifen or *o,p'*-DDT alone affected plasma T level, their combined exposure reduced plasma T levels. Then, in this case, tamoxifen might be behaving as an agonist of ER in fish brain or testes [30].

Generally, addressing potential impacts on more ecologically relevant responses, such as growth, gonad histopathology, sex ratios and reproduction, to chemical stressors is of key to ecological risk assessment process. As for gonad histopathology, exposure with tamoxifen resulted in histological lesions in the ovary including oocyte atresia with granulosa cell transformation, being consistent with the reduced egg production; while in testis of exposed male zebrafish, the observed asynchrony of stages within spermatogenic cysts may account for the decreased fertilization [21]. Williams et al. [19] reported that although exposure to tamoxifen citrate did not affect the histological appearance of the ovary, the increase in testicular Leydig cell hyperplasia was observed in the male fathead minnow. However, in our study, exposure to tamoxifen for 21 days did not cause any change in gonadosomatic indices (GSI) and gonadal histopathology, while only the liver histology was slightly altered in adult medaka [27].

Moreover, with regard to EDCs, gonad histology can be an important tool for phenoltypically sexing in the absence of genetic sex marker and provide more specific information in addressing the question of their environmental effects. By examining the gonad histology, as well as other secondary sex characteristics, exposure with tamoxifen was found to induce skewed sex ratios in aquatic organisms. As early as 1991, Lance and Bogart [31] found that, when injected into the alligator eggs incubated at a temperature which would normally result in 100% male hatchlings, tamoxifen reversed the embryos into apparently normal female hatchings. A similar result was also observed in the turtle (*Trachemys scripta*) [32]. This "sex-reverse" phenomenon showed a partial agonist action of tamoxifen, and was due to its SERM property. However, in terms of fish, tamoxifen displayed anti-estrogenic other than estrogenic activity. Dietary administration of 100 mg tamoxifen/kg feed during gonadal differentiation in a hybrid population of tilapia produced completely 100% male without producing an increased incidence of morphological abnormalities [33]. Kitano et al. [34] also reported tamoxifen dose-dependently induced masculinization of the genetic females, and the masculinization was counteracted by co-administration of E2, whereas enhanced by co-administration of MT. Similarly, in a partial life-cycle assay with zebrafish, exposure to tamoxifen significantly changed the sex ratio in F1 generation, with an increase ratio of males to females after exposure of F1 only or a higher proportion of undifferentiated gonads after exposure of P and F1. Exposure of P only, even at high concentrations, did not affect the sex ratio [21]. In our study, although no sex-reverse was observed in adult Japanese medaka (F0) after 21-day exposure to tamoxifen, there was a significant concentration-dependent increase in the proportion of F1 male relative to the controls by distinct coloration in male medaka caused by sex-linked genes [27]. However, Guiguen et al. [35] reported that tamoxifen had no effect on the masculinization of all-female populations of rainbow trout (at the dosage of 5 and 20 mg/kg) and tilapia (at the dosage of 25 mg/kg). Gonads from treated fish did not show any difference from those of the control all-female populations. Similarly, in a full life-cycle study using fathead minnows, histological examination of the gonads indicated that exposure of F1 fish to tamoxifen citrate did not result in any significant alteration in the expected sex ratio of males to females [19]. Moreover, it was also found that tamoxifen could mask many signs of estrogen (i.e. EE2) exposure, including secondary sexual characteristics, hypertrophy of ovaries and testes in the rainbow darter (*Etheostoma caeruleum*) [36]. Tamoxifen also decreased EE2-induced lipid accumulation in the liver, which demonstrated a clear protective effect [36]. Furthermore, the anti-estrogenic activity of tamoxifen was confirmed by other test systems. Kawamura et al. [37] established a transgenic medaka fish lines overexpressing estrogen receptor. Therefore, the embryo become hypersensitive to estrogen and failed to develop yolk veins while blood clots formed in the blood island within 3 days after exposure to the estrogen. When co-incubated with tamoxifen, the estrogen-induced developmental defects were recovered.

Reproduction and Growth

Most gonadal alternations will result in delaying or preventing reproduction from occurring. In fact, reproduction is dependent upon the appropriate coordination of the entire hypothalamic–pituitary–gonadal axis and therefore any interfering with this axis may result in adverse effects on reproduction. Also, as mentioned above, the evaluation of growth should not be ignored as it is a holistic parameter with population-level relevance. It was reported that exposure to tamoxifen in adult zebrafish reduced the number of clutches and egg produced in a concentration-dependent way [21]. Tamoxifen also reduced fertilization success, hatching and juvenile mortality. Although body length and weight were reduced with the highest concentration of tamoxifen depending on exposure of juveniles, the condition factor was never affected by treatment [21]. In a comprehensive study attempting to establish the acceptable concentrations of tamoxifen to fathead minnow, no significant reduction in F0 or F1 hatching success after exposure to tamoxifen citrate was found. Also, F0 fecundity was not reduced significantly by exposure. There was no evidence of biologically significant impairments in fathead minnow growth after 112 dph exposure to tamoxifen citrate in the full life-cycle study. Although there was a significant reduction in larval growth after 28 dph exposure, this effect was judged not to be adverse when taking into consideration comparison. Taking the survival, growth, hatching and spawning data from partial and full life-cycle studies as a whole, it was suggested that overall ^{adverse}NOEC and ^{adverse}LOEC values for tamoxifen citrate was 5.12 and 5.6 μg/L, respectively [19]. In our study with Japanese medaka, decreased hatchability and delayed time to hatching was observed in the exposure groups in the embryonic development study [27]. In the reproduction study of adult fish, fecundity and fertility were detrimentally affected only at the highest concentration. Hatching of the F1 generation eggs from the exposed F0 adults was decreased at the same concentration, while no effect was found for time to hatching or gross abnormalities [27]. Furthermore, we also investigated whether the adverse effects of estrogen could be ameliorated by co-exposure with tamoxifen. The data revealed that, even if tamoxifen could neutralize the effects of estrogen in some biomarkers (such as the VTG), the impaired reproductive capacity was not ameliorated, or even became more severe than exposure to each component alone [29]. However, it is surprising that tamoxifen has been proposed for use as a growth-promoting agent in aquaculture [38]. The juvenile bagrid catfish (*Pseudobagrus fulvidraco*) were fed with different concentrations of dietary tamoxifen (25, 50 or 100 mg/kg feed) for 180 days. The results showed that the administration of tamoxifen generally improved the growth and body composition of fish and the 50 mg/kg dietary tamoxifen was proved to be the optimal concentration. However, it was also found that the survival of tamoxifen groups significantly reduced compared with that of controls [38].

Gene Transcriptional Responses

Because the gene transcriptional responses represent the primary interaction site between chemical and organism, they provide essential clues for understanding how chemical exposure can affect organisms [39]. Therefore, more recently, the research into endocrine disruption has been conducted increasingly at the level of gene transcription. Through systematic monitoring of the gene transcriptional profiles, or a suite of functional relevant genes associated with the pathways of concern, it is anticipated that a better understanding of chemical-induced mechanisms of action can be achieved, which will ultimately aid in improving chemical risk assessment.

As early as 1996, Flouriot et al. [40] determined the *ER* and *VTG* mRNA accumulations by slot blot hybridization based on the cultured rainbow trout hepatocytes, and found that tamoxifen could inhibit estrogen-induced *ER* and *VTG* gene transcriptions, while resulted in no effects when treated alone. Using a relative RT-PCR technique, the *ERα* and *VTG* gene transcriptions in the liver of juvenile rainbow trout stimulated by E2 were reduced by the injection of tamoxifen, and the lower dose of tamoxifen seemed to block E2 activity more efficiently [41]. When fish were injected with tamoxifen alone, only the highest dose enhanced *VTG* mRNA level. However, with regard to the brain, tamoxifen did not induce any change in *ERα* and *GnRH* mRNA levels [41]. Also, with the quantitative real-time PCR assay, we found that exposure to tamoxifen reduced mRNA levels of the hepatic estrogen-response genes including *VTG1*, *VTG2* and *ERα* in female zebrafish both *in vivo* and *in vitro* [42]. With respect to males, only the lowest concentration of tamoxifen (30 μg/L) resulted in elevated expression of these genes, particularly *in vivo*, but higher concentrations slightly decreased it. All of this data confirmed the SERM properties of tamoxifen. Kitano et al. [34] demonstrated that the masculinization of the genetic females by tamoxifen was accompanied by suppression of ovary-type *P450arom* mRNA expression and induction of *Müllerian inhibiting substance* (*MIS*) mRNA expression by using RT-PCR, but no effects on mRNAs expression of *ERα* and *ERβ*. In contrast, 17β-estradiol counteracted masculinization of the genetic females by tamoxifen, upregulated *P450arom* mRNA expression and downregulated *MIS* mRNA expression.

In a more recent research conducted in our laboratory, the transcriptional responses of a set of functionally relevant genes associated with the pathways of the hypothalamic-pituitary-gonadal axis of Japanese medaka were investigated after treatment with waterborne tamoxifen at 30, 100 and 300 μg/L for 72 h [43]. As for hepatic *VTG* mRNA, the transcription level was elevated in exposed males, whereas decreased markedly in females which accompanied by the downregulated expression of *ERα*. In the brain, no effects on the expression of *ER* were observed, as previously observed, but with the exception of *ERα* which was induced by tamoxifen exposure in male. With regard to the gonad, the estrogen receptor remained unchanged following exposure, except for the highest concentration in males. Most steroid hormone synthesis-related genes in the gonad were not modulated significantly in the gonad of either gender, but the aromatase gene, i.e. *CYP19A*, was affected significantly with a gender-specific manner. More abundant expression of *CYP19A* was found in tamoxifen-exposed female relative to the control, which presumably compensating for the anti-estrogenic activity of tamoxifen. Conversely, tamoxifen suppressed *CYP19A* in the testes of males. However, as for the other aromatase isoform which is predominantly expressed in the brain, i.e. *CYP19B*, the effects caused by tamoxifen exposure displayed no gender-specificity, demonstrating a similar trend with the concentration-dependent decrease. The down-regulation observed in the brain in both sexes contrasting with the response to E2 and estrogen-mimicking compounds, may attribute to the anti-estrogenic activity of tamoxifen [43]. All of this data, when taken together, demonstrated that the mode of action of tamoxifen, as well as that of other pharmaceuticals, may be more complex than that realized currently.

Other Impacts to Aquatic Organisms

The endocrine disruption does not account for all of the adverse effects of tamoxifen on aquatic organisms. It was found that tamoxifen also induced developmental, reproductive and cytogenetic toxicity in sea urchin embryos [44]. These adverse effects were suggested to be corresponding to the induction of oxidative stress and subsequent oxidative damage to DNA and other biologically active molecules and cellular structures. It is thought that this pro-oxidant mode of action could partly explain carcinogenic effects in humans and rodents [44].

However, all of the above mentioned researches did not examine the mechanisms of toxicokinetic and toxicodynamic interaction in combinations of tamoxifen with other chemicals. Leanos-Castaneda et al. [45] determined whether tamoxifen affected plasma concentration of *o,p'*-DDT and its metabolites, *o,p'*-DDD and *o,p'*-DDE, in mature tilapia. A group of male fish treated concomitantly with tamoxifen and *o,p'*-DDT had significantly lower concentrations of plasma *o,p'*-DDT and its metabolites. It was suggested that tamoxifen, as well as other endocrine-active compounds, differentially modified the metabolism of *o,p'*- DDT through changes in the activity or the expression of cytochrome P450 detoxifying enzymes.

Conclusion

It was reported that less than 1% of pharmaceuticals data is available in the open literature or databases, and only a small number of new pharmaceuticals have undergone risk assessment using ecotoxicological tests [2]. Considering its potential effects of endocrine disruption as well as taking advantage of the considerable attention in research on EDCs, the currently available data about the ecotoxicity of tamoxifen is more comprehensive than most other human pharmaceuticals. As mentioned above, current investigations cover different biological levels of organism, ranging from the alternation of functional genes transcription to a suite of apical endpoints with more population-level relevance. Moreover, these investigations across an array of aquatic species, and the ^{adverse}NOEC and ^{adverse}LOEC values based on the chronic exposure were also suggested for certain fish [19]. All of these researches are helpful in advancing our understanding of the action of tamoxifen and informing the environmental risk assessment ultimately. However, it should be noted that some controversial results remain which may attribute to the difference between the aquatic organisms and test systems, and therefore conclusions concerning hazards to risks of pharmaceuticals to the aquatic ecosystem are premature.

Comparison of available toxicity data with environmental concentrations indicates that for tamoxifen, the concentration is too low in aquatic systems to induce adverse effects on the laboratory organism. However, just as other environmental pollutants, pharmaceuticals are present in the environment in mixtures. As we mentioned, even if tamoxifen can neutralize many signs induced by estrogen exposure, the impaired reproductive capacity become more severe than exposure to each component alone [29]. Such mixtures employing is only binary with different modes of action, which contrasting with the "real world" mixtures which are much more complex. Moreover, relevant information about the fate of tamoxifen in the aquatic systems as well as in the aquatic organisms is not sufficient. For example, although two-generation toxicity test has been performed, the data on bioaccumulation potential of tamoxifen is still lacking. Taking into account all of the above facts, more experimental data is needed for deriving an accurate and comprehensive profile of the possible environmental risk of tamoxifen and for concise regulatory decision-making in ecotoxicology. Additionally, another important aspect is to increase the knowledge about the fate of tamoxifen during the sewage treatment, and therefore to optimize STW process and ultimately solve the load of tamoxifen and its metabolites in wastewater and surface water.

Acknowledgments

We gratefully acknowledge the National Natural Science Foundation of China (No. 20907044, No.20837002), the National Basic Research Program of China (2010CB126100) and the Natural Science Foundation of Zhejiang Province (No.Y5090265) for supporting this research.

References

[1] Daughton, C.G. Cradle-to-cradle stewardship of drugs for minimizing their environmental disposition while promoting human health. I. Rationale for and avenues toward a green pharmacy. *Environ. Health Perspect.* 2003; 111(5):757-774.

[2] Fent, K., Weston, A.A., Caminada, D. Ecotoxicology of human pharmaceuticals. *Aquat. Toxicol.* 2006; 76(2):122-159.

[3] Santos, L.H.M.L.M., Araujo, A.N., Fachini, A., Pena, A., Delerue-Matos, C., Montenegro, M.C.B.S.M.. Ecotoxicological aspects related to the presence of pharmaceuticals in the aquatic environment. *J. Hazard Mater.* 2010; 175(1-3):45-95.

[4] Ashton, D., Hilton, M., Thomas, K.V. Investigating the environmental transport of human pharmaceuticals to streams in the United Kingdom. *Sci. Total Environ.* 2004; 333(1-3):167-184.

[5] Kolpin, D.W., Furlong, E.T., Meyer, M.T., Thurman, E.M., Zaugg, S.D., Barber, L.B., Buxton, H.T. Pharmaceuticals, hormones, and other organic wastewater contaminants in U.S. Streams, 1999-2000: A national reconnaissance. *Environ. Sci. Technol.* 2002; 36(6): 1202-1211.

[6] Owen, S.F., Giltrow, E., Huggett, D.B., Hutchinson, T.H., Saye, J., Winter, M.J., Sumpter, J.P. Comparative physiology, pharmacology and toxicology of β-blockers: Mammals versus fish. *Aquat. Toxicol.* 2007; 82(3):145-162.

[7] Carlson, R.W. Scientific review of tamoxifen: Overview from a medical oncologist. *Semin. Oncol.*1997; 24 (Suppl 1): 151-157.

[8] Jordan, V.C., Dix, C.J., Rowsby, L., Prestwich, G. Studies on the mechanism of action of the non-steroidal anti-estrogen tamoxifen (I.C.I. 46,474) in the rat. *Mol. Cell Endocrinol.* 1977; 7(2):177-192.

[9] U.S. EPA. Draft Detailed Review Paper on Fish Screening Assays for Endocrine Disruption. Columbus, Ohio. 2002

[10] Mueller, S.O., Korach, K.S. Mechanisms of Estrogen Receptor-Mediated Agonistic and Antagonistic Effects. Berlin Heidelberg: Springer-Verlag; 2001.

[11] MacCallum, J., Cummings, J., Dixon, J.M., Miller, W.R. Solid-phase extraction and high-performance liquid chromatographic determination of tamoxifen and its major metabolites in plasma. *J. Chromatogr. B.* 1996; 678(2):317-323.

[12] DellaGreca, M., Iesce, M.R., Isidori, M., Nardelli, A., Previtera, L., Rubino, M. Phototransformation products of tamoxifen by sunlight in water: Toxicity of the drug and its derivatives on aquatic organisms. *Chemosphere*. 2007; 67(10):1933-1939.

[13] Leguene, C., Clavere, P., Jore, D., Gardes-Albert, M. Radiolytic oxidation of tamoxifen using the free radicals OH and (or) HO_2. *Can. J. Physiol. Pharm*. 2001; 79(2):184-188.

[14] Thomas, K.V., Hilton, M.J. Targeted Monitoring Program for Pharmaceuticals in the Aquatic Environment, R&D Technical Report P6-012/6. Environment Agency. Bristol, UK. 2003.

[15] Hilton, M.J., Thomas, K.V. Determination of selected human pharmaceutical compounds in effluent and surface water samples by high-performance liquid chromatography-electrospray tandem mass spectrometry. *J. Chromatogr. A*. 2003; 1015(1-2):129-141.

[16] Thomas, K.V., Hilton, M.J. The occurrence of selected human pharmaceutical compounds in UK estuaries. *Mar. Pollut. Bull*. 2004; 49(5-6):436-444.

[17] Roberts, P.H., Thomas, K.V. The occurrence of selected pharmaceuticals in wastewater effluent and surface waters of the lower Tyne catchment. *Sci. Total Environ*. 2006; 356(1-3):143-153.

[18] Zhou, J.L., Zhang, Z.L., Banks, E., Grover, D., Jiang, J.Q. Pharmaceutical residues in wastewater treatment works effluents and their impact on receiving river water. *J. Hazard Mater*. 2009; 166(2-3):655-661.

[19] Williams, T.D., Caunter, J.E., Lillicrap, A.D., Hutchinson, T.H., Gillings, E.G., Duffell, S. Evaluation of the reproductive effects of tamoxifen citrate in partial and full life-cycle studies using fathead minnows (*Pimephales promelas*). *Environ. Toxicol. Chem*. 2007; 26(4):695-707.

[20] Andersen, H.R., Wollenberger, L., Halling-Sorensen, B., Kusk, K.O. Development of copepod nauplii to copepodites - A parameter for chronic toxicity including endocrine disruption. *Environ. Toxicol. Chem*. 2001; 20(12):2821-2829.

[21] van der Ven, L.T., van den Brandhof, E.J., Vos, J.H., Wester, P.W. Effects of the estrogen agonist 17β-estradiol and antagonist tamoxifen in a partial life-cycle assay with zebrafish (*Danio rerio*). *Environ. Toxicol. Chem*.2007; 26(1):92-99.

[22] Ankley, G., Black, M., Garric, J., Hutchinson, T., Iguchi, T. A framework for Assessing the Hazard of Pharmaceutical Materials to Aquatic Species. Pellston Workshop, Snowbird, Utah, USA, June 3-8, 2003, SETAC, Pensacola, FL, USA, 2005; 183-237.

[23] Iguchi, T., Irie, F., Urushitani, H., Tooi, O., Kawashima, Y., Roberts, M., Norrgren, L., Hutchinson, T. Availability of *in vitro* vitellogenin assay for screening of estrogenic and anti-estrogenic activities of environmental chemicals. *Environ. Sci*. 2006; 13(3):161-183.

[24] Pelissero, C., Flouriot, G., Foucher, J.L., Bennetau, B., Dunogues, J., Legac, F., Sumpter, J.P. Vitellogenin synthesis in cultured-hepatocytes - An *in vitro* test for the estrogenic potency of chemicals. *J. Steroid Biochem*. 1993; 44(3):263-272.

[25] Latonnelle, K., Le Menn, F., Kaushik, S.J., Bennetau-Pelissero, C. Effects of dietary phytoestrogens *in vivo* and *in vitro* in rainbow trout and Siberian sturgeon: Interests and limits of the in vitro studies of interspecies differences. *Gen. Comp. Endocrinol*. 2002; 126(1):39-51.

[26] Chikae, M., Ikeda, R., Hasan, Q., Morita, Y., Tamiya, E. Effects of tamoxifen, 17 α-ethynylestradiol, flutamide, and methyltestosterone on plasma vitellogenin levels of male and female Japanese medaka (*Oryzias latipes*). *Environ. Toxicol. Pharmacol.* 2004; 17(1):29-33.

[27] Sun, L.W., Zha, J.M., Spear, P.A., Wang, Z.J. Tamoxifen effects on the early life stages and reproduction of Japanese medaka (*Oryzias latipes*). *Environ. Toxicol. Pharmacol.* 2007; 24(1):23-29.

[28] MacGregor, J.I., Jordan, V.C. Basic guide to the mechanisms of anti-estrogen action. *Pharmacol. Rev.* 1998; 50(2):151-196.

[29] Sun, L.W., Zha, J.M., Wang, Z.J. Effects of binary mixtures of estrogen and anti-estrogens on Japanese medaka (*Oryzias latipes*). *Aquat. Toxicol.* 2009; 93(1):83-89.

[30] Leanos-Castaneda, O., Van Der Kraak, G., Lister, A., Sima-Alvarez, R., Gold-Bouchot, G. *o,p'*-DDT induction of vitellogenesis and its inhibition by tamoxifen in Nile tilapia (*Oreochromis niloticus*). *Mar. Environ. Res.* 2002; 54(3-5):703-707.

[31] Lance, V.A., Bogart, M.H. Tamoxifen sex reverses alligator embryos at male producing temperature, but is an anti-estrogen in female hatchlings. *Experientia*. 1991; 47(3):263-266.

[32] Wibbels, T., Crews, D. Specificity of steroid hormone-induced sex determination in a turtle. *J Endocrinol*. 1992; 133(1): 121-129.

[33] Hines, G.A., Watts, S.A. Non-steroidal chemical sex manipulation of tilapia. *J. World Aquacult. Soc*. 1995; 26(1):98-102.

[34] Kitano, T., Yoshinaga, N., Shiraishi, E., Koyanagi, T., Abe, S. Tamoxifen induces masculinization of genetic females and regulates P450 aromatase and Müllerian inhibiting substance mRNA expression in Japanese flounder (*Paralichthys olivaceus*). *Mol. Reprod. Dev*. 2007; 74(9):1171-1177.

[35] Guiguen, Y., Baroiller, J.F., Ricordel, M.J., Iseki, K., Mcmeel, O.M., Martin, S.A.M., Fostier, A. Involvement of estrogens in the process of sex differentiation in two fish species: The rainbow trout (*Oncorhynchus mykiss*) and a tilapia (*Oreochromis niloticus*). *Mol. Reprod. Develop*. 1999; 54(2):154-162.

[36] Elias, E.E., Kalombo, E., Mercurio, S.D. Tamoxifen protects against 17α-ethynylestradiol-induced liver damage and the development of urogenital papillae in the rainbow darter (*Etheostoma caeruleum*). *Environ. Toxicol. Chem*. 2007; 26(9):1879-1889.

[37] Kawamura, T., Sakai, S., Omura, S., Hori-e, R., Kawahara, T., Kinoshita, M., Yamashita, I. Estrogen inhibits development of yolk veins and causes blood clotting in transgenic medaka fish overexpressing estrogen receptor. *Zool. Sci*. 2002; 19(12):1355-1361.

[38] Park, I.S., Oh, H.S., Koo, J.G. Effect of oral tamoxifen on growth and survival in the bagrid catfish *Pseudobagrus fulvidraco*. *Aquacult Res*. 2003; 34(4):1471-1474.

[39] Moens, L.N., Smolders, R., van der Ven, K., van Remortel, P., Del-Favero, J., De Coen, W.M. Effluent impact assessment using micro array-based analysis in common carp: A systems toxicology approach. *Chemosphere* 2007; 67(11):2293-2304.

[40] Flouriot, G., Pakdel, F., Valotaire, Y. Transcriptional and post-transcriptional regulation of rainbow trout estrogen receptor and vitellogenin gene expression. *Mol. Cell Endocrinol*. 1996; 124(1-2):173-183.

[41] Vetillard, A., Bailhache, T. Effects of 4-n-nonylphenol and tamoxifen on salmon gonadotropin-releasing hormone, estrogen receptor, and vitellogenin gene expression in juvenile rainbow trout. *Toxicol. Sci*. 2006; 92(2):537-544.

[42] Sun, L.W., Wen, L.L., Shao, X.L., Qian, H.F., Jin, Y.X., Liu, W.P., Fu, Z.W. Screening of chemicals with anti-estrogenic activity using *in vitro* and *in vivo* vitellogenin induction responses in zebrafish (*Danio rerio*). *Chemosphere*. 2010; 78(7):793-799.

[43] Sun, L.W., Shao, X.L., Chi, J.A., Hu, X.H., Jin, Y.X., Fu, Z.W. Transcriptional responses in the brain, liver and gonad of Japanese ricefish (*Oryzias latipes*) exposed to two anti-estrogens. *Comp. Biochem. Physiol. C*. 2011; 153(4):392-401.

[44] Pagano, G., de Biase, A., Deeva, I.B., Degan, P., Doronin, Y.K., Iaccarino, M., Oral, R., Trieff, N.M., Warnau, M., Korkina, L.G. The role of oxidative stress in developmental and reproductive toxicity of tamoxifen. Life Sci. 2001; 68(15), 1735-1749

[45] Leanos-Castaneda, A., Gold-Bouchot, G., Van Der Kraak, G., Lister, A., Ceja-Moreno, V., Sima-Alvarez, R. An aromatase inhibitor and tamoxifen decrease plasma levels of *o,p*'-DDT and its metabolites in Nile tilapia (*Oreochromis niloticus*). *Mar. Environ. Res*. 2004; 58(2-5):337-342.

In: Tamoxifen Concepts and Cancer: New Paradigms
Editor: Ramon Andrade de Mello
ISBN: 978-1-62081-520-5

Chapter V

Innovative Approaches to Tamoxifen Administration for Breast Cancer Prevention

Brandy M. Heckman-Stoddard[1], Oukseub Lee[2], Matteo Lazzeroni[3], Seema Khan[2], Andrea DeCensi[4] and Barbara K. Dunn[1,*]
[1]Division of Cancer Prevention, National Cancer Institute, Bethesda, MD, US
[2]Department of Surgery, Robert H. Lurie Comprehensive Cancer Center, Northwestern University, Chicago, IL, US
[3]Divisions of Cancer Prevention and Genetics, European Institute of Oncology, Milan, Italy
[4]Division of Medical Oncology, E.O. Ospedali Galliera, Genoa, Italy

Abstract

Tamoxifen has long been a mainstay of treatment of estrogen receptor (ER)-positive breast cancer in both the metastatic and adjuvant settings. In 1998, results from the large phase III Breast Cancer Prevention Trial (conducted by the National Surgical Adjuvant Breast and Bowel Project/NSABP) led to the Food and Drug Administration's approval of tamoxifen for reduction of breast cancer incidence in high-risk women. The toxicities associated with tamoxifen, particularly endometrial cancer and thromboembolic events, have hampered the drug's uptake by high-risk women who should benefit from its preventive effects. Among the strategies to overcome such obstacles to preventive tamoxifen use is the investigation of novel, and potentially safer, modes of delivery of this agent. Two novel approaches are discussed in this paper. Low-dose tamoxifen, expected to confer fewer adverse events, is being examined by varying both dose and interval of administration. Low-dose tamoxifen is being investigated in in both clinical biomarker-based trials and observational studies. Modulation of systemic biomarkers, including lipid and IGF levels, and tissue biomarkers, including Ki-67, which are known

* Corresponding author: Barbara Dunn, PhD, MD, Division of Cancer Prevention, 6130 Executive Blvd. EPN 2056, Bethesda, MD 20892-7340; Phone: (301) 402-1209; Fax: (301) 480-1342; E-mail: dunnb@mail.nih.gov.

to be favorably affected by conventional tamoxifen dosing, has been observed. These findings suggest possible beneficial clinical prevention effects from novel low-dose tamoxifen regimens. An alternative approach is administration of topical forms of tamoxifen directly to breast tissue in high-risk women. Avoidance of systemic administration is expected to limit the distribution of drug to tissues susceptible to tamoxifen-induced toxicity. While clinical trials of topical tamoxifen are still ongoing, laboratory data suggest that appropriate formulations of drug successfully penetrate the skin to reach breast tissue, where a preventive effect is expected.

Introduction

For more than three decades, oral administration of tamoxifen, a triphenylethylene (TPE), has been a standard component of the treatment of estrogen receptor (ERα)-positive breast cancer [1,2]. More recently, because of its proven effectiveness and well understood side effect profile, tamoxifen has been used for prevention, for both pre- and postmenopausal women who are at increased risk of breast cancer [2]. Its use as a preventive agent is especially appropriate for premenopausal women or those with atypical hyperplasia (AH) or lobular carcinoma in situ (LCIS), who are at very high risk and who benefit the most in terms of risk reduction [2-4]. For a postmenopausal woman with an elevated risk of breast cancer, the net benefit is most pronounced if she has had a hysterectomy and, thus, is not at risk of developing endometrial cancer. However, the toxicities of tamoxifen, such as thromboembolic events and endometrial cancers, still pose a clinically significant problem overall.

Despite the strong evidence supporting preventive tamoxifen, as well as its approval for risk reduction by the US Food and Drug Administration (FDA) and endorsement for this purpose in specific categories of women by the American Society of Clinical Oncology Clinical Practice Guidelines committee [2-4], the acceptability of tamoxifen to the community of high-risk women and their physicians has been low [5-10]. The limited uptake of tamoxifen for prevention in oncology has been attributed primarily to concern about drug toxicities and a perceived unfavorable balance between risks and benefits. These concerns about drug toxicity are exacerbated by the lack of experience with oncology drugs among the internists, gynecologists and family practitioners who generally manage high-risk women. These primary care physicians are often reluctant to prescribe tamoxifen, which they perceive as a "cancer drug" with challenging side effects.

To reduce the risk of these adverse events, effective, yet safe drugs are being developed that could replace tamoxifen. Indeed, novel endocrine agents including both newer selective ER modulators (SERMs) and aromatase inhibitors are being evaluated as alternatives to tamoxifen for the treatment [11-13] and prevention [8] of breast cancer. A major caveat to the use of these newer agents is their limitation to postmenopausal high-risk women; tamoxifen remains the preventive agent of choice for premenopausal women at increased risk of breast cancer. The reluctance to prescribe tamoxifen for risk reduction due to concerns that this clearly effective agent has toxicities that are unacceptable in the prevention setting has sparked interest in developing additional approaches to its use. One strategy to reduce the side effects of tamoxifen, and thereby improve the risk: benefit profile of this preventive agent, has been to examine the efficacy of lower doses, which are anticipated to be associated with lower toxicity. Another novel approach, topical application of tamoxifen, addresses not only the limitations due to systemic toxicity but also additional problems of efficacy related to metabolism of tamoxifen when administered systemically. These promising alternatives are discussed in this chapter.

Low-Dose Tamoxifen for Breast Cancer Prevention

The efforts to circumvent the concerning side effects of tamoxifen while maintaining its beneficial impact on breast cancer risk reduction using doses lower than the standard 20 mg/day are discussed in the following paragraphs. Here we present an analysis of the rationale that justifies the use of tamoxifen at low doses in clinical trials, results of several phase II trials (listed in Table 1), a description of ongoing phase III trials, and the future perspectives using this approach.

Rationale

Although tamoxifen is a prototypical designer drug that binds to a specific molecular target, the ER, following saturation kinetics [9], its early clinical development has been characterized by the search for the maximum tolerated dose rather than the optimal biologic dose. Yet, comparison of a 20 mg/day dose of tamoxifen with higher doses indicates comparable efficacy with respect to lowering recurrence of and mortality from breast cancer [1]. In addition, data from animal studies have indicated that reducing the tamoxifen dose to the equivalent of 1 mg/day for humans did not diminish the drug's inhibitory activity on mammary tumor formation [10]. In fact, no dose–response relationship for doses between 20 and 40 mg/day has been observed for efficacy endpoints in adjuvant treatment trials [1]. Conversely, with respect to toxicity, the endometrial effect of tamoxifen is known to be both time [1]- and dose [13]-dependent, Together, all these data suggest that the use of lower doses of the drug offers a reasonable approach to minimizing toxicity while retaining activity.

Clinical Trials of Low-Dose Tamoxifen

In 1998 Breuer et al. evaluated the association between tamoxifen treatment and rate of bone fractures in older, nursing home residents [14]. A total of 93,031 women, aged 65 years and older, whose data were part of thc 1993 New York State Minimum Data Set (MDS) and for whom there was documentation of treatment with at least one medication were included in the analysis. This cross-sectional study involved a secondary analysis of 1385 matched sets of residents, where each set included one resident who was receiving tamoxifen treatment and up to four residents who were not. During the 1.5-year period for which bone fractures were documented in the 1993 MDS, the fracture rates were: 7.62% in women not treated with tamoxifen, 3.20% in women receiving tamoxifen 10 mg/day, and 6.73% in women receiving tamoxifen 20 mg/day.

Table 1. Clinical Trials using novel approaches for tamoxifen administration including alternative dosing and topical formulations

Experimental Agent, ClinicalTrials.gov Number or EudraCT #	Study Design	Study Population	Target Accrual	Primary Endpoint	Results
Low Dose (LD) Tamoxifen					
Multi-dose Tamoxifen[24,25]	20mg/d vs. 5mg/d vs. 1mg/d for 4 wks	Presurgical ER+ IBC	120	% Change in Ki-67	Ki-67 LI at lower doses of tamoxifen was comparable to those achieved with the standard dose. Secondary analysis showed Ki-67 response after short-term neoadjuvant tamoxifen is a good predictor of recurrence-free survival and overall survival
LD Tamoxifen[29], NCT01196936	5mg/d vs. placebo for 2 yrs	5 yr survivors of HL treated with chest RT of 15 Gy or more prior to age 30	300	% Change in MD	Ongoing
LD Tamoxifen/ Fenretinide[30,31]	5mg/d Tam, 200mg/d Fen, combination, vs. placebo for 2 yrs followed for an additional yr	Premenopausal DCIS or early IBC in previous 3 yrs or High Risk	235	% Change in MD and IGF-1at 24 mos	Despite favorable effects on plasma IGF-I levels and mammographic density, the combination of low-dose tamoxifen plus fenretinide did not reduce breast neoplastic events
LD Tamoxifen/ Anastrozole[42]	1mg/d Ana, 10mg/wk Tam, vs. combination for 1 yr	Postmenopausal DCIS	75	Plasma anastrozole, cardiovascular risk, C-telopeptide, estrogens, SHBG, IGF-I, endometrial Ki-67	The addition of a weekly tamoxifen administration did not impair anastrozole bioavailability and modulated favorably its safety profile
LD Tamoxifen[43] in HRT users	1 mg/d Tam and placebo/wk, placebo/d and 10 mg/wk Tam, 5 mg/d Tam and placebo/wk, or both placebos for 1 yr	Current or *de novo* HRT Users	210	% Change IGF-1	IGF-I declined in all tamoxifen arms ($p = .005$), with a greater change on 5 mg/day. Tamoxifen did not increase endometrial Ki-67 LI.

Experimental Agent, ClinicalTrials.gov Number or EudraCT #	Study Design	Study Population	Target Accrual	Primary Endpoint	Results
LD Tamoxifen (HOT)[44,45]	5 mg/d Tam vs. placebo for 5 yrs	Current or *de novo* HRT Users	1886	Incidence of IBC and DIN	Sub-study of 120 women showed a non-significant reduction of MD, with a significant trend in women aged <55 (relative difference between HRT+placebo and HRT+Tam = +5.5 vs -2.8; p=.001).
LD Tamoxifen[49,50]	Observational study of 20mg/wk or 5mg/d	Women with previous DIN	680	Second Primary IBC	High ER or PgR expression is a significant adverse prognostic indicator of DIN. LD Tam appears to be an active treatment. Women with low-expression ER or PgR DIN do not seem to benefit from tamoxifen.
LD Tamoxifen[51], NCT01357772 2007-007740-10	5mg/d Tam vs. placebo for 3 yrs	Women operated on for LIN 2 and 3, or ER+ intraepithelial neoplasia or DIN 1-3, excluding DIN 1a	1400	Incidence of IBC	Ongoing
Topical 4-Hydroxy Tamoxifen					
Tamoxifen/ Topical 4-OHT[81]	20mg/d Tam and placebo gel 1x/d vs. placebo tablet and 4-OHT gel for 2-3 wks	Presurgical – ER+ IBC	55	% Change in Ki-67	See Table 2
Tamoxifen/ Topical 4-OHT[84], NCT00952731	20mg/d Tam and placebo gel 1x/d vs. placebo tablet and 4-OHT gel 1x/d for 4-10 wks	Presurgical – HR+ DCIS	112	% Change in Ki-67	Ongoing

Ana-Anastrozole, BL- baseline, CB- core biopsy, DCIS- ductal carcinoma in situ, DIN- ductal intraepithelial neoplasia, ER- estrogen receptor, Fen- Fenretinide, HL- Hodgkin Lymphoma, HR- hormone receptor (estrogen receptor and/or progesterone receptor), HRT- hormone replacement therapy, IBC- invasive breast cancer, IGF-1-insulin-like growth factor, LD- Low dose, LI- labeling index, LIN- lobular intraepithelial neoplasia , MD- mammographic density, RPFNA- random periaveolar fine needle aspiration, RT- radiation therapy, SHBG- serum hormone binding globulin, Tam-Tamoxifen, 4-OHT- 4-hydroxy-tamoxifen.

The odds ratio (OR) for bone fractures among women receiving tamoxifen 20 mg/day compared with women who were not treated was 0.916 [95% confidence interval (CI), 0.720-1.164; p = .472] and was 0.312 (95% CI, 0.112-0.865; p = .025) for those receiving 10 mg/day. The rates of hip fracture were 4.98%, 2.40%, and 4.57% for controls and women receiving tamoxifen 10 mg and 20 mg/day, respectively. Whereas the hip fracture rate for women receiving 20 mg/day was statistically similar to that of the controls (OR=0.963; 95% CI, 0.718-1.291; p = .800), the difference between the controls and those receiving 10 mg daily approached significance (OR=0.313; 95% CI, 0.096-1.018; p = .054) and seemed to be protective.

In the same year, DeCensi et al. performed two experiments to assess the effect of low-dose tamoxifen in 127 healthy hysterectomized women aged 35-70 years, randomly assigned to one of the following four treatment arms: placebo (n = 31) or tamoxifen 20 mg/day (n = 30) (first experiment); or tamoxifen 10 mg/day (n = 34) or tamoxifen 10 mg/alternate days (n = 32) (second experiment) [15]. Baseline and 2-month measurements were compared for the following parameters: 1) total cholesterol (primary endpoint) and other surrogate markers of cardiovascular disease, e.g., low-density lipoprotein cholesterol, high-density lipoprotein cholesterol, triglycerides, and lipoprotein(a); 2) blood cell count; 3) fibrinogen; 4) antithrombin III; 5) osteocalcin; and 6) in a subgroup of 103 women, insulin-like growth factor (IGF)-I . Reduction in the conventional dose of tamoxifen (20 mg/day) by up to 75% did not affect the activity of the drug on a large number of biomarkers, most of which are surrogate markers of cardiovascular disease. In particular, after adjustment for the baseline values, there were reductions in circulating levels of total cholesterol and IGF-I of the same magnitude in all three tamoxifen treatment arms.

To provide further insight into the effect of tamoxifen at low doses on the IGF system, the drug serum levels attained after 2 months of either placebo (n = 32), tamoxifen 20 mg/day (n = 26), 10 mg/day (n = 23) or 10 mg/every other day (n = 29) were correlated with the changes in IGF-I, IGF-II, IGF Binding Protein (IGFBP)-1, IGFBP-3, and IGF-I/IGFBP-3 ratio [16]. Compared with placebo, tamoxifen induced the following mean (+/- standard error) percent changes in biomarkers: reduction of IGF-I (-16.9+/- 7.8%; p < .05), a non-significant increase in IGF-II (22.9+/- 12.2%), an increase in IGFBP-1 (49.3+/- 22.7%; p < .05), and a non-significant change in IGFBP-3 (-4.0%+/- 9.2%). No significant concentration-response relationship was observed between serum tamoxifen concentration and the biomarker changes except for the ratio of IGF-I/IGFBP-3, which decreased by 1.53 (-1.53+/- 0.68%) for each increase of 10 ng/ml in serum tamoxifen concentration (p = .02) [16]. A previous analysis evaluating blood concentrations of tamoxifen and its main metabolites demonstrated that an 80% reduction in blood concentrations does not seem to affect the activity of tamoxifen on biomarkers of cardiovascular or breast cancer risk [17]. Furthermore, biomarker recovery was slower than serum tamoxifen elimination, suggesting that the biological effect outlasts the presence of drug, even at low tamoxifen concentrations [18]. This prolonged pharmacodynamic half-life of tamoxifen and its metabolites provided the rationale for weekly administration of the drug in a preventive context.

A further investigation of the pharmacodynamic properties of tamoxifen at lower doses in a prevention setting involved a study of the effect on levels of ultrasensitive C-reactive protein (CRP), an index of low-grade vascular inflammation and important risk marker for cardiovascular disease (CVD) [19], in a population of healthy women [20]. This biomarker had been shown to be lowered by standard-dose tamoxifen in a previous study [21]. Changes in CRP were compared after 2 months of either placebo (n = 24), tamoxifen 10 mg on alternate days (n = 26), 10 mg/day (n = 22), or 20 mg/day (n = 19) in healthy women aged 35-70 years. Low doses were observed to decrease ultrasensitive CRP levels, with a possible beneficial effect on CVD. The median percent change was -2.2% (95% CI, -23.3- 42.8%) with placebo, -39.1% (95% CI, -59.9- -28.7%) with 10 mg on alternate days, -56.9% (95% CI, -68.6- -38.4%) with 10 mg/day and -42.9% (95% CI, -62.6- -1.6%) with 20 mg/day (p = .291 for the linear dose-response trend). Similar results were obtained when the data were classified according to blood tamoxifen concentrations, with a median reduction of 47% (95% CI, 36.3-65.5%) for women with low tamoxifen concentrations (< 30 ng/mL).

Subsequent trials have investigated the effect of low-dose tamoxifen alone and in combination with other drugs on breast cancer proliferation biomarkers. Ki-67 labeling index (LI) is one of the most studied surrogate biomarkers of cell proliferation. It is commonly used to screen drugs' therapeutic and preventive potential in clinical models of short-term presurgical therapy for breast cancer, in as much as the decrease in this proliferation-related antigen after short-term presurgical treatment has shown prognostic significance for progression-free and overall survival in several studies [22-24].

DeCensi et al. analyzed the effects of tamoxifen at 1 mg/day and 5 mg/day relative to those of the standard dose of 20 mg/day on Ki-67 LI levels in breast tumor specimens [25]. One hundred and twenty women with ER-positive breast cancer were randomly assigned to tamoxifen at 1, 5, or 20 mg/day for 4 weeks before surgery. Expression of the tumor proliferation marker Ki-67 was determined before (baseline) and after treatment. All levels were compared with those in the tumors of two nonrandomized control groups (34 women with ER-negative breast cancer and 29 additional women with ER-positive breast cancer). Expression of Ki-67 decreased in all three tamoxifen groups, with no difference in the magnitude of reduction among the groups (p =.81). Relative to baseline, Ki-67 expression decreased by a median of 15.0% (95% CI, 0.0-24.1%) among the tamoxifen groups but increased by 12.8% (95% CI, 0.0-19.6%) among the nonrandomized control groups. We observed dose-concentration relationships for measurements of tamoxifen and its metabolites in serum and cancer tissue. The high tamoxifen concentration in breast tissue suggested that the drug preferentially accumulates in this tissue, with the drug and metabolite concentrations being 2–15 times those of the corresponding serum levels. Importantly, with a tamoxifen dose of 1 mg/day, levels of 4-hydroxytamoxifen (4-OHT) in tissue were approximately 10–20 times greater than the 50% inhibitory concentration range observed in a number of MCF-7 breast cancer cell clones after 48–72 hours, namely, 0.5–5 n*M*, or 0.2–2 ng/mL [26].

The concentrations of tamoxifen, 4-OHT, N-desmethyltamoxifen, and N-didesmethyltamoxifen in serum, normal breast tissue and breast cancer tissue following the conventional dosage and two low-dose regimens were examined in the same preoperative population that had been randomized to multiple doses of tamoxifen versus placebo [27]. Tamoxifen levels exhibited a dose-concentration relationship, and the concentrations of tamoxifen and its metabolites were related to each other. Serum and tissue concentrations of tamoxifen were associated with baseline-to-post-treatment changes in SHBG levels but not with changes in Ki-67 levels. Together with a >10-fold variation in serum tamoxifen concentrations and a consistent serum-to-tissue concentration relationship at all doses, this lack of association of Ki-67 levels with dose suggested once again that tamoxifen treatment would be improved by administration of lower doses coupled with therapeutic drug monitoring.

Recently, the prognostic and predictive value of baseline and post-treatment Ki-67 labeling indices (percent of cells showing positive labeling for Ki-67) were evaluated using long-term follow-up data from the presurgical multi-dose tamoxifen study of 120 pre- and postmenopausal women with early-stage ER-positive breast cancer [25]. After 7.2 years of follow-up [24], women whose post-treatment Ki-67 labeling indices were in the second (14–19%), third (20–29%) and top (≥30%) quartiles had a hazard ratio (HR) for recurrence of 2.92 (95% CI, 0.95–8.96), 4.37 (95% CI, 1.56–12.25) and 6.05 (95% CI, 2.07–17.65), respectively, when compared with those in the bottom quartile (<14%) (p-trend = .001). The risk of invasive disease recurrence was 2.2% (95% CI, 0.9–5.0%) per point increase in baseline Ki-67 (p-trend = .076) and 5.0% (95% CI, 2.3–7.7%) per point increase in post-tamoxifen Ki-67 (p-trend < .001). The risk of death was 5.5 (95% CI, 1.26–23.16) times higher in patients with post-drug Ki-67 ≥20% than in those with Ki-67 <20% (p-trend = .006). Ki-67 response after short-term neoadjuvant tamoxifen was a good predictor of recurrence-free survival and overall survival, further supporting its use as a surrogate endpoint biomarker to tailor adjuvant treatment to the individual patient and to screen novel drugs in a cost-effective manner.

Nuclear receptor coactivator expression and activity may partly explain the complex agonist/antagonist effects that are seen with tamoxifen at the clinical level. In 2010 Haugan Moi et al. assessed the gene expression of the steroid receptor coactivators SRC-1, SRC-2/transcription intermediary factor 2, and SRC-3/amplified in breast cancer 1 (AIB1) and the growth factor receptor HER-2/neu in response to three tamoxifen dose regimens [28]. Surgical specimens from ER-positive breast cancer and adjacent normal breast tissue from 64 patients treated for 4 weeks preoperatively with tamoxifen 20, 5, or 1 mg/day and 28 nontreated breast cancer controls were analyzed for coactivator and HER-2/neu mRNA expression using real-time reverse transcription-PCR. The gene expression levels were related to immunohistochemical expression of Ki-67, serum levels of IGF-I and SHBG, other prognostic factors, and clinical outcome. The coactivators and HER-2/neu mRNA levels were higher in malignant compared with normal tissue (p < .001). Tamoxifen significantly increased the expression of coactivators in normal and malignant tissue irrespective of dose, especially for SRC-3/AIB1 (p < .001 tamoxifen-treated versus nontreated subjects). SRC-3/AIB1 and HER-2/neu mRNA levels were positively correlated with each other (p = .016), but the coactivators could not explain the variability of Ki-67, IGF- I, and SHBG. Although not significant, SRC-3/AIB1 tended to be higher in subjects with poor clinical outcome and unfavorable prognostic factors. Increases in coactivator mRNA levels seem to reflect an early response to tamoxifen that occurs without a dose-response relationship in the 1- to 20-mg dose range of tamoxifen.

The utility of preventive low-dose tamoxifen is currently being evaluated in an entirely different cohort of high-risk women: female survivors of Hodgkin lymphoma (HL) who were previously treated with ≥15 Gy of mantle irradiation to the chest before age 30 (NCT01196936) [29]. The 20- to 55-fold increased risk of developing breast cancer seen in these women is comparable to that associated with a *BRCA1/2* mutation. In addition to prior chest irradiation for HL, eligible women must be ≥25 years of age and have been diagnosed with HL at least 5 years prior to study participation, without any evidence of active HL during that period, and have a well-defined menopausal status, either pre- or postmenopausal. In this phase IIb randomized, double-blind, placebo-controlled trial, 300 eligible women are being randomized to tamoxifen 5 mg/day or to placebo for 2 years. Breast tissue is sampled using random peri-areolar fine needle aspiration both before and at the end of the 2-year treatment period. The primary endpoint of the trial is change in mammographic density. Additional outcomes to be analyzed include (1) surrogate biomarkers of efficacy: breast cytomorphologic and proliferation measures and insulin growth factors; (2) safety and tolerability using both patient-reported outcomes as well as the objective outcomes of lipid profiles, clotting factors, and markers of bone turnover; and (3) a series of risk modifiers: age, menopausal status, body mass index, prior hormone use, personal history of benign breast disease, family history of cancer, and parameters of radiation exposure including dose, age at exposure, and latency from chest irradiation.

Trials of Low Dose Tamoxifen in Combination with Other Agents

Tamoxifen and Fenretinide

Low-dose tamoxifen has been evaluated in combination with other agents, specifically fenretinide, a synthetic retinoid derivative, in a randomized double-blind 2 x 2 trial in high-risk premenopausal women [30,31]. The rationale for combining these agents was based on animal studies that showed a synergistic effect in inhibiting mammary carcinogenesis [32,33]. A total of 235 premenopausal women with pT1mic/pT1a breast cancer (n = 21), intraepithelial neoplasia (IEN; n = 160), or 5-year Gail model risk $\geq$ 1.3% (n = 54) were randomly allocated to either tamoxifen 5 mg/day, fenretinide 200 mg/day, a combination of the two, or placebo. During the 2-year intervention, tamoxifen significantly lowered IGF-I and mammographic density relative to placebo by 12% and 20%, respectively; fenretinide by 4% and 10% (not significant); and the combination by 20% and 22%, with no evidence for a synergistic interaction. Tamoxifen increased endometrial thickness principally in women becoming postmenopausal, whereas fenretinide decreased endometrial thickness significantly. The annual rate of breast neoplastic events [including invasive breast cancer and ductal carcinoma in situ (DCIS), but not lobular carcinoma in situ (LCIS); n = 48] was 3.5% +/- 1.0%, 2.1% +/- 0.8%, 4.7% +/- 1.3%, and 5.2% +/- 1.3% in the tamoxifen, fenretinide, combination, and placebo arms, respectively; with HRs of 0.70 (95% CI, 0.32-1.52), 0.38 (95% CI, 0.15-0.90), and 0.96 (95% CI, 0.46-1.99) relative to placebo (tamoxifen x fenretinide adverse interaction p = .03). No clear association with tumor receptor type was noted. Baseline IGF-I and mammographic density did not predict breast neoplastic events, nor did change in mammographic density. Thus, despite favorable effects on plasma IGF-I levels and mammographic density, the combination of low-dose tamoxifen plus fenretinide did not reduce breast neoplastic events compared to placebo, whereas both single agents, particularly fenretinide, showed numerical reduction in annual odds of breast neoplasms. Next, the effect of tamoxifen and fenretinide on features linked to insulin resistance was evaluated, using the homeostasis model assessment (HOMA; fasting insulin x glucose/22.5) to estimate insulin sensitivity [34]. Women were considered as showing improved insulin sensitivity when their HOMA shifted from $\geq$2.8 to $<$2.8. Women taking tamoxifen showed a decrease in insulin sensitivity by almost 7 times compared with subjects not taking tamoxifen (OR, 0.15; 95% CI, 0.03-0.88). In the tamoxifen group, only 5% showed improvements in insulin sensitivity. Interestingly, women with intraepithelial or microinvasive neoplasia exhibited higher HOMA values (3.0) than unaffected subjects (2.8) with a p = .07), suggesting that features of the metabolic syndrome should be taken into consideration before proposing tamoxifen for breast cancer prevention.

Tamoxifen and Aromatase Inhibitors

Aromatase inhibitors are a standard treatment for ER–positive breast cancer in postmenopausal patients [11,35-38]and are being tested and have recently been shown to be effective as chemopreventive agents in at-risk women [39,40] . However, these agents are associated with increased rates of bone fracture, joint and tendon disorders, and possibly increased cardiovascular risk due to their profound estrogen-suppressive effect, raising concern as to their long-term safety, especially in the prevention setting. Moreover, prolonged aromatase inhibitor treatment may lead to the onset of endocrine resistance with the emergence of estrogen hypersensitive cell clones [41]. One potential approach to counteracting these phenomena is to supplement the aromatase inhibitor with tamoxifen in order to exploit its partial estrogenicity. Accordingly, Bonanni et al. assessed whether the addition of a low dose of tamoxifen influenced anastrozole bioavailability and favorably modulated biomarkers of bone fracture, breast cancer, cardiovascular disease, and endometrial cancer risk (42). The influence of *CYP2D6* genotype on tamoxifen effects was also determined. Seventy-five postmenopausal women with breast IEN were randomly allocated to either anastrozole 1 mg/day or tamoxifen 10 mg/week or a combination of the two for 12 months. Study endpoints were plasma drug concentrations and changes of C-telopeptide, osteocalcin, estradiol/SHBG ratio, estrone sulfate, IGF-I/IGFBP-3, C-reactive protein, antithrombin-III, and endometrial Ki-67 expression and thickness. Anastrozole concentrations were not affected by the combination with low-dose tamoxifen, whereas endoxifen levels were lower in poor CYP2D6 metabolizers. C-telopeptide levels increased by 20% with anastrozole and decreased by 16% with tamoxifen and by 7% with their combination ($p < .001$); osteocalcin showed similar changes. With respect to markers of breast cancer risk, compared with anastrozole, the combination arm was associated with a greater reduction in the ratio of IGF-I/IGFBP-3 levels (-17% versus -9%; $p = .004$) and lower reductions in the ratio of estradiol/SHBG levels and estrone sulfate levels (-15% versus -29% and -30% versus -38%, respectively). However, the IGF-I/IGFBP-3 and estradiol/SHBG ratios did not decrease in poor CYP2D6 metabolizers. Endometrial thickness was not greater in the combination than in the anastrozole arm. In conclusion, the addition of a weekly low-dose tamoxifen administration did not impair anastrozole bioavailability and modulated favorably its safety profile, providing the rationale for larger studies of this combination treatment.

Tamoxifen and Hormone Replacement Therapy

The safety and the activity of the combination of low-dose tamoxifen with hormone replacement therapy (HRT) were studied in a dose ranging trial [43]. Two hundred and ten current or de novo HRT users were randomly assigned to one of the following four arms: tamoxifen 1 mg/day and placebo/week, tamoxifen 10 mg/week and placebo/day, tamoxifen 5 mg/day and placebo/week, or both placebos (per day and per week) for 12 months. The primary endpoint was the change of plasma IGF-I over the 12 months, and secondary endpoints included changes in IGFBP-3, IGF-1/IGFBP ratio, fibrinogen, antithrombin III, CRP, C-telopeptide, mammographic percent density, and endometrial thickness. Endometrial proliferation was assessed by pipelle biopsy in superficial, deep glandular, and stromal compartments after 12 months. Compared with placebo, IGF-I declined in all tamoxifen arms ($p = .005$), with a greater change on 5 mg/day compared to 10 mg/week or 1 mg/day ($p = .019$). Tamoxifen increased IGFBP-3 and lowered antithrombin-III, CRP, and mammographic density, with the greatest effects seen with 5 mg/day. Tamoxifen increased endometrial thickness but not Ki-67 expression, which was lowest at the 5 mg/day dose. Menopausal symptoms were not significantly worsened by tamoxifen. In conclusion, doses of tamoxifen ≤ 5 mg/day favorably modulated biomarkers of breast carcinogenesis and cardiovascular risk in HRT users with no increase in endometrial proliferation and menopausal symptoms. A dose of 5 mg/day was the most effective and was then selected for a phase III trial in HRT users.

The Hormone Replacement Therapy Opposed by Low Dose Tamoxifen (HOT) study is a multicenter phase III trial in postmenopausal healthy women on HRT and is designed to assess whether the combination of HRT and low-dose tamoxifen retains the benefits while reducing the risks of either agent [44]. The rationale was based primarily on the findings of the Italian Tamoxifen Prevention Study, where 5,408 healthy hysterectomized women aged 35-70 years were randomized to tamoxifen 20 mg/day or placebo for 5 years [45]. After 81.2 months median follow-up, 79 breast cancers occurred (34 on tamoxifen versus 45 on placebo, $p = .215$) [46]. In the subgroup of 1,580 women who used estrogen replacement therapy (ERT) at some point during the study, 23 breast cancers were observed: 17 on placebo and 6 on tamoxifen (HR=0.35, 95% CI, 0.14-0.89). The HOT trial completed its accrual in 2007, with 1884 subjects enrolled [44]. The clinical results of the main clinical trial are expected shortly. Hopefully this trial will be able to assess whether the combination of HRT and low-dose tamoxifen retains the benefits while reducing the risks of either agent while maintaining a high compliance rate. A recent presentation provided preliminary results regarding mammographic density modifications and transvaginal ultrasound-determined endometrial changes in a subgroup of HOT study participants [47]. Mammographic density was measured at baseline and after 1 year using a computer-assisted method that was centrally implemented by a single trained radiologist [48]. Transvaginal ultrasound was performed at baseline and repeated together with an endometrial biopsy after 3 years of treatment. As evaluated in 120 subjects, at 12 months tamoxifen was shown to induce a non-significant reduction in mammographic density, with a significant trend toward reduction in women aged ≤55 years (relative difference between HRT + placebo and HRT + tamoxifen = +5.5 versus -2.8; $p = .01$). Transvaginal ultrasound was performed in 173 subjects. Endometrial thickness increased in the tamoxifen arm compared to placebo, with a reduction of -0.6 mm in the placebo arm and an increase of 1.5 mm in the tamoxifen arm ($p<.0001$). Only 4 endometrial polyps were seen in the tamoxifen arm, and no cases of endometrial hyperplasia or cancer were observed in the 173 biopsies performed.

Low-Dose Tamoxifen and Intraepithelial Neoplasia

Based on the aforementioned studies, the use of low-dose tamoxifen in different forms, be it 5 mg/day or 10 mg on alternate days or 20 mg per week, was introduced in the European Institute of Oncology (EIO) clinical guidelines for DCIS in 2004, where this dosing approach is now routinely used. Recently the cancer prevention group at the EIO investigated the postsurgical treatment outcomes of women undergoing surgery for ductal intraepithelial neoplasia (DIN) at the EIO between 1996 and 2005, with follow-up until December 2006. In this study, 974 women underwent breast conserving surgery (BCS) and 293 patients mastectomy [49]. The administration of any medical treatment including a variety of hormonal and retinoid agents was shown to be associated with a borderline significant 45% lower risk of breast cancer events in women with ER-positive, HER-2-negative DIN. In order to provide additional clues as to the best treatment of women with DIN a subsequent analysis assessed the effect of low-dose tamoxifen on the occurrence of breast cancer events according to the expression level of ER and progesterone receptor (PgR) [50]. A total of 309 patients with DIN received low-dose tamoxifen according to institutional guidelines and were compared with 371 patients with DIN who received no systemic treatment. Women with DIN characterized by both ER and PgR > 50% who were not treated had a higher incidence of breast events than similar women on tamoxifen (HR=1.76; 95% CI, 1.00–3.12) or women with ER and PgR <50% DIN (HR=1.72; 95% CI, 1.14–2.58). Among untreated patients with ER >50% DIN, recurrence was higher in PgR ≥ 50% DIN than in PgR < 50% DIN, whereas recurrence was similar among women with low PgR (<50%) DIN regardless of treatment; tamoxifen had no beneficial effect in the latter subgroup. No difference in endometrial cancer incidence was noted. These observations led the authors to conclude that high ER and especially high PgR expression is a significant adverse prognostic indicator for DIN, and that low-dose tamoxifen appeared to be an active treatment in women with high ER or PgR expression, whereas women with low-expression ER or PgR (<50%) DIN did not seem to benefit from tamoxifen.

At present no standard treatment exists to treat these women, particularly in Europe, where tamoxifen is not approved for women with prior DCIS (DIN 2-3). Accordingly, a large multicenter phase III trial is currently ongoing to evaluate the efficacy and safety of tamoxifen 5 mg/day for reducing breast cancer incidence in 1400 women operated on for lobular intraepithelial neoplasia (LIN 2, 3) or ER-positive DIN (DIN 1-3; 1a is excluded) (NCT01357772) [51]. In addition to the primary endpoint of incidence of invasive breast cancer and ductal carcinoma in situ (DIN 1c, 2, 3) of the breast the study is also examining endometrial cancer, clinical bone fractures, cardiovascular events, venous thromboembolic events, and clinically manifest cataracts and overall mortality. To improve patient selectivity and provide meaningful clinical results in a 3-year period, a genotype analysis of *CYP2D6* will be performed and serum levels of tamoxifen and its metabolites will be measured and correlated with surrogate biomarkers of tamoxifen activity. The hypothesis is that poor CYP2D6 metabolizers might show lower modulation of surrogate biomarkers with tamoxifen treatment, including a smaller decrease in IGF-I levels and percent mammographic density, compared with normal/fast CYP2D6 metabolizers. The rationale comes from a previous nested case-control study from the Italian Tamoxifen Prevention Trial study in which a pharmacogenomic interaction between tamoxifen and several polymorphisms of the *CYP2D6* and *SULT1A1* genes was demonstrated [52]. The study included 182 Caucasian subjects, 47 breast cancer cases and 135 matched controls. Using the AmpliChip CYP450 Test, among the 182 subjects, these investigators identified 8 poor metabolizers (PM), 17 intermediate metabolizers (IM), 151 extensive metabolizers (EM) and 3 ultrarapid metabolizers (UM). Among women allocated to the tamoxifen arm, PM women showed a higher risk of developing breast cancer compared to the remaining phenotypes (p = .035). In an exploratory analysis, among 58 women with a *CYP2D6*2A* allele, 9 breast cancers were diagnosed in the placebo arm and only 1 in the tamoxifen arm (p = .0001). *CYP2C19* and *SULT1A1* polymorphisms did not show any correlation with tamoxifen efficacy. Tamoxifen exhibited reduced efficacy in CYP2D6 PMs in the chemoprevention setting. Conversely, the authors suggested that the *CYP2D6*2A* allele may be associated with increased efficacy of tamoxifen, supporting the relevance of pharmacogenomic analyses to the tailoring of tamoxifen treatment to the individual woman. While recent studies have discounted this hypothesis in the adjuvant setting [53,54], further studies are necessary to assess the role that may be played by tailoring tamoxifen dosing to genotypes of tamoxifen metabolizing enzymes, especially in a prevention setting.

In conclusion, while tamoxifen is currently considered for primary risk reduction therapy for any woman with a Gail risk score ≥ 1.66% or those with prior atypical hyperplasia or in situ cancer [3,4,55], one possible strategy for reducing toxicity is to decrease the dose of drug, especially in selected subjects based on genetic and clinical factors. Validation of low-dose tamoxifen both in terms of efficacy and safety may provide an advantage from a public health perspective, as a reduction of breast cancer incidence would translate into a decrease in the number of costly health procedures, which would, in turn, be replaced by an inexpensive drug.

Topical Tamoxifen for Breast Cancer Prevention

Clinical Concerns about Oral Tamoxifen for Breast Cancer Prevention

As alluded to in the previous section, tamoxifen is a prodrug and requires conversion by the phase I drug metabolizing cytochrome P450 enzymes, including CYP2D6 and CYP3A4/5, to its major anti-estrogenic metabolites [56]. The *N*-desmethyltamoxifen (*N*-desT) metabolite is present in high concentrations and the 4-hydroxytamoxifen (4-OHT) metabolite has high affinity for ERα, implying high activity. Both of these molecules are converted to *N*-desmethyl-4-hydroxytamoxifen (endoxifen, ENX), which resembles *N*-desT in being present in high concentration (10-fold higher than that of 4-OHT in serum) and has an affinity for ERα that is equivalent to that of 4-OHT (100-fold greater than the affinity of tamoxifen) [57-59]. Recent reports suggest that ENX is the dominant metabolite responsible for the therapeutic effect of tamoxifen because of its high abundance combined with its high affinity for ERα as well as its ability to cause proteasomic degradation of ERα [60-62]. An important corollary of this metabolic requirement is that the effectiveness of tamoxifen may be compromised in about one-third of women because of enzyme polymorphisms which result in decreased production, and thus availability, of ENX [56]. This constitutional variability in genes encoding tamoxifen-metabolizing enzymes is probably a major contributor to the resistance of some ER-positive breast cancers to tamoxifen. Such resistance was demonstrated in the NSABP P-1: BCPT trial where only 50% of ER-positive breast cancers were prevented by oral tamoxifen [55] and in an overview of the four tamoxifen prevention trials which showed a 48% reduction in ER-positive breast cancers [63]. Importantly, constitutional genetic variability is expected to influence tamoxifen metabolism regardless of the route of administration. This is true not only because the genetic variants are present in all cells in the body but also because drug activation via the phase I enzyme system occurs in organs other than the liver, including the breast.

In addition, certain challenges to the preventive efficacy of tamoxifen are specifically related to its oral use. Tamoxifen's hepatic metabolism, for example, allows for excretion of a considerable fraction of orally ingested drug before it reaches the target organ, contributing to reduced efficacy. Problems with toxicity can also result from systemic administration, due to the activity of tamoxifen in non-breast tissues. This off-target action, often seen with long-term systemic exposure to tamoxifen, is associated with hot flashes, night sweats, and menstrual irregularity, as well as the more serious risks of thromboembolism and endometrial cancer [55]. Thus, the systemic delivery of tamoxifen is problematic both from the perspective of efficacy through inefficient metabolism, and toxicity through high systemic exposure. In women with DCIS and those at high risk of breast cancer, effective concentrations are required only in breast tissue; systemic exposure is redundant, and minimization of side effects is essential, since agents offered to healthy high-risk women need to be both safe and well tolerated.

Local Percutaneous Administration of Drugs to the Breasts

Transdermal delivery has long been recognized as an effective alternative form of therapy that avoids some of the pitfalls of conventional systemic therapy, including oral administration. When delivered transdermally, a drug is characterized by distinct pharmacokinetics. This includes longer retention in the local tissue and delayed excretion due to detouring around hepatic metabolism, which results in excretion of a large fraction of orally ingested agents. For example, the percutaneous route has provided an effective method for delivery of reproductive hormones. Several transdermal therapeutic systems releasing estrogens, progestogens and androgens from patches applied to the skin are currently in clinical use. For women, transdermal systems have been developed for HRT and contraception. However, due to the effectiveness of the barrier function of the stratum corneum, only a relatively small number of lipophilic drugs with low molecular weights (< 500 Da) have been successfully formulated for these purposes.

The idea of topical administration of a drug locally to the breast was first tested with progesterone for local treatment of benign (nonmalignant) breast diseases [64,65]. Topical daily application of progesterone, 50 mg in hydroalcoholic gel for three months, was efficacious in treating benign breast diseases (mastodynia, fibroadnomas, etc.) [66,67]: this benefit resulted from local antiestrogenic activity of progesterone in the breast [68,69]. In fact, progesterone has been observed to concentrate in the breast before its diffusion to systemic circulation [64,65].

Subsequently, Mauvais-Jarvis et al. expanded the topical treatment of hormone-dependent benign breast diseases to include 4-OHT hydroalcoholic gel. The feasibility of this approach is due to the fact that 4-OHT is an active metabolite suitable for local delivery and in addition, shows greater antiestrogenic activity than tamoxifen in vitro. Furthermore, topical administration avoids the metabolic sequelae that occur when 4-OHT produced in the liver following ingestion of oral tamoxifen is readily conjugated and inactivated by hepatic enzymes [70]. Prior to initiating their treatment study, Mauvais-Jarvis et al. determined whether 4-OHT could be concentrated directly in the breast like progesterone. A pre-surgical study of 12 women with ER-positive breast cancer was undertaken to compare the concentration and metabolism of ^{3}H-labeled *trans*-4-OHT with that of tamoxifen following topical administration to the affected breast for up to 7 days [70]. Surgically resected breast tissue obtained 12-24 hrs after one topical dose (80 μCi in 60% alcoholic solution for each drug) showed that both 4-OHT and tamoxifen were detectable in both the breast tumor tissue and surrounding normal mammary tissue. Both drugs remained unmetabolized except that 20% of the administered *trans*-4-OHT had been isomerized to *cis*-4-OHT when the tissue was obtained after 7 days. Although the maximal concentration of both 4-OHT and tamoxifen in the breast tissue was reached 24 hours after a topical application, 4-OHT was retained for a much longer period in the breast than was tamoxifen. Plasma kinetics for 4-OHT and tamoxifen revealed that tamoxifen appeared in plasma more rapidly and decreased faster than did 4-OHT, possibly related to the lower affinity of tamoxifen for the ER present in breast tumors and breast epithelium. Next, 4-OHT was applied topically to two different anatomical sites (breast versus abdomen) to compare whether the breast tissue retention of 4-OHT is dependent on the site of application. The plasma and urine concentrations of 4-OHT during the first three days were much lower when 4-OHT was applied to the breast than the abdomen. Based on these observations, the authors postulated that 4-OHT was retained longer in sites containing ERs than in sites lacking ERs.

Subsequently, Pujol et al. showed that 4-OHT applied through the skin of the breast concentrates in the breast at 10-fold higher levels than when it is applied to the arm or shoulder [71]. The investigators attributed this differential accumulation to the binding of 4-OHT to ERs present in breast tumors and breast epithelium. In actuality, ERα expression in non-malignant breast tissue is very low but ERβ is high and may account for at least some of the localization in the normal breast. However, receptor binding alone is insufficient to explain 4-OHT retention in the breast [72,73]. A more plausible explanation relates to the embryological origin of the breast as a skin appendage (i.e. a modified sweat or apocrine gland). Studies of the embryological development of the breast suggest that the breast gland (parenchyma) and its skin envelope are a single unit with a well developed internal lymphatic (and venous) circulation [74]. The conclusions of these embryological studies are supported by the fact that the skin and parenchyma of the breast drain to the same sentinel lymph nodes [75,76]. These common drainage patterns predict that other drugs applied to the skin of the breast should also concentrate in the parenchyma to a greater degree than can be expected based on systemic absorption and delivery through the circulation. Therefore, this model of transdermal local pharmacotherapy for breast cancer prevention and for DCIS therapy should be applicable to a variety of agents as long as they show sufficient dermal permeation. It is important to emphasize, however, that the issue of whether transdermal delivery to the breast is a local or a systemic treatment deserves further investigation.

By bypassing first-pass metabolism in the liver, the delivery of active metabolites directly to the breast through its skin envelope potentially avoids changes in the clotting cascade, which may contribute to the pro-thrombotic effects of tamoxifen and raloxifene [63,77,78]. Since the risk of thromboembolism is a major concern not only with tamoxifen use, but with all SERMs tested clinically to date, the avoidance of this toxicity would offer a considerable advantage for women considering SERM therapy for breast cancer prevention, and for treatment of DCIS. Additionally, the very low plasma concentrations observed following transdermal application of 4-OHT in the studies conducted so far suggest that uterine toxicity and hot flashes are likely to be reduced by the transdermal delivery of active tamoxifen metabolites to the breast [70,71,79]. Furthermore, by circumventing the need for prodrug activation, the limitations due to low bioavailability of active metabolites caused by polymorphisms in tamoxifen metabolizing genes should be overcome [60,61].

Topical Tamoxifen in Studies of Mastalgia

A number of studies addressing relief of breast pain or tenderness have been performed in Europe using a hydro-alcoholic gel of 4-OHT (Besins, France). This topical 4-OHT gel was applied in daily doses ranging from 0.25 mg to 4 mg, divided equally between the two breasts[71]. In the most recent report [79], a randomized phase II study of a 4-month intervention compared a placebo control group to two treated groups (4 mg/day and 2 mg/day). The primary efficacy endpoint, change in mean pain intensity as measured by the Visual Analog Scale (VAS) showed a statistically significant improvement with the 4-OHT gel at a concentration of 4 mg/day for 4 menstrual cycles, despite the fact that average plasma levels of 4-OHT gel were 50 ± 64 pg/ml (mean ± SD), much lower than those seen with oral tamoxifen. The benefit was greatest in the fourth cycle, with a 32 mm reduction in the VAS in the 4 mg/day group, compared to a 26 mm reduction in the 2 mg/day group, and a 19 mm reduction in the control group (p = .0034). Of relevance to the discussion of this delivery approach in the setting of chemoprevention, the frequency of hot flushes was low in these premenopausal women with a mean age of 36 years; in the last month of the study, 1/38 participants reported 6-10 flushes in the placebo group, none was reported by the 41 women in the 2 mg/day group, and 2/45 women reported flushes in the 4 mg/day group (1-5 flushes in one individual, and 16+ in the other). In contrast, 58% of the 35-49 year-old women in the P-1 trial reported hot flushes after 3 months on tamoxifen, with a relative risk of 1.6 compared to placebo [80]. Headaches occurred in 10% of women taking placebo, 15% of the 2 mg/day group, and 20% of the 4 mg/day group. Application-site skin irritation was observed in 7% of the lower dose and 4% of the higher dose group.

Clinical Efficacy of Topical 4-OHT in Chemoprevention

Topical application of 4-OHT has also been tested as a potential chemoprevention agent. Rouanet et al have reported promising results from a pre-surgical study of 55 postmenopausal women with T1 or T2 invasive ER-positive breast cancer (Table 1) [81]. Patients were randomized into five groups and treated for two to three weeks; three groups were treated with topical 4-OHT gels (0.5, 1, or 2 mg/breast/day), one group received oral tamoxifen (20mg/day), and the fifth group received no treatment. The primary endpoints of the study were reductions in the tumor tissue proliferation indices, Ki-67 and PCNA (proliferating cell nuclear antigen). For the 45 patients assessable for efficacy, the differences in tumor tissue Ki-67 levels between baseline and following 2-3 weeks of treatment were compared among treatment groups (Table 2) [81]. Drug-treated groups (topical 4-OHT gels and oral tamoxifen) demonstrated a significant decrease in median Ki-67 levels as compared with the no-treatment group (p = .0055). No significant dose-dependent difference in reduction of Ki-67 levels was observed among the three topical 4-OHT groups (p = .07; median values of reduction in Ki-67 level were -3.8 for oral tamoxifen (20mg/day, n=10) and -0.8, -4.5, -3.9 for 4-OHT gels 0.5mg/day (n=8), 1 mg/day (n=9), and 2 mg/day (n=8), respectively. Thus, the daily topical application of 1 or 2 mg 4-OHT hydroalcoholic gel to the breast skin resulted in sufficient breast tissue concentrations to achieve inhibition of tumor cell proliferation to the same degree as that seen with the standard dose of oral tamoxifen (20 mg/day) but with much lower plasma levels, 2-11% of the levels achieved with oral tamoxifen. The no-treatment group and the 0.5mg/day group experienced no adverse effects. Although hot flushes were reported in the oral tamoxifen group and the 1 and 2 mg/day gel treatment groups, all patients were postmenopausal women with some level of baseline hot flushing. Despite this, an exacerbation related to systemic exposure to 4-OHT cannot be ruled out in this very short-term study. Of note, the lowest plasma level of tamoxifen metabolite exposure that is associated with hot flushes has not been defined, and the possibility remains that the low-level exposure (2-11% of the levels seen with oral tamoxifen) observed in this study may still exert a systemic effect.

Table 2. Proliferative Markers Evolution According to the Treatment (labeling index)[81]

	No Treatment Control	Oral Tamoxifen (20mg/day)	4-OHT Gel (0.5 mg/day)	4-OHT Gel (1 mg/day)	4-OHT Gel (2 mg/day)	p**	p†	p‡
Ki67*	N=10	N=10	N=8	N=9	N=8			
Tru-Cut								
Median	5	6.7	4.1	6.8	6.7	0.44	0.48	0.24
Range	2.4-9.0	2.5-11.6	0.99-12.8	3.2-11.3	3.5-10.3			
Tumor								
Median	5.8	2.8	3.3	3.3	3.2	0.0054	0.42	0.98
Range	2.7-12.4	1.2-3.7	0.8-8.99	0.9-6.7	2.05-4.8			
Change from baseline								
Median	0.28	−3.8	−0.8	−4.5	−3.9	0.0055	0.11	0.07
Range	−2.5-8.4	−10.2-1.0	−4.1-1.9	−5.9-1.1	−7.0-0.6			
PCNA*	N=10	N=11	N=8	N=8	N=9			
Tru-Cut								
Median	11.4	7.8	7.2	11	6.9	0.12	0.11	0.04
Range	3.3-15.2	1.4-7.6	2.3-5.3	4.0-8.2	0.7-9.1			
Tumor								
Median	11.9	3.0	4.6	6.3	4.5	0.002	0.19	0.19
Range	3.6-15.2	1.4-7.6	2.3-5.3	4.0-8.2	0.7-9.1			
Change from baseline								
Median	0.54	−2.9	−2.2	−4.4	−4.2	0.0019	0.42	0.22
Range	−0.81-2.9	−9.4-0.12	−7.3-0.61	−11-2.9	−7.4-2.2			

Abbreviation: 4-OHT, 4-hydroxy-tamoxifen; PCNA, proliferating cell nuclear antigen.
* Count is a labeling index calculated by stained cells/counterstained elements.
** Kruskal-Wallis test among the five groups.
† Kruskal-Wallis test among the four groups with oral tamoxifen.
‡ Kruskal-Wallis test among the three groups with 4-OHT gel.
Reprinted with permission from American Society of Clinical Oncology.

Besins laboratory and an affiliated company Ascend hold multiple patents for 4-OHT including indications for benign breast disease and reduction in breast density [82,83]. A phase I trial was conducted to examine tolerance and pharmacokinetics in healthy premenopausal women age 18-45 with application of the gel daily for two menstrual cycles. Multiple dosages, including 0.5, 1, and 2 mg/day, and multiple concentrations were examined. Topical 4-OHT was well tolerated in all 36 patients with no systemic effect on FSH, LH, estradiol, or progesterone hormone levels. Additionally a phase II randomized, placebo-controlled study examined the efficacy of 4-OHT to reduce mammographic density in women on continuous HRT. After a period of 4 months mammographic density was significantly reduced in the 1.5 and 2 mg/day treatment groups. A phase II randomized, double blind, placebo-controlled trial has been completed in 100 premenopausal women ages 30-50 examining the effect of 4-OHT on breast density. These trials provided preliminary data to examine the efficacy of 4-OHT in women with DCIS.

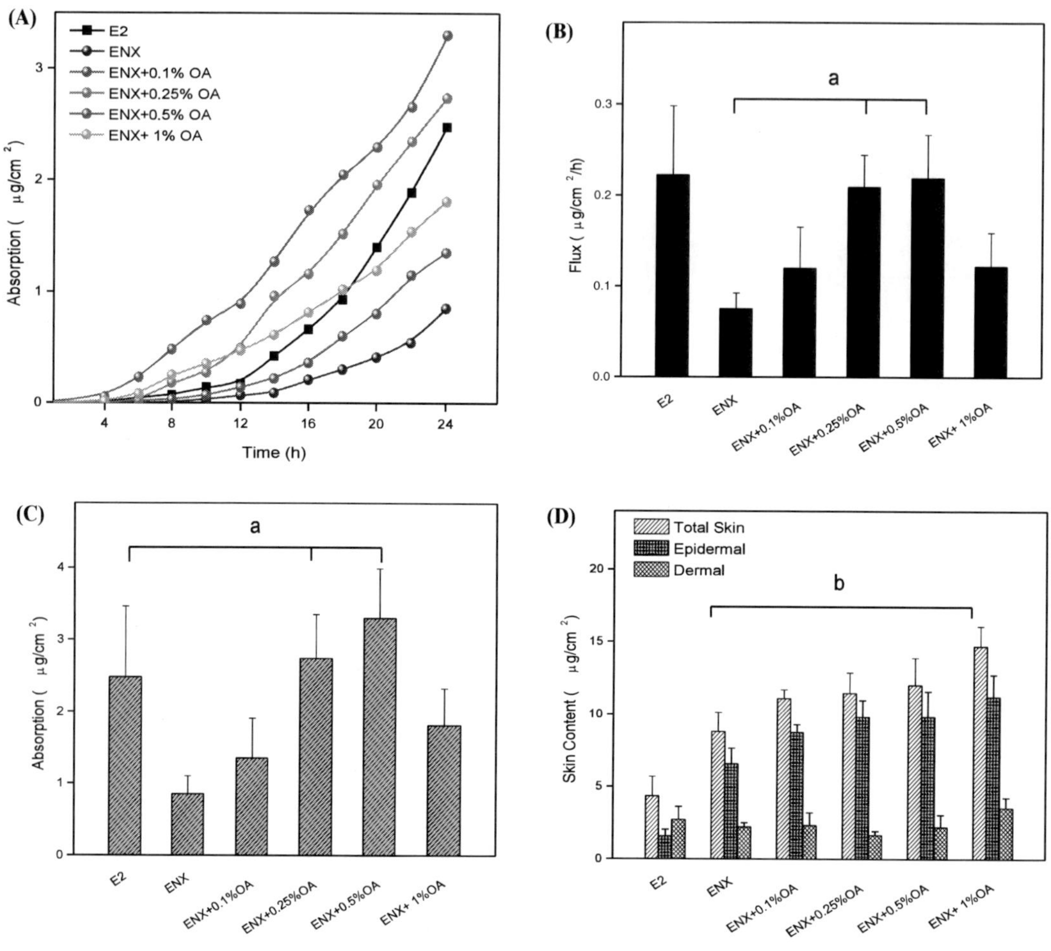

Figure 1. *Permeation parameters of ENX compared with E2.* The applied dose of the compounds was 78.9 (µg/cm2). The skin samples from three subjects were used and each treatment condition was tested in duplicate on the skin samples from a subject in each experiment. (A) permeation profile, (B) flux (µg/cm2/h) (C) absorption at 24 h (µg/cm2) and (D) Skin content (µg/cm2) of the compounds was measured separately from epidermis and dermis and was combined as total skin content after 24 h. All measurements were expressed as the mean ± SEM, n = 5–6. Notes: [a] $P < 0.05$ and [b] $P = 0.045$. The P-values were determined using the Wilcoxon rank sum test. Abbreviations: ENX, endoxifen; E2, estradiol; OA, oleic acid; SEM, standard error of the mean. *Reprinted with permission from Dove Medical Press Ltd.* [87].

Ongoing Phase II-B Study of 4-OHT Gel in Women with DCIS

Using the same formulation of 4-OHT as in prior studies [79,81] (Besins, France), Khan et al. have initiated an NCI/DCP supported multi-center presurgical study in women with

DCIS (NCT00952731) [84] in the US. Women with a core-biopsy diagnosis of ER-positive DCIS are being randomized to either oral tamoxifen at 20 mg/day or application of a 4-OHT gel at a dose of 2 mg/breast/day applied once daily for 6-10 weeks. The primary endpoint is decreased cell proliferation in the DCIS lesion (as reflected in the Ki-67 labeling index), but additional parameters of interest include breast versus systemic concentrations of 4-OHT and its isomers, effects on the coagulation cascade, and the presence of hot flushes. The planned sample size is 112 women. This study should provide information about the efficacy and tolerability of topical 4-OHT at a dose twice that used in the prior study by Rouanet et. al. [81], with more extensive data on toxicity relating to hot flushes and hypercoagulability. In addition, exploratory analyses are planned of tamoxifen metabolism genotypes relative to efficacy, tolerability and coagulability. The treatment interval is too short to assess uterine effects.

Preclinical Study of Transdermal Delivery of Endoxifen

Given the encouraging early results with transdermal 4-OHT, the other important tamoxifen metabolite, endoxifen, is an attractive candidate for local transdermal therapy for the breast for several reasons. Wu et al. have reported that endoxifen has an advantage over 4-OHT in that it causes proteasomic degradation of ERα and may have more selective anti-estrogenic effects [62]. Therefore, endoxifen is expected to give better therapeutic efficacy than 4-OHT, but its specific toxicity profile is currently unknown. If it shares even some of the toxicity of the parent drug, tamoxifen, and its percutaneous absorption in the human is equivalent to (or better than) that of 4-OHT, it would be an excellent candidate for transdermal delivery. Additionally, the chemical structure of endoxifen would render it more promising for transdermal application because it is more amenable to conjugation to nanoparticles for controlled release. For these reasons and because the binding affinities of 4-OHT and endoxifen are both 25-fold greater for ERα and 56-fold greater for ERβ than that of tamoxifen [85,86], Lee et al. have investigated the relative permeation of 4-OHT and endoxifen using human split-thickness skin (STS) [87]. They found that the permeation of endoxifen into human skin was not as efficient as that of 4-OHT in a vehicle of 60 % (v/v) ethanol-phosphate buffer (PB), but the addition of 1% (v/v) oleic acid greatly improved permeation of endoxifen over 24 hours. Although significant increases in permeation parameters were also seen for 4-OHT with the addition of oleic acid, the increase in endoxifen permeation was larger, bringing endoxifen permeation into a range which is very compatible with transdermal therapy [87]. An ethanol-based vehicle is necessary to solubilize TPEs, but ethanol is also a widely used skin permeation enhancer; ethanol is used in topical drug delivery systems for estradiol, progesterone, fentanyl, and other drugs. Oleic acid is also a well-known permeation enhancer, which has been employed to increase absorption of TPEs in the 60 % (v/v) ethanol-PB vehicle [88]. Several researchers have observed a permeation enhancing effect with oleic acid in ethanol-water systems across hairless rodent skin [89-91]. It is not clear why endoxifen benefits more from the addition of oleic acid than 4-OHT but this may be related to a difference in their structure. Endoxifen is smaller and more polar than 4-OHT because one methyl group at a tertiary amine is replaced with a hydrogen, resulting in a secondary amine, which is more hydrophilic than the tertiary amine of 4-OHT. Because oleic acid appears to make the stratum corneum fluidic [92,93] and ethanol gives a continuous driving force [88,94], endoxifen may move faster through the skin than 4-OHT. The amine group of endoxifen may provide a favorable balance of hydrophilic and hydrophobic properties, allowing endoxifen to traverse the stratum corneum more easily. In support of this, the results reported in the hairless rat skin model showed that the co-solvent system of oleic acid-ethanol-water efficiently increased skin permeation of both lipophilic and hydrophilic drugs [90].

The permeation enhancing effect of oleic acid for endoxifen appears to be optimal at concentrations of 0.25% to 0.5% in 60% ethanolic solution, with estradiol (E2) as a reference transdermal compound to determine whether the permeation of endoxifen with oleic acid can be improved to a level consistent with effective transdermal delivery. Furthermore, although endoxifen alone permeates human skin more slowly than E2, the addition of oleic acid improves the permeation of endoxifen to a level similar to that of E2 (Figure 1) [87]. Together, these results suggest that endoxifen is an excellent candidate for transdermal delivery, providing strong justification for the development of endoxifen for local transdermal delivery to the breast. Khan et al. have initiated an in vivo preclinical study to assess mammary gland and systemic distribution of endoxifen by transdermal delivery and to evaluate the in vivo therapeutic efficacy of endoxifen, compared to standard doses of oral tamoxifen in the athymic nude rat model with xenograft tumors of ERα-positive breast cancer [95]. These studies will guide the development of a clinical study to evaluate the efficacy of this approach for prevention of ER-positive breast cancer in the near future.

In addition to studies of transdermal delivery of SERMs, the Khan laboratory has initiated a study of the cyclooxygenase (COX) inhibitor drug diclofenac as a patch of diclofenac epolamine (diclofenac hydroxyethylpyrrolidine) (NCT01380353) [96], to be applied to the skin of the breast or the abdomen for three days prior to mastectomy, followed by measurement of drug concentration in tissue samples from eight different locations of the mastectomy specimen. Epolamine is a pharmacologically inactive salt but improves solubility and adjusts the hydrophilic and lipophilic properties of diclofenac for better topical delivery [97,98]. In a manner similar to the studies by Mauvais-Jarvis and colleagues using 4-OHT [70], this study is anticipated to demonstrate selective concentration of drugs in the breast when applied to its skin envelope, compared to application elsewhere. Accordingly, the diclofenac study is expected to validate the specific local concentration of drugs delivered through the breast skin.

In summary, serious consideration needs to be given to the topical transdermal approach as an alternative to oral therapy for breast cancer prevention agents. The recognition that the breast is a target for local rather than systemic transdermal therapy needs to be confirmed in additional studies. Once proven, however, these studies of transdermal approaches should open the way for the development of a number of drugs that target different pathways to be tested for breast cancer prevention efficacy.

Conclusion

Both low dose tamoxifen and topical transdermal application of tamoxifen metabolites show promise for breast cancer prevention with reduced side effects relative to standard dose oral tamoxifen. In the setting of low dose tamoxifen, *CYP2D6* genotyping may assume particular importance, given the potential complicity of impaired metabolism with limited available concentration of drug. Topical applications are of great interest but drug formulation and dosage require close examination. Furthermore, the feasibility of a long-term intervention needs to be determined as a daily gel application may pose a potential challenge to patient compliance. Transdermal delivery through a patch may be a superior formulation as long as it doesn't compromise efficacy. An additional localized approach might involve intraductal instillation of 4-OHT or endoxifen. Support of the feasibility of this method comes from the treatment setting. A recently completed phase I study examining the potential of intraductal administration of pegylated liposomal doxorubicin (PLD), with successful administration in 15 of the 17 women 2-4 weeks prior to surgery for early stage breast cancer with the failures due to the extent of disease or previous excisional biopsy [99]. Of interest, preclinical intraductal administration of 4-OHT has been shown in the N-methyl-N-nitrosourea–induced rat model of ER-positive breast cancer to be effective at significantly preventing tumorigenesis [100]. The same intraductal approach is being applied in the prevention setting in a pilot study of women with core biopsy-documented DCIS using a intraductal injection of PLD followed by 4-6 weeks of observation prior to definitive surgery (NCT00671476) [101,102]. Finally, future studies must evaluate these alternative approaches to tamoxifen administration in the correct high-risk populations in order to optimize the benefit/risk ratio relative to that observed with standard dose oral tamoxifen.

References

[1] Early Breast Cancer Trialists' Collaborative Group, *Lancet.* 351, 1451 (1998).

[2] B. Fisher, J. P. Costantino, D. L. Wickerham, R. S. Cecchini, W. M. Cronin, A. Robidoux, T. B. Bevers, M. T. Kavanah, J. N. Atkins, R. G. Margolese, C. D. Runowicz, J. M. James, L. G. Ford, and N. Wolmark, *J. Natl. Cancer Inst.* 97, 1652 (2005).

[3] R. T. Chlebowski, N. Col, E. P. Winer EP, *J. Clin. Oncol.* 20, 3328 (2002).

[4] K. Visvanathan, R.T. Chlebowski, P. Hurley, N. F. Col, M. Ropka, D. Collyar, M. Morrow, C. Runowicz, K. I. Pritchard, K. Hagerty, B. Arun, J. Garber, V. G. Vogel, J. L. Wade, P. Brown, J. Cuzick, B. S. Kramer, and S. M. Lippman, *J. Clin. Oncol.* 27, 3235 (2009).

[5] J. Tchou, N. Hou, A. Rademaker, V. C. Jordan, M. Morrow, *Cancer.*100, 1800 (2004).

[6] E. A. Waters, K. A. Cronin, B. I. Graubard, P. K. Han and A. N. Freedman, *Cancer Epidemiol Biomarkers Prev.* 19, 443 (2010).

[7] P. M. Ravdin, *Cancer Prev Res (Phila).* 3, 686 (2010).

[8] S. R. Cummings, S. Eckert, K. A. Krueger, D. Grady, T. J. Powles, J. A. Cauley, L. Norton, T. Nickelsen, N. H. Bjarnason, M. Morrow, M. E. Lippman, D. Black, J. E. Glusman, A. Costa, and V. C. Jordan, *JAMA.* 281, 2189 (1999).

[9] E. Coezy, J. L. Borgna, H. Rochefort, *Cancer Res.* 42, 317 (1982).

[10] C. Maltoni, F. Minardi, F. Belpoggi, C. Pinto, A. Lenzi, and F. Filippini, Experimental results on the chemopreventive and side effects of tamoxifen using a human-equivalent animal model. In: C. Maltoni, M. Soffritti and D. Walter, editors. *The Scientific bases of cancer chemoprevention.* New York; Elsevier Science; 1996:197-207.

[11] M. Baum, A. U. Budzar, J. Cuzick, J. Forbes, J. H. Houghton, J. G. Klijn and T. Sahmoud, *Lancet.* 359, 2131 (2002).

[12] M. Dowsett, J.M. Dixon, K. Horgan, J. Salter, M. Hills and E. Harvey, *Clin Cancer Res.* Jun 2000;6(6):2260-2267.

[13] L. E. Rutqvist, H. Johansson, T. Signomklao, U. Johansson, T. Fornander and N. Wilking, *J. Natl. Cancer Inst.* 87, 645 (1995).

[14] B. Breuer, S. Wallenstein, R. Anderson, *J. Am. Geriatr Soc.* 46, 968 (1998).

[15] A. Decensi, B. Bonanni, A. Guerrieri-Gonzaga, S. Gandini, C. Robertson, H. Johansson, R. Travaglini, M. T. Sandri, A. Tessadrelli, G. Farante, F. Salinaro, D. Bettega, A. Barreca, P. Boyle, A. Costa, and U. Veronesi, *Journal of the National Cancer Institute.* 90, 1461 (1998).

[16] B. Bonanni, H. Johansson, S. Gandini, A. Guerrieri-Gonzaga, R. Torrisi, M. T. Sandri, M. Cazzaniga, S. Mora, C. Robertson, E. A. Lien and A. Decens, *Breast Cancer Res. Treat.* 69, 21 (2001).

[17] A. Decensi, S. Gandini, A. Guerrieri-Gonzaga, H. Johansson, L. Manetti, B. Bonanni, M. T. Sandri, A. Barreca, A. Costa, C. Robertson and E. A. Lien, *J. Clin. Oncol.* 17, 2633 (1999).

[18] A. Guerrieri-Gonzaga, L. Baglietto, H. Johansson, B. Bonanni, C. Robertson, M. T. Sandri, L. Canigiula, C. Lampreda, S. Diani, E. A. Lien and A. Decensi, *Cancer Epidemiology Biomarkers and Prevention.* 10, 967 (2001).

[19] P. M. Ridker N. Rifai, L. Rose, J. E. Buring, N. R. Cook, *N. Engl. J. Med.* 347, 1557 (2002).

[20] B. Bonanni, H. Johansson, S. Gandini, A. Guerrieri-Gonzaga, M. T. Sandri, F. Mariette, E. A. Lien and A. Decensi, *Journal of Thrombosis and Haemostasis.* 1, 2149 (2003).

[21] M. Cushman, J. P. Costantino, R. P. Tracy, K. Song, L. Buckley, J. D. Roberts and D. N. Krag, *Arteriosclerosis, Thrombosis, and Vascular Biology.* 21, 255 (2001).

[22] M. Dowsett, I. E. Smith, S. R. Ebbs, J. M. Dixon, A. Skene, R. A'Hern, J. Salter, S. Detre, M. Hills and G. Walsh, *J. Natl. Cancer Inst.* 99, 167 (2007).

[23] M. J. Ellis, Y. Tao, J. Luo, R. A'Hern, D. B. Evans, A. S. Bhatnagar, H. A. Chaudri Ross, A. von Kameke, W. R. Miller, I. Smith, W. Eiermann and M. Dowsett, *J. Natl. Cancer Inst.*100, 1380 (2008).

[24] A. DeCensi, A. Guerrieri-Gonzaga, S. Gandini, D. Serrano, M. Cazzaniga, S. Mora, H. Johansson, E. A. Lien, G. Pruneri, G. Viale, and B. Bonanni, *Ann. Oncol.* 22, 582 (2011).

[25] A. Decensi, C. Robertson, G. Viale, F. Pigatto, H. Johansson, E. R. Kisanga, P. Veronesi, R. Torrisi, M. Cazzaniga, S. Mora, M. T. Sandri, G. Pelosi, A. Luini, A. Goldhirsch, E. A. Lien and U. Veronesi, *J. Natl. Cancer Inst.*95, 779 (2003).

[26] L. M. Greenberger, T. Annable, K. I. Collins, B. S. Komm, C. R. Lyttle, C. P. Miller, P. G. Satyaswaroop, Y. Zhang and P. Frost, *Clinical Cancer Research.* 7, 3166 (2001).

[27] E. R. Kisanga, J. Gjerde, A. Guerrieri-Gonzaga, F. Pigatto, A. Pesci-Feltri, C. Robertson, D. Serrano, G. Pelosi, A. Decensi and E. A. Lien, *Clinical Cancer Research.* 10, 2336 (2004).

[28] L. L. Haugan Moi, M. Hauglid Flageng, S. Gandini, A. Guerrieri-Gonzaga, B. Bonanni, M. Lazzeroni, J. Gjerde, E. A. Lien, A. DeCensi and G. Mellgren, *Clinical Cancer Research.* 16, 2176 (2010).

[29] City of Hope Medical Center. Low Dose Tamoxifen in Hodgkin Lymphoma Survivors for Breast Cancer Risk Reduction (LDTam). 2011; http://clinicaltrials.gov/ct2/show/NCT01196936, Accessed October 12, 2011.

[30] A. C. Guerrieri-Gonzaga, C. Robertson, B. Bonanni, D. Serrano, M. Cazzaniga, S. Mora, M. Gulisano, H. Johansson, F. Formelli, M. Intra, A. Latronico, D. Franchi, G. Pelosi, K. Johnson and A. Decensi, *J. Clin. Oncol.* 24, 129 (2006).

[31] A. Decensi, C. Robertson, A. Guerrieri-Gonzaga, D. Serrano, M. Cazzaniga, S. Mora, M. Gulisano, H. Johansson, V. Galimberti, E. Cassano, S. M. Moroni, F. Formelli, E. A. Lien, G. Pelosi, K. A. Johnson and B. Bonanni, *J. Clin. Oncol.* 27, 3749 (2009).

[32] T. A. Ratko, C. J. Detrisac, N. M. Dinger, C. F. Thomas, G. J. Kelloff and R. C. Moon, *Cancer Res.* 49, 4472 (1989).

[33] R. C. Moon RC, G. J. Kelloff, C. J. Detrisac, V. E. Steele, C. F. Thomas and C.C. Sigman, *Anticancer Res.*12, 1147 (1992).

[34] H. Johansson, S. Gandini, A. Guerrieri-Gonzaga, S. Iodice, M. Ruscica, B. Bonanni, M. Gulisano, P. Magni, F. Formelli and A. Decensi, *Cancer Research.* 68, 9512 (2008).

[35] B. Thurlimann, A. Keshaviah, A. S. Coates, H. Mouridsen, L. Mauriac, J. F. Forbes, R. Paridaens, M. Castiglione-Gertsch, R. D. Gelber, M. Rabaglio, I. Smith, A. Wardley, K. N. Price and A. Goldhirsch, *N. Engl. J. Med.* 353, 2747 (2005).

[36] P. E. Goss, J. N. Ingle, S. Martino, N. J. Robert, H. B. Muss, M. J. Piccart, M. Castiglione, D. Tu, L. E. Shepherd, K. I. Pritchard, R. B. Livingston, N. E. Davidson, L. Norton, E. A. Perez, J. S. Abrams, P. Therasse, M. J. Palmer, and J. L. Pater, *N. Engl. J. Med.* 349, 1793 (2003).

[37] R. Jakesz, W. Jonat, M. Gnant, M. Mittlboeck, R. Greil, C. Tausch, J. Hilfrich, W. Kwasny, C. Menzel, H. Samonigg, M. Seifert, G. Gademann, M. Kaufmann and J. Wolfgang, *Lancet.* 366, 455 (2005).

[38] R. C. Coombes, E. Hall, L. J. Gibson, R. Paridaens, J. Jassem, T. Delozier, S. E. Jones, I. Alvarez, G. Bertelli, O. Ortmann, A. S. Coates, E. Bajetta, D. Dodwell, R. E. Coleman, L. J. Fallowfield, E. Mickiewicz, J. Andersen, P. E. Lonning, G. Cocconi, A. Stewart, N. Stuart, C. F. Snowdon, M. Carpentieri, G. Massimini, J. M. Bliss and C. van de Velde, *N. Engl. J. Med.* 350, 1081 (2004).

[39] J. Cuzick, *Breast Cancer.*15, 10 (2008).

[40] P. E. Goss, J. N. Ingle, J. E. Ales-Martinez, A. M. Cheung, R. T. Chlebowski, J. Wactawski-Wende, A. McTiernan, J. Robbins, K. C. Johnson, L. W. Martin, E. Winquist, G. E. Sarto, J. E. Garber, C. J. Fabian, P. Pujol, E. Maunsell, P. Farmer, K. A. Gelmon, D. Tu and H. Richardson, *N. Engl. J. Med.* 364, 2381 (2011).

[41] M. Dowsett, L. A. Martin, I. Smith and S. Johnston, *J. Steroid Biochem. Mol. Biol.* 95, 167 (2005).

[42] B. Bonanni, D. Serrano, S. Gandini, A. Guerrieri-Gonzaga, H. Johansson, D. Macis, M. Cazzaniga, A. Luini, E. Cassano, S. Oldani, E. A. Lien, G. Pelosi and A. Decensi, *Clin. Cancer Res.* 15, 7053 (2009).

[43] A. Decensi, S. Gandini, D. Serrano, M. Cazzaniga, M. Pizzamiglio, F. Maffini, G. Pelosi, C. Daldoss, U. Omodei, H. Johansson, D. Macis, M. Lazzeroni, M. Penotti, L. Sironi, S. Moroni, V. Bianco, G. Rondanina, J. Gjerde, A. Guerrieri-Gonzaga and B. Bonanni, *J. Clin. Oncol.* 25, 4201 (2007).

[44] A. Decensi, A. Galli and Veronesi U, *Recent Results Cancer Res.* 163, 104 (2003).

[45] U. Veronesi, P. Maisonneuve, A. Costa, V. Sacchini, C. Maltoni, C. Robertson, N. Rotmensz and P. Boyle, *Lancet.* 352, 93 (1998).

[46] U. Veronesi, P. Maisonneuve, N. Rotmensz, B. Bonanni, P. Boyle, G. Viale, A. Costa, V. Sacchini, R. Travaglini, G. D'Aiuto, P. Oliviero, F. Lovison, G. Gucciardo, M. R. del Turco, M. G. Muraca, M. A. Pizzichetta, S. Conforti and A. Decensi, *J. Natl. Cancer Inst.* 99, 727 (2007).

[47] B. Bonanni, P. Maisonneuve, D. Serrano, C. Varricchio, M. Cazzaniga, M. Lazzeroni, B. Santillo, R. Di Pace, L. Meneghetti, A. Tagliafico, U. Veronesi and A. De Censi, *ASCO Meet Abstr.* 29, Abstr. 1527 (2011).

[48] A. Tagliafico, A., G. Tagliafico, S. Tosto, F. Chiesa, C. Martinoli, L. E. Derchi and M. Calabrese, *Breast.* 18, 35 (2009).

[49] A. Guerrieri-Gonzaga, E. Botteri, N. Rotmensz, F. Bassi, M. Intra, D. Serrano, G. Renne, A. Luini, M. Cazzaniga, A. Goldhirsch, M. Colleoni, G. Viale, G. Ivaldi, V. Bagnardi, M. Lazzeroni, A. Decensi, U. Veronesi and B. Bonanni, *Oncologist.* 14, 201 (2009).

[50] Guerrieri-Gonzaga A, Botteri E, Lazzeroni M, et al. Low-dose tamoxifen in the treatment of breast ductal intraepithelial neoplasia: results of a large observational study. *Ann. Oncol.* May 2010;21(5):949-954.

[51] Ente Ospedaliero Ospedali Galliera. Trial of Low Dose Tamoxifen in Women With Breast Intraepithelial Neoplasia (TAM-01), 2011, http://clinicaltrials.gov/ct2/show/NCT01357772. Accessed October 12, 2011.

[52] D. Serrano, D. Macis, S. Gandini, H. Johansson, A. Guerrieri-Gonzaga, G. Mellgren, E. A. Lien, F. Mariett, M. Sandri, A. Decensi and B. Bonanni *J. Clin. Oncol. 2007 ASCO Annu. Meet Proc.* 25, 503 (2007).

[53] J. M. *Rae, S. Drury, D. F. Hayes, V. Stearns, J. N. Thibert, B. P. Haynes, J. Salter, S. Pineda, J. Cuzick and Dowsett M, Cancer Res.* 70, S1 (2011).

[54] B. *Leyland-Jones, M. M. Regan, M. Bouzyk, R. Kammler, W. Tang, O Pagani, R. Maibach, P. Dell'Orto, B. Thürlimann, K. N. Price and G. Viale, Cancer Res.* 70, S1 (2011).

[55] B. Fisher, J. P. Costantino, D. L. Wickerham, C. K. Redmond, M. Kavanah, W. M. Cronin, V. Vogel, A. Robidoux, N. Dimitrov, J. Atkins, M. Daly, S. Wieand, E. Tan-Chiu, L. Ford and N. Wolmark, *J. Natl. Cancer Inst.* 90, 1371 (1998).

[56] B. K. Dunn, M. H. Greene, J. M. Kelley, J. P. Costantino, R. J. Clifford, Y. Hu, G. Tang, N. Kazerouni, P. S. Rosenberg, D. M. Meerzaman and K. H. Buetow, *Int. J. Mol. Epidemiol. Genet.* 1, 332 (2010).

[57] V. C. Jordan and K. E. Allen, *Eur. J. Cancer.* 16, 239 (1980).

[58] K. E. Allen, E. R. Clark and V. C. Jordan, *Br. J. Pharmacol.* 71, 83 (1980).

[59] B. S. Katzenellenbogen, M. J. Norman, R. L. Eckert, S. W. Peltz and W. F. Mangel, *Cancer Res.* 44, 112 (1984).

[60] M. P. Goetz, J. M. Rae, V. J. Suman, S. L. Safgren, M. M. Ames, D. W. Visscher, C. Reynolds, F. J. Couch, W. L. Lingle, D. A. Flockhart, Z. Desta, E. A. Perez and J. N. Ingle, *J. Clin. Oncol.* 23, 9312 (2005).

[61] M. P. Goetz, S. K. Knox, V. J. Suman, J. M. Rae, S. L. Safgren, M. M. Ames, D. W. Visscher, C. Reynolds, F. J. Couch, W. L. Lingle, R. M. Weinshilboum, E. G. Fritcher, A. M. Nibbe, Z. Desta, A. Nguyen, D. A. Flockhart, E. A. Perez and J. N. Ingle, *Breast Cancer Res. Treat.* 101, 113 (2007).

[62] X. Wu, J. R. Hawse, M. Subramaniam, M. P. Goetz, J. N. Ingle and T. C. Spelsberg, *Cancer Res.* 69, 1722 (2009).

[63] J. Cuzick T. Powles, U. Veronesi, J. Forbes, R. Edwards, S. Ashley and P. Boyle, *Lancet.* 361, 296 (2003).

[64] R. Sitruk-Ware R, B. Seradour B and C. Lafaye. (1980). Treatment of benign breast disease by progesterone applied topically. In: P. V. C. Mauvais-Jarvis and J. Wepierre editors. *Percutaneous Absorption of Steroids.* 219-229. New York, Academic Press.

[65] J. De Boever, C. Verheugen C and G. Van Maele. (1983). Steroid concentrations in serum, glandular breast tissue, and breast cyst fluid of control and P-treated patients. In: A. Angeli, H. L. Bradlow and L. Dogliotti, editors. *Endocrinology of cystic breast disease.* 93-99. New York, Raven Press.

[66] P. Mauvais-Jarvis, N. Sterkers, F. Kuttenn and J. Beauvais, *J. Gynecol. Obstet. Reprod. Biol. (Paris).* 7, 477 (1978).

[67] P. Mauvais-Jarvis. (1983). Hormonal therapy of benign breast disease. In: D. T. Krieger and C. W. Bardin, editors. *Current Therapy in Endocrinology.* Philadelphia: B.C. Decker; 1983:428-432.

[68] S. Fournier, F. Kuttenn, F. de Cicco, N. Baudot, C. Malet and P. Mauvais-Jarvis, *J. Clin. Endocrinol. Metab.*55, 428 (1982).

[69] P. Mauvais-Jarvis, F. Kuttenn and A. Gompel, *Breast Cancer Res. Treat.* 8, 179 (1986).

[70] P. Mauvais-Javis, N. Baudot N, D. Castaigne, P. Banzet and F. Kuttenn, *Cancer Res.* 46, 1521 (1986).

[71] H. Pujol, J. Girault, P. Rouanet, S. Fournier, J. Grenier, J. Simony, J. B. Fourtillan and J. L. Pujol, *Cancer Chemother. Pharmacol.* 36, 493 (1995).

[72] S. A.Khan, M. A. Rogers, K. K. Khurana, M. M. Meguid and P. J. Numann, *J. Natl. Cancer Inst.* 90, 37 (1998).

[73] D. Ricketts, L. Turnbull, G. Ryall, R. Bakhshi, N. S. Rawson, J. C. Gazet, C. Nolan and R. C. Coombes, *Cancer Res.* 51, 1817 (1991).

[74] A. Ackerman, G. Kessler, T. Gyorfi, H. Tsou H and G. Gottlieb, *Am. J. Dermatopathol.* 29, 211 (2007).

[75] S. P. Povoski, J. O. Olsen, D. C. Young, J. Clarke, W. E. Burak, M. J. Walker, W. E. Carson, L. D. Yee, D. M. Agnese, R. V. Pozderac, N. C. Hall and W. B. Farrar, *Ann. Surg. Oncol.* 13, 1412 (2006).

[76] V. S. Klimberg, I. T. Rubio, R. Henry, C. Cowan, M. Colvert and S. Korourian, *Ann. Surg.* 229, 860 (1999).

[77] F. Cosman, M. Baz-Hecht, M. Cushman, M. D. Vardy, J. D. Cruz, J. W. Nieves, M. Zion and R. Lindsay, *Thromb. Res.* 116, 1 (2005).

[78] J. Cuzick, J. Forbes, R. Edwards, M. Baum, S. Cawthorn, A. Coates, A. Hamed, A. Howell and T. Powles, *Lancet.* 360, 817 (2002).

[79] R. Mansel, A. Goyal, E. L. Nestour, V. Masini-Eteve and K. O'Connell, *Breast Cancer Res. Treat.* 106, 389 (2007).

[80] R. Day, P. A. Ganz, J. P. Costantino, W. M. Cronin, D. L. Wickerham and B. Fisher, *J. Clin. Oncol.* 17, 2659 (1999).

[81] P. Rouanet, G. Linares-Cruz, F. Dravet, S. Poujol, S. Gourgou, J. Simony-Lafontaine, J. Grenier, A. Kramar, J. Girault, E. Le Nestour and T. Maudelonde, *J. Clin. Oncol.* 23, 2980 (2005).

[82] Jay Bua, *United States Patent* No. 7,485,623, Feb. 3, 2009.

[83] Elizabeth Le Nestour, *United States Patent* No.7,507,769, Mar. 24, 2009.

[84] Robert H. Lurie Cancer Center. 4-Hydroxytamoxifen or Tamoxifen Citrate in Treating Women With Newly Diagnosed Ductal Breast Carcinoma in Situ. 2011; http://clinicaltrials.gov/ct2/show/NCT00952731. Accessed October 12, 2011.

[85] Y. C. Lim, Z. Desta, D. A. Flockhart and T. C. Skaar, *Cancer Chemother Pharmacol.* 55, 472 (2005).

[86] Y. C. Lim, L. Li, Z. Desta, Q. Zhao, J. M. Rae, D. A. Flockhart and T. C. Skaar, *J. Pharmacol. Exp. Ther.* 318, 503 (2006).

[87] O. Lee, D. Ivancic, R. J. Chatterton, A. Rademaker and S. Khan, *Breast Cancer (London)* 3, 61 (2011).

[88] A. C. Williams and B. W. Barry, *Adv. Drug Deliv. Rev.* 56, 603 (2004).

[89] M.Goodman and B. W. Barry, *J. Invest. Dermatol.* 91, 323 (1988).

[90] D. D. Kim, J. L. Kim and Y. W. Chien, *J. Pharm. Sci.* 85, 1191 (1996).

[91] M. J. Kim, H. J. Doh, M. K. Choi, S. J. Chung, C. K. Shim, D. D. Kim, J. S. Kim, C. S. Yong and H. G. Choi, *Drug Deliv.* 15, 373 (2008).

[92] J. Y. Fang, T. L. Hwang and Y. L. Leu, *Int. J. Pharm.* 250, 313 (2003).

[93] B. Yu, C. Y. Dong, P. T. So, D. Blankschtein and R. Langer, *J. Invest. Dermatol.* 117, 16 (2001).

[94] T. Ogiso, T. Paku, M. Iwaki and T. Tanino, *Biol. Pharm. Bull.* 18, 1566 (1995).

[95] E. A. Lien, E. Solheim and P. M. Ueland. *Cancer Res.*51, 4837 (1991).

[96] Northwestern University. Test Uniformity of Transdermal Drug Delivery to Breast Using Diclofenac Epolamine. 2011; http://clinicaltrials.gov/ct2/show/NCT01380353. Accessed October 12, 2011.

[97] C. A. Heyneman, C.Lawless-Liday and G. C. Wall, *Drugs.*60, 555 (2000).

[98] A. Fini A, G. Fazio and I. Rapaport, *Drugs Exp. Clin. Res.* 19, 81 (1993).

[99] V. Stearns, T. Mori, L. K. Jacobs, N. F. Khouri, E. Gabrielson, T. Yoshida, S. L. Kominsky, D. L. Huso, S. Jeter, P. Powers, K. Tarpinian, R. J. Brown, J. R. Lange, M. A. Rudek, Z. Zhang, T. N. Tsangaris and S. Sukumar, *Sci. Transl. Med.* 3, 106ra108 (2011).

[100] S. Murata, S. L. Kominsky, M. Vali, Z. Zhang, E. Garrett-Mayer, D. Korz, D. Huso, S. D. Baker, J. Barber, E. Jaffee, R. T. Reilly and S. Sukumar, *Cancer Res.* 66, 638 (2006).

[101] Doctor Susan Love Research Foundation. Doxorubicin Hydrochloride Liposome in Treating Women With Ductal Carcinoma in Situ Undergoing Surgery. 2011; http://clinicaltrials.gov/ct2/show/NCT00671476. Accessed November 7, 2011.

[102] M. Flanagan, S. Love nad E. S. Hwang, *Curr. Breast Cancer Rep.* 2, 75 (2010).

In: Tamoxifen Concepts and Cancer: New Paradigms
Editor: Ramon Andrade de Mello
ISBN: 978-1-62081-520-5

Chapter VI

The Use of Tamoxifen in an Estrogen-Independent Manner for Various Neoplasms

Andrew Trister and Shilpen Patel*
University of Washington, Department of Radiation Oncology,
Seattle, WA, US

Abstract

Tamoxifen has been shown to be an excellent treatment against neoplasms with increased expression of the estrogen receptor. In addition, tamoxifen and its metabolites have been shown to have antineoplastic activity through estrogen-independent inhibition of protein kinase C (PKC) pathways and MAP kinase cascades. This pathway has been used to treat a number of neoplasms including hepatocellular carcinoma, metastatic melanoma, prostate cancer and high-grade gliomas.

Early trials of the addition of tamoxifen to best available therapies for hepatocellular carcinoma and metastatic melanoma in small cohorts have shown improved survival. Additionally, studies of patients with recurrent high-grade gliomas demonstrated accumulation of tamoxifen in malignant cells by biopsy. Intracellular transport of tamoxifen in micromolar concentrations is sufficient to inhibit the PKC activity in glioma cell lines in vitro. These low doses are sufficient to induce apoptosis in these cell lines. Recent studies of the genomic and proteomic perturbations in high grade gliomas have shown an increased activity of protein kinase C (PKC) dependent pathways. Furthermore, tamoxifen and its metabolite, N-desmethyltamoxifen, have been shown to cross the blood-brain barrier and accumulate within tumors to therapeutic levels.

Through estrogen-independent modification of PKC, tamoxifen may present an additional treatment in the armamentarium against neoplastic diseases including high grade gliomas when used in conjunction with the standard of care. This chapter will review the pathways of tamoxifen induced apoptosis that are estrogen-independent as

* Shilpen Patel, MD, Assistant Professor, University of Washington Medical Center, Department of Radiation Oncology, NN146L, 1959 NE Pacific Street, Box 356043, Seattle, WA 98195-6043; Tel: 206-598-4100; Fax: 206-598-3786; E-mail: shilpenp@u.washington.edu.

well as results from studies of the utility of tamoxifen in the treatment of various estrogen receptor negative cancers.

Introduction

Tamoxifen is a ligand of the estrogen receptor (ER) that selectively modulates its activity. It additionally has activity on the estrogen related receptors (ERR) and on G-protein coupled estrogen receptors (GPER) which have related binding domains for estrogens, however are more selective for the form and downstream activity. [1] The activity of the active metabolites of tamoxifen, 4-hydroxytamoxifen (OHT) and N-desmethyltamoxifen (DMT), have been used to great effect in neoplasms with an increased expression of estrogen receptor. In addition, there has been seen to be some effect of tamoxifen in breast cancer that are not ER amplified. The mechanism for this ER independent action has been tied to the role of tamoxifen on estrogen-independent apoptotic pathways that are linked to Myc expression. [2] More recent work has elucidated non-estrogen related pathways that are mediated through protein kinase C (PKC), TGF-β, calmodulin, ceramide, and MAP kinases. [3] In much higher doses than needed in ER-positive tumors, tamoxifen can induce apoptosis through one or more of these pathways. This has led to investigation of tamoxifen in treating hepatocellular, renal cell, pancreatic, malignancies in addition to melanoma and high grade gliomas.

This chapter will briefly review the effects of tamoxifen on the PKC pathways that lead to apoptosis as well as a discussion of c-myc and MAP kinase pathways. The estrogen independent effects will be the basis for a discussion of clinical results of the utility of tamoxifen in ER-negative tumors.

Protein Kinase C

Like many kinases, protein kinase C (PKC) has many effectors and has been implicated in a host of cell responses to stress and signal transduction. PKC is active in regulating cell proliferation and malignant transformation as well as in regulating cell survival and apoptosis. [4] There are many isoforms of PKC that exert differing effects on cell cycle functions. [5] Due to the complexity of the interactions with these different isoforms, it is unclear whether tamoxifen induces an activation or degradation of PKC activity, [6] though it is thought that a decrease in PKC activity can largely be attributed to tamoxifen. [7] Tamoxifen has been shown to induce down-regulation of PKC followed by an increase in the same PKC pathway that is related to oxidative stress. [8]

The exact interaction of tamoxifen with PKC has been difficult to elucidate. Tamoxifen has been seen to directly bind to PKC at the triphenylethylene binding site which may modulate its activity. [9] There are also both upstream and downstream targets such as phospholipase C and phosphoinositide kinase as well as activation of caspases that lead to oxidative stress pathways resulting in apoptosis. [10] Tamoxifen may also induce the translocation of PKC to mitochondrial surface resulting in cytochrome c release, which is another trigger for the cell to undergo apoptosis. [11]

Myc

Myc is a transcription factor that regulates the expression of a large number of genes. [12] One of the first effects of Myc was the downregulation of Bcl-2 which leads to apoptosis. Just like with PKC, Myc is a proto-oncogene, and dysregulation of the Myc transcription factor can lead to changes in cell cycle checkpoint control and gene overexpression. Myc is thought to prime the cell to undergo apoptosis through interactions with adaptor and ligand gene products that may lead to the increase in apoptotic machinery required for the cell to undergo apoptosis.

Apoptotic death induced by tamoxifen has been linked to an overexpression of Myc. [2] It is not clear whether the change in expression is due to a conserved pathway from cell stress or if there are direct effects of tamoxifen on the expression of Myc. The direct action of tamoxifen on the upregulation of Myc, and the subsequent role of Myc in tamoxifen-induced apoptosis remains a subject of investigation.

MAP Kinase

Mitogen-activated protein kinases (MAPK) are serine-threonine kinases that are organized in a cascade of multiple phosphorylation events leading to their activation. Much like the PKC and Myc pathways, MAPK has a number of upstream regulators and downstream effectors that lead to a host of cellular functions. The direct role of MAPK on apoptosis is cell and context specific, and activation may or may not lead to apoptosis.

A study of ER-negative MDA MB-231 breast cancer cells in culture treated with tamoxifen at various concentrations demonstrated an increase in the MAP kinase JNK1 one hour after treatment which persisted for four hours. [13] Interestingly, treatment with vitamin-E prior to tamoxifen reduced this up-regulation of activity, perhaps demonstrating a need for oxidative stress to induce the MAPK pathway. A separate study of ER-positive breast cancer cells demonstrated a rescue from tamoxifen induced apoptosis with a selective inhibitor of a MAP kinase, p38, [14] demonstrating that MAPK cascades may play a crucial role in cell death from tamoxifen exposure.

Clinical Implications

Tamoxifen has a role in cell death that goes beyond the estrogen-receptor dependent mechanisms and leads to apoptotic signal cascades under various circumstances. While these mechanisms have not been fully elucidated, a number of different effectors have been implicated in leading to tamoxifen induced apoptosis. As these effectors are also often implicated in carcinogenesis, tamoxifen has been used as both a primary and adjuvant treatment in a number of different cancers.

Hepatocellular Carcinoma

Hepatocellular carcinoma (HCC) is a relatively rare tumor that is usually seen secondary to viral hepatitis infections. Liver transplantation remains the only curative approach for HCC, however transplantation is performed only in highly selected patients. Resection of tumors, radiofrequency ablation, radiation treatment, chemical embolization have all been used to varying degrees of efficacy to slow the progression of disease. Chemotherapy has largely been disappointing with little evidence for more than palliation of symptoms. Estrogen receptors were thought to be involved with the progression of HCC, and given the clinical efficacy of tamoxifen in breast cancers, a number of trials attempted the use of tamoxifen in the treatment of HCC.

Trials of tamoxifen in hCC during the late 1980s demonstrated no antitumor effect with the addition of tamoxifen to the regimen for patients with HCC. [15,16] Two small followup studies that were open-label and non-randomized did show a small improvement in the survival of patients with unresectable and advanced HCC who were treated with tamoxifen. [17,18] A randomized trial of tamoxifen in patients with unresectable HCC who were not candidates for other interventional therapies demonstrated no benefit of the addition of tamoxifen. [19] A critique of these initial trials is that the doses of tamoxifen used were significantly lower than the doses required to induce apoptosis through the intracellular pathways enumerated above (20-60mg/day).

A more recent multicenter randomized controlled study of 329 patients with unresectable advanced HCC attempted to induce apoptosis through the use of high doses of tamoxifen (60 or 120 mg/day). [20] This trial followed the patient's quality of life index as well as the survival on this intervention with no difference on either endpoint of overall survival or quality of life.

A meta-analysis of trials for patients with hepatocellular carcinoma who were in the placebo arm demonstrated a variety of responses. [21] The differences in survival in the untreated patients may be representative of heterogeneity in the biology of hepatocellular carcinoma patients. Greater effort in determining the biochemical pathways that may be dysregulated in a particular patient's tumor may lead to better use of known drugs like tamoxifen.

Renal Cell Carcinoma

Renal cell carcinoma is the most lethal of the genitourinary tumors with a 5 year survival of 60-70%. Treatment for localized disease focuses on surgical resection (nephrectomy) if there is unilateral disease, however when the disease has become metastatic, a systemic approach is favored. An early observation that renal cell cancer occasionally regressed spontaneously introduced the idea of an immune-modulated mechanism of apoptosis within the cancer cells. Given the effect of tamoxifen on upregulation of MAPK cascades that lead to apoptosis, high dose tamoxifen treatment was shown to have some improvement in tumor progression and overall survival with little toxicity. [22] A similar study showed opposite effect of high dose tamoxifen on advanced renal cell patients where it was felt that any benefit that was seen in the tamoxifen group was largely due to spontaneous remission of disease with no true therapeutic benefit of tamoxifen. [23]

Many of the early trials of tamoxifen in renal cell cancer have been superseded by the use of targeted agents that work against tyrosine kinases directly. Many of these agents have shown great efficacy in renal cell carcinoma, and have had superiority to tamoxifen or alkylating agents.

High Grade Glioma

High-grade gliomas are the most common primary brain tumor in adults, and patients often have a poor prognosis despite multiple modality treatment. The current standard of care for high-grade gliomas is the use of post-operative radiation therapy with concurrent temozolomide. Temozolomide is a novel oral methylating agent that is 100% bioavailable and has been shown to improve survival when used in conjunction with radiation and surgery. Multiple cooperative group trials have attempted the use of additional chemotherapeutic agents which have largely been unsuccessful in improving survival.

We have undertaken a phase I clinical trial to study the maximal tolerated dose of tamoxifen when administered with the standard of care radiation therapy and concurrent temozolomide (75 mg/m^2) for patients with high grade glioma. In our study, 17 patients took an escalating dose of tamoxifen, beginning at 50 mg/m^2 divided twice daily with increments of 25 mg/m^2 until a dose limiting toxicity was encountered. We found that a dose of 100 mg/m^2 was well tolerated. Consistent with RTOG 00-21 trial, this dose is sufficient to lead to PKC inactivation, and we have now shown that it can be safely combined with radiation and temozolomide. Furthermore, there is a concern that lower doses of tamoxifen ($<75 mg/m^2$) may not be sufficient to affect the PKC pathway.

Conclusion

Tamoxifen is an important drug in the arsenal against cancers. While the greatest target of this medication remains the estrogen receptor, tamoxifen induces apoptosis in malignant cells through a variety of pathways that are induced when the drug is given in doses up to eight times greater than needed to bind to estrogen receptors. There have been a number of trials for the utility of tamoxifen in a variety of ER-negative cancers that largely aimed to take advantage of PKC and MAPK induced apoptosis in the cells. While a number of trials showed equivocal or slightly improved results with tamoxifen in the single agent setting more contemporary studies utilizing this drug as an adjuvant demonstrated promising results.

One of the limitations of tamoxifen as an agent against PKC or MAPK pathways is that the direct mechanism of action is unknown, and while the toxicity profile of higher dose treatments is favorable, there is still not conclusive evidence that the pharmacokinetics favors significant inhibition of pathways in vivo. The possibility of using tamoxifen as an adjuvant agent in the setting of standard treatments with other chemotherapies and/or radiation therapy, makes the question of toxicities of high dose tamoxifen one that may require further investigation. With poor prognosis in diseases like glioblastoma and metastatic melanoma, there may increasingly be a role for additional therapies that modulate cell cycle control. Further investigation is warranted into the direct mechanisms of action for tamoxifen in the estrogen independent cell. A greater delineation of the effects of tamoxifen can lead to even better directed adjuvant therapies.

References

[1] Fitts JM, Klein RM, Powers CA: Tamoxifen Regulation of Bone Growth and Endocrine Function in the Ovariectomized Rat: Discrimination of Responses Involving Estrogen Receptor {alpha}/Estrogen Receptor {beta}, G Protein-Coupled Estrogen Receptor, or Estrogen-Related Receptor {gamma} Using Fulvestrant (ICI 182780). *J. Pharmacol. Exp. Ther.* 338:246-54, 2011.

[2] Kang Y, Cortina R, Perry RR: Role of c-myc in tamoxifen-induced apoptosis estrogen-independent breast cancer cells. *J. Natl. Cancer Inst.* 88:279-84, 1996.

[3] Mandlekar S, Kong AN: Mechanisms of tamoxifen-induced apoptosis. *Apoptosis* 6:469-77, 2001.

[4] Gonzalez-Guerrico AM, Meshki J, Xiao L, et al: Molecular mechanisms of protein kinase C-induced apoptosis in prostate cancer cells. *J. Biochem. Mol. Biol.* 38:639-45, 2005.

[5] Musashi M, Ota S, Shiroshita N: The role of protein kinase C isoforms in cell proliferation and apoptosis. *Int. J. Hematol.* 72:12-9, 2000.

[6] Cheng AL, Chuang SE, Fine RL, et al: Inhibition of the membrane translocation and activation of protein kinase C, and potentiation of doxorubicin-induced apoptosis of hepatocellular carcinoma cells by tamoxifen. *Biochem. Pharmacol.* 55:523-31, 1998.

[7] O'Brian CA, Liskamp RM, Solomon DH, et al: Inhibition of protein kinase C by tamoxifen. *Cancer Res.* 45:2462-5, 1985.

[8] Gundimeda U, Chen ZH, Gopalakrishna R: Tamoxifen modulates protein kinase C via oxidative stress in estrogen receptor-negative breast cancer cells. *J. Biol. Chem.* 271: 13504-14, 1996.

[9] O'Brian CA, Ward NE, Anderson BW: Role of specific interactions between protein kinase C and triphenylethylenes in inhibition of the enzyme. *J. Natl. Cancer Inst.* 80: 1628-33, 1988.

[10] Cabot MC, Zhang Z, Cao H, et al: Tamoxifen activates cellular phospholipase C and D and elicits protein kinase C translocation. *Int. J. Cancer* 70:567-74, 1997.

[11] Majumder PK, Pandey P, Sun X, et al: Mitochondrial translocation of protein kinase C delta in phorbol ester-induced cytochrome c release and apoptosis. *J. Biol. Chem.* 275: 21793-6, 2000.

[12] Gearhart J, Pashos EE, Prasad MK: Pluripotency redux--advances in stem-cell research. *N. Engl. J. Med.* 357:1469-72, 2007.

[13] Mandlekar S, Hebbar V, Christov K, et al: Pharmacodynamics of tamoxifen and its 4-hydroxy and N-desmethyl metabolites: activation of caspases and induction of apoptosis in rat mammary tumors and in human breast cancer cell lines. *Cancer Res.* 60:6601-6, 2000.

[14] Zhang CC, Shapiro DJ: Activation of the p38 mitogen-activated protein kinase pathway by estrogen or by 4-hydroxytamoxifen is coupled to estrogen receptor-induced apoptosis. *J. Biol. Chem.* 275:479-86, 2000.

[15] Melia WM, Johnson PJ, Williams R: Controlled clinical trial of doxorubicin and tamoxifen versus doxorubicin alone in hepatocellular carcinoma. *Cancer Treat Rep*. 71: 1213-6, 1987.

[16] Engstrom PF, Levin B, Moertel CG, et al: A phase II trial of tamoxifen in hepatocellular carcinoma. *Cancer* 65:2641-3, 1990.

[17] Farinati F, Salvagnini M, de Maria N, et al: Unresectable hepatocellular carcinoma: a prospective controlled trial with tamoxifen. *J. Hepatol*. 11:297-301, 1990.

[18] Martinez Cerezo FJ, Tomas A, Donoso L, et al: Controlled trial of tamoxifen in patients with advanced hepatocellular carcinoma. *J. Hepatol*. 20:702-6, 1994.

[19] Castells A, Bruix J, Bru C, et al: Treatment of hepatocellular carcinoma with tamoxifen: a double-blind placebo-controlled trial in 120 patients. *Gastroenterology* 109:917-22, 1995.

[20] Chow PK, Tai BC, Tan CK, et al: High-dose tamoxifen in the treatment of inoperable hepatocellular carcinoma: A multicenter randomized controlled trial. *Hepatology* 36:1221-6, 2002.

[21] Cabibbo G, Enea M, Attanasio M, et al: A meta-analysis of survival rates of untreated patients in randomized clinical trials of hepatocellular carcinoma. *Hepatology* 51:1274-83, 2010.

[22] Stahl M, Wilke H, Schmoll HJ, et al: A phase II study of high dose tamoxifen in progressive, metastatic renal cell carcinoma. *Ann. Oncol*. 3:167-8, 1992.

[23] Schomburg A, Kirchner H, Fenner M, et al: Lack of therapeutic efficacy of tamoxifen in advanced renal cell carcinoma. *Eur. J. Cancer* 29A:737-40, 1993.

In: Tamoxifen Concepts and Cancer: New Paradigms
Editor: Ramon Andrade de Mello
ISBN: 978-1-62081-520-5

Chapter VII

Tamoxifen: More Than an ER Antagonist

D. H. McGuinness and J. Edwards*
Institute of Cancer, College of Medical, Veterinary and Life Sciences, McGregor Building, Western Infirmary, Glasgow, Scotland

Abstract

Tamoxifen has become the drug of choice for the treatment of estrogen receptor positive (ER^{+ve}) early breast cancer; it has also gained recognition for its potential in the treatment of other disorders, including PCOS and bipolar mania. The duality of Tamoxifen action, acting as an antagonist in ER^{+ve} breast cancer and a partial agonist in other tissues, was originally unexpected as it was believed it would act as an antagonist throughout the body. This dual action has led to some highly beneficial effects, for example, prevention of osteoporosis, and some extreme side effects including increasing the risk for endometrial cancer. Tamoxifen has also found a role as a component of many complex treatments for various cancers and disorders, giving this drug new life and new expanded limitations. However, Tamoxifen faces stiff competition in the form of aromatase inhibitors that have been touted as being both more effective and having fewer side effects, although it has been proposed that some side effects, for example, memory impairment, may be even more severe for aromatase inhibitors. The undesired effects of aromatase inhibitors have been suggested to act through other mechanisms to produce some effects both intentional and undesired. Yet in the face of this competition and the unwanted side effects, Tamoxifen still holds the title of drug of choice.

The mechanisms of action, the side effects and the broad range of applications have led to Tamoxifen being intensively studied. While its target, the estrogen receptor (ER), explains many of the pathways Tamoxifen influences, its effects in other pathways are not so obvious. Recent studies have suggested that the number of signaling pathways affected by or affecting its action is very broad. The involvement of a wide range of

* Corresponding Author: Dr. J. Edwards, Institute of Cancer Science; College of Medical, Veterinary and Life Sciences; McGregor Building; Glasgow Western Infirmary; Glasgow; G11 6NT; E-mail: joanne.edwards@glasgow.ac.uk; Tel: +141 211 5441; Fax: *+141 211 5432*

signaling molecules has the potential to explain the effects, side effects and limitations of this drug. Furthermore, insight into these intracellular effects may unlock more surprises in the capabilities of this drug. The efficacy this drug demonstrates and its broad range of applications have been at the core of its success. This chapter seeks to examine the signaling pathways associated with Tamoxifen action and resistance and relate these to its effects on cancer and other disorders, as well as discussing the future implications for this drug.

Introduction

Tamoxifen, originally called Nolvadex from Astra Zeneca, is the drug of choice for estrogen-dependent breast cancer and has been in use for over 30 years. Tamoxifen is well established as the drug of choice for estrogen receptor positive (ER^{+ve}) breast cancer, although it has also been used for estrogen receptor negative (ER^{-ve}) breast cancer and it has been employed for the prevention of breast cancer. In fact, it is one of only two drugs fully approved for preventative therapy of which it is the more efficacious and can be used in premenstrual women [1].

It has found great service in the treatment of breast cancer from treating early stage disease, metastatic disease and as an adjuvant therapy following surgery or radiotherapy. A pro-drug, Tamoxifen is metabolized into its active components by the Cytochrome P450 family of enzymes. This is reinforced by studies demonstrating that the administration of a strong CYP2D6 inhibitor, for example, the antidepressant paroxetine, should be avoided in patients using Tamoxifen [2].

Originally believed to be an estrogen antagonist, Tamoxifen is now known to be a partial non-steroidal estrogen agonist that competitively inhibits estradiol at the receptor level. There are some functions that Tamoxifen appears to be unable to affect, for example, the estrogen-induced Ca^{2+} influx in cells is not inhibited by Tamoxifen action [3]. Furthermore, the inability of Tamoxifen to inhibit some estradiol actions in a neuroblastoma cell line is further evidence of its selective nature [4].

Due to Tamoxifen and its selective action, able to function as both an agonist and an antagonist while being unable to affect some estradiol based functions, it is now well accepted as the original selective estrogen receptor modulator (SERM) and is considered the prototype for all other SERMs in use today [5].

The success of Tamoxifen has led to the introduction of several generations of new SERMs, none of which have been conclusively shown to be superior to Tamoxifen although many are still undergoing clinical trials [6]. Furthermore, research into the action and effects of Tamoxifen has led to the development of SERDs (selective estrogen receptor downregulators) and aromatase inhibitors, the use of which has improved the outcome for many breast cancer patients particularly those with advanced ER^{+ve} disease [7].

In fact, Tamoxifen is still so popular and well used that dose, timing and duration of treatment is still studied and reviewed to this day [8]. This may be critical to the efficacy and potential side effects seen due to some functions being dose-dependent [9].

The mRNA profiles seen in cells between this and other anti-estrogens, for example, letrozole, is quite different [10], indicating a different mode of action for each of these drugs. This in combination with the fact that the anti-cancer effect of Tamoxifen in ER^{-ve} breast cancer can only be explained by effects on signaling pathways suggests that the selective action and specificity of this drug may result in a much broader reach for this aging, humble estrogen antagonist [11].

Tamoxifen Action

It is well accepted that Tamoxifen is mostly effective in ER^{+ve} breast cancer, recent studies have suggested that only the lowest levels of ER positivity are associated with an increase in breast cancer mortality and recurrence after tumor removal by surgery and adjuvant treatment with Tamoxifen [12]. One of the active metabolites of Tamoxifen, N-desmethyl Tamoxifen, binds competitively to the ER and competes out endogenous estrogen; in fact, the mode of action has been compared to that of phytoestrogens. Alpha-hydroxy-, N-desmethyl- and N-didesmethyl- Tamoxifen is predominantly mediated via CYP3A4 and can be highly variable and dependant on genetic variability [13]. Allelic variation in CYP2D6 has also been demonstrated to be key to the effective metabolism of Tamoxifen and its toxicity [14, 15]. Whereas, variants of CYP3A, CYP2B6 and CYP2C19 do not appear to influence the efficacy or toxicity of Tamoxifen at all [16]. Additionally, it has been suggested that another metabolite, 4-HydroxyTamoxifen (OHT) which can be found in patient plasma, also has a role to play in the overall effect of Tamoxifen. Formation of these active compounds is inhibited by erythromycin and diltiazem both of which are activated by and inhibit the Cytochrome family of enzymes.

Originally, it was believed that Tamoxifen acted purely as an estrogen antagonist by binding directly to membrane-bound estrogen receptor alpha (ERα), further research has revealed that it can act through both ERα and estrogen receptor beta (ERβ). The action of Tamoxifen on the different receptor isotypes has long been recognized, it is believed that the greater efficacy seen in ERα positive breast cancer may be due to its ability to recruit steroid receptor co-activator, SRC-3 (also know as amplified in breast cancer 1 AIB1) when under the influence of Tamoxifen. It was also noted that silencing of SRC-3 resensitized endocrine resistant cells and that the presence of the different isotypes of ER associated with differences in recurrence rates [17]. The fact that Tamoxifen has been shown to be effective in ER^{-ve} breast cancer and as more research has been conducted into the action and effects of Tamoxifen, it has become increasingly evident that interaction with ERα alone is not fully responsible for all of the actions, side effects and therapeutic abilities of Tamoxifen. The only way to elucidate the full action of this drug is to examine its interactions within the cell and map out the signaling pathways involved. Furthermore, investigation into the cellular actions of this drug may provide new insights into future uses and methods of controlling the side effects.

OHT has been shown to directly activate GPR30, the estrogen G-protein coupled receptor also known as the membrane estrogen receptor (mER), signaling in ER^{-ve} human breast cancer cells; this, in turn, induces a series of transcription factor in a similar fashion to that found in fibroblasts. This activity has been proposed as the mechanism behind the aggressive behavior found in some breast cancers in response to endocrine treatment [18]. It also represents selective action of Tamoxifen through the various isoforms of ER.

Estrogen has also been shown to increases levels of several members of the insulin growth factor (IGF) pathway in breast cancer tissues, which stimulates growth, Tamoxifen inhibits this pathway [19].

Oxytocin is also controlled by estrogen and is involved in stimulating uterine contractions during labor, neuromodulation, breastfeeding and maternal behaviors as well as some social bonding. Its receptors are G-protein coupled, it is believed that it is at this level, via an increase in expression of G-proteins and/or phospholipase C that estrogen acts increasing the cell responsiveness to oxytocin. Tamoxifen has been shown to reverse the estrogen effect, although whether this is by directly reversing the increase in G-protein expression or via up-regulation of protein kinase C (PKC) which inhibits the oxytocin pathway remains to be seen [20].

It has been demonstrated that estradiol causes degradation of both ERα and ERβ via the proteasome in breast cancer tissue, whereas Tamoxifen has the opposite effect, protecting both receptor isoforms, thus potentiating the receptor effects. In endometrial cancer cells, both estradiol and Tamoxifen stabilize ERα and cause the degradation of ERβ by the proteasome indicating that Tamoxifen acts as an antagonist in breast cancer and an agonist in uterine cancers. This is most likely due to the activation of the AKT pathway in breast tumors and the ERK pathway in uterine cancer [21], which may result in differential phosphorylation patterns of ER in these two tissues. Many of the effects of ERα are mediated through activation of various signaling pathways. One of the most important of these is the mitogen-activated protein kinase (MAPK) signaling cascade which has a major influence in many vital cellular functions and at least one component of this pathway or its activators has been implicated in almost all forms of cancer. It is also known that MAPK phosphorylates ERα on S118. Studies have demonstrated that in breast cancer, this occurs via EGFR signaling into the MAPK pathway. Furthermore, it has been shown that this signaling is bi-directional with this pathway reducing the level of phosphorylation, and thus lowering the activation state, of ERα[22].

Both estrogen and Tamoxifen are capable of inducing AP-1, a transcription factor comprising a homo- or heterodimer of phosphorylated *c*-jun and c-fos, transcription with ERs present in the cytoplasm, however, when ERs are present in the nucleus this transcription is repressed. This indicates that ER is capable of interacting with other molecules and activates them in a non-genomic fashion [23]. Allowing for direct activation at the protein level, this massively increases the possibilities for Tamoxifen action by not limiting its abilities to ER response elements in the genome, these interactions can be explained by activation of the androgen receptor (AR).

Cell line studies have demonstrated that Tamoxifen can affect the levels of C-X-C chemokine receptor type 4 (CXCR4), also known as CD184 and is modulated by tumor necrosis factor alpha (TNFα), which may result in reduced immune surveillance of cancer cells helping to protect them from the immune system [24], this molecule is also up-regulated during implantation in the endometrium. This receptor and its reciprocal chemokine, stromal cell-derived factor-1 (CXCL12) are responsible for activating pathways involved in proliferation, survival and migration of cancer cells, thus when they are downregulated, as they are in breast cancer, the ability of the tumor to grow and metastasize is restricted. However, other studies have shown that Tamoxifen can increase the levels of both CXCR4 and CXCL12 in endometrial cancer models, providing a potential explanation for the increased risk of endometrial cancer in patients taking Tamoxifen [25]. Interestingly, studies using breast cancer cell lines demonstrate that CXCL12 is not upregulated by Tamoxifen [26]. Additionally, it has been shown that Tamoxifen can lower levels of monocyte chemotactic protein-1 (MCP-1), which can be induced by TNFα, in endometrial cancer thus reducing the ability of monocytes to penetrate into the tumor, which further reduces the ability of the immune system to attack this type of cancer when under the influence of this drug [27]. The action of Tamoxifen on the immune system extends further by being able to antagonize the effects of estrogen on dendritic cells, reducing the expression of CD40, major histocompatability complex (MHC) class II and increasing expression of several cytokines including TNFα [28].

Tamoxifen reduces the levels of the phosphorylated form of NEDD9, which is a key component in adhesion-dependent signaling pathways in breast tumors [29]. NEDD9 is more than likely activated via Src kinase/protein tyrosine kinase 2 (PTK2), and ultimately via the AR. It has also been suggested that in instances of poor cell-cell contact, Tamoxifen treatment may encourage invasion through its action on Src kinase, via the AR, this has implications for individuals who have inherent problems with cellular adhesion [30].

Side Effects

Adjuvant therapy with Tamoxifen is generally taken for 5 years, this reduces the risk of the same cancer recurring and lowers the risks for developing another primary cancer in the other breast. There is a suggestion that women become resistant to the effects of Tamoxifen after 5 years and that the risks may outweigh the benefits in long-term treatments. This long-term usage makes consideration of possible side-effects critical for treatment and requires close monitoring to ensure the risks don't outweigh the benefits. Like most medications, there are side effects, some of which are reasonably minor and others are closely linked to other anti-cancer treatments.

The most common side effects are hot flashes and sweats which affect approximately 45% of patients, painful joints and fatigue which are apparent in 25% of cases, vomiting affects around 20% and abnormal menstrual cycles. Abnormal menstrual cycles may stem from the ability of Tamoxifen to hold the diestrus phase and prevent pregnancy in rats [31, 32]. To date, the effect on the ability of women to get pregnant while taking Tamoxifen has not been addressed, this is probably due to the circumstances under which it is normally administered. It has also been demonstrated that estradiol can increase the phosphorylation of transient receptor potential vanilloid receptor 1 (TRPV1) thus reducing transduction in nociceptors; Tamoxifen has the opposite effect [33]. This may explain the pain some patients experience in joints. As a Calmodulin antagonist, Tamoxifen appears to be capable of causing platelet apoptosis [34], no adverse side effect has, as yet, been attributed to this phenomenon; however, it may be linked to some other less common side effects including increased risk of thrombosis, rashes and eye problems. More seriously, Tamoxifen use has been linked to an increased risk of other hormonally affected cancers including uterine and hepatic.

Given that estrogens protect females from aging through the upregulation of anti-oxidants via MAPK and NFκB [35], it may be possible that the increase in risk of developing other cancers while receiving Tamoxifen may be due to reactive oxygen species (ROS) alone or in combination with differential expression of estradiol-controlled genes. Furthermore, administering natural free radical scavengers with Tamoxifen can negate much of the hepatotoxicity encountered, suggesting that much of the damage done is caused by the downregulation of anti-oxidants and adding more weight to the possibility that these free radicals increase cancer risk [36]. Furthermore, it may just be possible that treatment with Tamoxifen may speed up the aging process in women by reversing the effect of estrogen, however, given the timescales involved and the alternatives the overall significance of this may be minimal. Hepatic steatosis is also a major issue, where abnormal lipid deposits build up around the liver adding further insult. This has been studied in mice where it was discovered that a large number of genes differentially regulated by Tamoxifen in the liver were involved in lipid and carbohydrate metabolism [37]. The increased risk of endometrial cancer found in patients taking Tamoxifen may be related to src kinase which stabilizes ERα in endometrial cells and potentiates Tamoxifen agonist action by phosphorylation of Serine 167 (S167), this is also believed to be in conjunction with activation of AKT kinase, which is also known as PKB and is known to phosphorylate ERα directly at S167 [38].

It has been reported that estradiol increases sensitivity to radiotherapy for cancer and can increase the bystander effect, where the effect of the radiation therapy is passed on via cell-cell communication in ER^{+ve} breast cancer. It has also been suggested that, in line with its role as an antagonist, Tamoxifen can negate any beneficial effect that estradiol exerts in ER^{+ve} breast cancer. Whereas neither estradiol nor Tamoxifen have any influence in ER^{-ve} breast cancer [39].

Not all side effects have a negative impact. One such side effect is the preservation of bone.I In fact, Tamoxifen actually increases bone density, whereas aromatase inhibitors have the opposite effect. Although these effects on the skeleton do not directly relate to cancer survival and treatment, they do have a beneficial effect for patients helping improve their quality of life compared to alternative treatments [40]. It has also been demonstrated that this ability to increase bone mineral density is not associated with genetic variations in ER, but is, in fact, a general effect that is more pronounced in post-menopausal women [41]. This effect appears to be mediated via COX-2 induction of PGE-2 which results in an increase in osteoblast proliferation [42]. These facts have led to Tamoxifen being hailed as a treatment for osteoporosis.

Another potentially beneficial side effect is that Tamoxifen may slow down weight loss, in a study conducted in rats Tamoxifen appeared to be able to partially counter the slimming effects of oleoyl-estrone [43], indicating that it can have a direct influence on the storage and/or usage of lipids.

Tamoxifen Resistance

Interestingly, ER levels are usually maintained when Tamoxifen resistance is acquired, indicating that other mechanisms are taking over to subvert the action that Tamoxifen is blocking. Despite this, it is also apparent that ER activation can still influence the efficiency of the MAPK signaling pathway, believed to be mediated via TGFα [44]. However, it is apparent that these tumors are largely estrogen-independent with the ability to replicate and grow independent of the hormone signal. It is estimated that 50% of patients with advanced

ER^{+ve} breast cancer do not respond to Tamoxifen and the other 50% will ultimately develop resistance, the reason and mechanisms behind this are still not fully understood, although the breast cancer anti-estrogen resistance (BCAR) genes are a strong candidate [45].

It has been observed that members of the fibroblast growth factor (FGF) and fibroblast growth factor receptor (FGFR) families are involved in the development and progression of some breast cancers. It has been demonstrated in cell lines that high levels of FGFs, in particular FGF1 result in reduced sensitivity to Tamoxifen. This data is further confirmed by the finding that increased expression of FGFR3 is present in Tamoxifen resistant breast cancer [46]. Focal adhesion kinase (FAK) is also associated with endocrine resistance in breast tumors [47]. Additionally, high levels of cytosolic phospholipase A(2)α (cPLA(2)α) are correlated with reduced effect of Tamoxifen treatment and overall survival.I In fact, this can be considered an independent marker for poor response to endocrine therapy [48].

Recently, high levels of Sphingosine 1-phosphate receptors (S1P1 and S1P3), Sphingosine kinase 1 and extracellular signal-regulated kinase (erk)-1/2 have been shown to be associated with development of Tamoxifen resistance in ER^{+ve} breast cancer [49]. It has also been suggested that measurement of ERα or downstream signaling targets of Tamoxifen, including Her2, epidermal growth factor receptor (EGFR), insulin-like growth factor -1 (IGF-1) and insulin-like growth factor receptor (IGF-1R) can predict Tamoxifen resistance [50]. Her2 has been further implicated by its association with cyclin D1, which is vital for regulation in G1 phase of the cell cycle, it has been demonstrated that moderate expression of cyclin D1 associates with Tamoxifen sensitivity whereas strong or weak levels associate with resistance [51]. The involvement of cyclin D1 and EGFR in this pathway also directly implicates AR as a key player in the response and resistance to Tamoxifen. It has also been noted that administration of Tamoxifen can induce higher levels of Her2, driving towards the development of resistance as part of its own action [52]. Further studies suggest that the effects of Tamoxifen on the IGF pathway may be insulin-dependent [53]. Recent evidence suggests that other members of the Her family, Her3 and Her4, may also play a role in the development of endocrine resistance [54].

Poor prognosis in ERα positive breast cancer is associated with high levels of BCAR4, which also associates with Tamoxifen resistance. This appears to be mediated through extracellular signal-regulated kinase (ERK) 1/2 and/or Akt1/2 activation [55]. Activated ERK1/2 phosphorylation in ER^{+ve} tumors has been directly linked to reduced Tamoxifen effect [56] and is probably directly mediated through EGFR. Caveolin-1 has been related to resistance; however, it appears to be more of a casualty than a causative effect as the levels are suppressed by EGFR and ERK [57]. Growth factor signaling appears to be critical in cases of insensitivity to Tamoxifen and in acquired Tamoxifen resistance, this resistance can be immediate or can occur in as little as 3 months [58] and suggests that the primary action of Tamoxifen is via growth factor activation by direct interaction with the ER. In fact, EGFR/Her2 have been shown to be very important in acquired resistance to Tamoxifen [59], through interactions with IGF-R1. It appears that the cross-talk between ER and the EGFR pathway, resulting in dephosphorylation of Serine 118 (S118) of ERα is also found in acquired Tamoxifen resistance [60]. High levels of Her2 have been found to correlate with poor response to Tamoxifen [61]. It has also been suggested that EGFR/Her2 increase the phosphorylation state of Akt [62], indicating that the PI3 kinase pathway downstream of the MAPK pathways may play a vital role in restoring tumor growth and expansion in

Tamoxifen-resistant tumors. P21-activated kinase (Pak1) has also been suggested as a player in Tamoxifen resistance where Tamoxifen appears to cause an increase in the direct interaction between Pak1 and ER in Tamoxifen resistant, but not sensitive, breast cancer cells. This mechanism of resistance is believed to induce a conformational change in ER that prevents Tamoxifen binding to the ER [63], this could explain isolated incidents of Tamoxifen resistance, but cannot account for the large number of cases where the tumour becomes resistant to all hormone therapy.

High levels of cAMP-dependent protein kinase A (PKA) are found in a large number of cancers, including breast cancer, it has also been demonstrated that phosphorylation of ER by PKA may lead to Tamoxifen resistance and that this may be linked to hereditary forms of breast cancer [64]. In fact, it has been proposed that cyclooxygenase-2 (COX-2), acting through prostaglandin E2 (PGE2), acts to stimulate the activity of PKA and protein kinase C (PKC), resulting in Tamoxifen resistance [65]. The presence of COX-2 may be explained by the inflammation caused by tumors or may be a direct result of Tamoxifen interaction with the immune system.

It has also been suggested that the adhesion related p130Cas/BCAR1 is associated with the development of Tamoxifen resistance; in this case, Tamoxifen acts as an anti-estrogen increasing the phosphorylation levels of p130Cas/BCAR1. This appears to be mediated through Src kinase and FAK [66]. Activity of Src kinase has been shown to be increased in Tamoxifen resistant breast cancer cells, however, this activity does not appear to be due to increased expression at either gene or protein level [67]. Furthermore, Src kinase control of FAK activity may play a key role in the increased invasiveness of breast tumours that have become Tamoxifen resistant [68]. The EGFR pathway has also been implicated in increasing motility and invasiveness in Tamoxifen resistant breast cancer [69], indicating that the development of endocrine resistance may well be an escalation of tumorigenesis rather than just a sidestep to maintain the status quo.

Ultimately, Tamoxifen resistance is associated with overexpression and/or activation in the EGFR and MAPK pathways. This is demonstrated by studies that inhibit AKT and or MAPK in Tamoxifen-resistant tissues which restore Tamoxifen sensitivity [70].

Alternative Uses

Tamoxifen has become the drug of choice for treatment of ER^{+ve} breast cancer. Its uses, however, don't stop there. Thirty years of research into the structure and function of this drug has led to suggestions that it may be highly useful in other areas. For example, the opposing effects of estradiol and Tamoxifen on the regulation of an amyloid-beta neurotoxicity related plasmalemmal anion channel and the generally accepted belief that estradiol has neuroprotective effects has led to the belief that this drug may find a new use in dissecting the processes involved in neurodegenerative disorders [71]. In addition to these findings, it has also been shown that SERMs, but not estradiol, induce an anti-inflammatory response in rat and mouse brain cells and this activity was believed to be mediated through AP-1 which can be activated via the MAPK pathway [72]. Furthermore, galanin, which is believed to have neuroprotective activity and may be involved in Alzheimer's Disease (AD) [73], is influenced by estradiol and Tamoxifen [74]. Ultimately, this may lead to breakthroughs in the treatment and/or prevention of neurodegenerative disorders, in particular AD. Tamoxifen has also been shown to be a relatively selective PKC inhibitor, which suggests that this drug may have a role to play in diseases or disorders that involve overactive PKC. For example, it has been suggested that Tamoxifen may be useful in the treatment of bipolar disorder, where high levels of PKC are associated with mania [75, 76]. Interestingly, Tamoxifen is a mild inhibitor of muscle cell depolarization, which is also due to its PKC inhibiting action, however no function or side effect has yet been attributed to this activity [77].

Given that Tamoxifen is effective in both ERα and estrogen receptor beta ERβ positive breast cancers and the broader range of tissues expressing ERβ, it is possible that the range of Tamoxifen effect on cancers in other tissue types, as yet unexplored, may prove to be highly successful [78].

Due to its SERM activity, the use of Tamoxifen in hormone-related disorders is also a possibility. In fact, its use in Polycystic Ovarian Syndrome (PCOS) is already recommended [79]. It has also been used to treat male infertility, as an estrogen blocker, it can solve some fertility problems, however, some research suggests that this avenue may need further investigation as it can cause chromosomal abnormalities in mice [80]. This issue is further compounded by the suggestion that prenatal exposure to Tamoxifen may cause abnormalities in neural development, highlighted by studies in rats [81].

Estrogen has been shown to be protective against early atherosclerosis and this is believed to be due to its ability to regulate MCP-1. It has also been demonstrated that some SERMs, including Tamoxifen, are able to mimic this ability of estrogen, however, they are not as potent as estrogen itself [82]. This suggests that Tamoxifen may find a new role in the research and/or prevention of heart disease.

Tamoxifen has also become broadly used and highly successful in the establishment of mouse models, in this context it is used to selectively silence genes in specifically bred mice using Tamoxifen-dependent Cre recombinase in a Cre-Lox system. This allows studies on genes that are lethal at embryogenesis to be studied in an adult model and/or tissue specific manner. It also allows knock in mutations where Tamoxifen, or one of its metabolites, can be used to activate normally silent gene expression. An example of this is the use of 4-OHT to activated telomerase in a mouse model to show the ability of telomerase to reverse tissue regeneration [83]. Furthermore, Tamoxifen is also used regularly as a research tool, not only in identifying pathways involved in its own action or in resistance to its action but also as an aid to elucidate the roles of oestradiol, ERα and ERβ.

In addition to all of these alternative functions, Tamoxifen may also have a role to play in the regulation of the immune system and infection control. Recent studies have suggested that Tamoxifen, through its role as an ERβ antagonist, can reduce the infectivity of *Chlamydia trachomatis* by 30-90% in cell line models of infection [84].

Future Possibilities

Aromatase inhibitors (AIs), which block estrogen biosynthesis have been shown to be more effective at treating breast cancer with less side effects than Tamoxifen and have been approved for use [85], it would have been logical to assume that the future of Tamoxifen was limited. Further research has proven that AIs have just as many issues as Tamoxifen, including aromatase inhibitor (AI)-associated musculoskeletal syndrome (AIMSS), which occurs in approximately 50% of cases [86]. Despite this, and associated bone mineral density issues, AIs have largely replaced Tamoxifen as the drug of choice for post-menopausal women with breast cancer. Although, it has also been suggested that using Tamoxifen in combination with AIs in a sequential manner may provide even greater benefits for patients, including better treatment for early disease and prevention of recurrence [87].

Some studies have described methods for using Tamoxifen in combination with natural phytoestrogens, resulting in an enhanced tumour fighting ability with increased tumor cell apoptosis and decreased proliferation in breast tumors; whereas it results in a reduction of the tumor-promoting ability in hepatocytes, indicating that the efficacy can be improved and the side effects reduced by combining it with phytoestrogens [88]. However, other studies have demonstrated that this effect may be dose-dependent, high doses of phytoestrogens and Tamoxifen have a synergistic effect, whereas low doses of phytoestrogens actually have a negative impact on the efficacy of Tamoxifen [89]. Caffeic acid phenethyl ester, from propolis, also protects against hepatotoxicity by reversing many of the ill effects of Tamoxifen including normalizing the activity of glutathione reductase, glutathione peroxidise, superoxide dismutase and catalase as well as reducing the elevated levels of TNFα [90]. Conversely, some natural substances can have a negative effect on Tamoxifen, for example, sesame seeds can inhibit the anti-tumor effects [91]. Vitamin E alone can inhibit breast cancer cell growth, however, it also reduces the efficacy of Tamoxifen [92], indicating too much of a good thing may interfere with effective medication. Other studies have demonstrated the ability of chlorpromazine to enhance the cytotoxic effect of Tamoxifen in breast cancer cell lines [93]. Histone deacetylase inhibition has also been demonstrated to be a key co-factor with Tamoxifen treatment, the use of histone deacetylase inhibitors alongside Tamoxifen resulted in an increase of its anti-proliferative action and also blocked its induction of proliferation in uterine cells [94]. The fact that inhibition at the later stages of the MAPK pathway can restore Tamoxifen sensitivity suggests that Tamoxifen action is at the receptor or entry level of the MAPK pathway and that if it was given in conjunction with an inhibitor, it may be effective in nearly all cases. This may indicate that the future of this drug in the treatment of cancer may lie in combinatorial ventures rather than solo efforts making it both safer and more effective.

The possibility of effectiveness in the treatment of cancer in other tissues has opened up new avenues of exploration and may ultimately unveil new territory for Tamoxifen to conquer. This exploration has already begun with non-small cell lung cancer being assessed for ERα and ERβ expression and the anti-tumor effects of Tamoxifen [95]. There is also some evidence to suggest that Tamoxifen may find a future role in the treatment of chemo-resistant melanoma, which is notoriously difficult to treat. One such study used Tamoxifen in combination with curcumin to increase reactive oxygen species (ROS) and thus induce apoptosis [96].

As would be expected, polymorphisms in Cytochrome P450 genes can reduce the effect of Tamoxifen in individuals [16]. This, in combination with all of the other factors that can affect the function of Tamoxifen, suggests that individualized and tailored treatments may be an important factor in the future of this highly successful drug that has already withstood the test of time. However, with new possibilities opening up for its use, its continued importance in research, the side effects of aromatase inhibitors and the continued high usage in treatment of both early and advanced ER^{+ve} breast cancer, it is obvious that it is here to stay.

Conclusion

Collectively, the information presented here allows several conclusions about the action of Tamoxifen.

Firstly, it suggests that Tamoxifen action and its side effects are dose-dependent, this is emphasized by the effect of Ca^{2+} levels in the treatment of neuroblastoma cells where Tamoxifen action can shift from growth promoting to growth inhibitory in a dose-dependent fashion and that serum factors can cause this dose dependency to shift requiring a higher or lower dose to achieve optimal effect [97]. Taken in combination with the high variability in the production of active metabolites by the CYP family of enzymes due to allelic variance this further suggests that the individual genetic code and personal health and well-being may play a much larger role in the efficacy of this drug than has ever been suggested before. Furthermore, this dose dependency may explain the duality of function seen in the human body. Low doses act as an estrogen agonist, whereas high doses act as an antagonist. The dose may be more dependent on the tissue requirements than on the actual physical level, for example, ER^{+ve} breast cancer tissue has an absolute requirement for estrogen, in this circumstance, demand is high therefore lower levels of Tamoxifen are required to engage its antagonist function. Whereas the same physical level in tissues with lower demand, for example, the liver, will exhibit the agonist behavior of Tamoxifen. Tamoxifen is a weak agonist and a poor substitute for estrogen, and it may be plausible that higher doses act more by blocking estrogen action than by antagonizing it. In fact, there is no available data to dispute this hypothesis as most research is conducted under the circumstances of reversing changes made by oestrogen.

Secondly, the most important signaling pathway that is influenced by this drug is the MAPK pathway, through differential stimulus this pathway can control and/or influence almost all functions within the cell. This gives Tamoxifen access and control to all of these functions, however, its influence appears to be mostly limited to cell cycle control, slowing growth, and apoptosis. It has been suggested that the production of ROS by Tamoxifen is a result of direct action on the mitochondria, however, this is more likely to be due to its influence on glutathione enzymes, the mechanism of action on these enzymes remains unknown but it is more likely to be a knock on effect from activation of MAPK and ultimately PKA, AKT and PKC than a direct effect. Despite the large amount of data presented on the influence of Tamoxifen on various signaling components and the belief that it affects many signaling pathways individually, it has yet to be conclusively shown that these effects are entirely independent of the main EGFR/MAPK axis.In fact, many of the functions exhibited are under the direct control of the androgen receptor (AR) which is directly influenced by EGFR. This axis can exert its influence over a large number of key transcription factors and effectors within the cell and can ultimately influence all of the signaling mechanisms described thus far. This is reinforced by the ability of MAPK inhibitors to restore sensitivity to Tamoxifen, as this pathway is also key to subverting the effects of Tamoxifen. However, independent effects cannot be completely denied, the IGF pathway does not have very close links to EGFR although it does exert some influence through the MAPK pathway, it may be that this is an alternative pathway used by Tamoxifen. Whether activation of either pathway is specific to one particular metabolite and/or the various isoforms of ER, or whether environmental circumstances play a role in determining

Tamoxifen action remains to be seen. Direct interactions with other pathways would be required to demonstrate that direct action is taking place and not a knock on effect from either of these two pathways, to date the only direct interactions that have been demonstrated are between Tamoxifen metabolites and the ERs, which then activate EGFR and IGFR, as well as translocating to the nucleus to interact with ER response elements.

Thirdly, the interactions between Tamoxifen and various natural substances found in the normal human diet suggest that closer control of diet may have a major impact on the efficacy of this drug. It is apparent from these studies that these compounds cause a disturbance to the cellular environment and may further influence the required dosage levels of Tamoxifen possibly even pushing the drug from tumor-inhibiting to tumor-promoting activities. This has serious implications for individual treatments and may require dosages to be revisited due to lifestyle choices, these would be extremely challenging calculations to make and ultimately would prove too costly to implement. However, simple advice on foods to avoid may pay large dividends in the outcome of treatment. Furthermore, interaction with other drugs appears to be a double-edged sword, with some beneficial associations and other not so helpful interactions. Despite this, the way forward for this drug may well be in the form of combinatorial treatments, with the potential for sequential treatments with AIs for treating breast cancer, the possibilities of mixing with other drugs to reduce side effects and toxicity and the opportunity to treat various cancers as well as completely unrelated disease in combination with other compounds.

What is certain about Tamoxifen is that it established itself quickly, gave up its secrets and still managed to remain king of the hill. Not only will this drug stick around, but it will continue to drive research into its own actions as well as the disorders it can influence. This drug is here to stay and it has opened up whole new avenues for exploration.

References

[1] Cuzick, J., et al., Preventive therapy for breast cancer: a consensus statement. *Lancet Oncol.,* 2011. 12(5): p. 496-503.

[2] Zembutsu, H., et al., Should CYP2D6 inhibitors be administered in conjunction with tamoxifen? *Expert Rev. Anticancer Ther.*, 2011. 11(2): p. 185-93.

[3] Benten, W.P., et al., Estradiol binding to cell surface raises cytosolic free calcium in T cells. *FEBS Lett*, 1998. 422(3): p. 349-53.

[4] Watters, J.J., et al., Rapid membrane effects of steroids in neuroblastoma cells: effects of estrogen on mitogen activated protein kinase signaling cascade and c-fos immediate early gene transcription. *Endocrinology*, 1997. 138(9): p. 4030-3.

[5] Lumachi, F., et al., Endocrine therapy of breast cancer. *Curr. Med. Chem.*, 2011. 18(4): p. 513-22.

[6] Uray, I.P., P.H. Brown, Prevention of breast cancer: current state of the science and future opportunities. *Expert Opin. Investig. Drugs*, 2006. 15(12): p. 1583-600.

[7] Orlando, L., et al., Molecularly targeted endocrine therapies for breast cancer. *Cancer Treat. Rev.,* 2010. 36 Suppl 3: p. S67-71.

[8] Karn, A., et al., Tamoxifen for breast cancer. *JNMA J. Nepal Med. Assoc.*, 2010. 49(177): p. 62-7.

[9] Childs, E.W., et al., 17beta-estradiol mediated protection against vascular leak after hemorrhagic shock: role of estrogen receptors and apoptotic signaling. *Shock,* 2010. 34(3): p. 229-35.
[10] Sun, L., et al., Transcriptional responses in the brain, liver and gonad of Japanese ricefish (Oryzias latipes) exposed to two anti-estrogens. *Comp. Biochem. Physiol. C Toxicol. Pharmacol.*, 2011. 153(4): p. 392-401.
[11] Rivera-Guevara, C., Camacho, J. Tamoxifen and its new derivatives in cancer research. *Recent Pat. Anti-cancer Drug Discov.,* 2011. 6(2): p. 237-45.
[12] Morgan, D.A., Refalo, N.A.,Cheung, K.L. Strength of ER-positivity in relation to survival in ER-positive breast cancer treated by adjuvant tamoxifen as sole systemic therapy. *Breast*, 2011. 20(3): p. 215-9.
[13] Coller, J.K., et al., Large interindividual variability in the in vitro formation of tamoxifen metabolites related to the development of genotoxicity. *Br. J. Clin. Pharmacol.*, 2004. 57(1): p. 105-11.
[14] de Souza, J.A., Olopade, O.I. CYP2D6 genotyping and tamoxifen: an unfinished story in the quest for personalized medicine. *Semin. Oncol.*, 2011. 38(2): p. 263-73.
[15] Higgins, M.J., Stearns, V. Pharmacogenetics of endocrine therapy for breast cancer. *Annu. Rev. Med.*, 2011. 62: p. 281-93.
[16] Singh, M.S., Francis, P.A., Michael, M. Tamoxifen, cytochrome P450 genes and breast cancer clinical outcomes. *Breast*, 2011. 20(2): p. 111-8.
[17] Mc Ilroy, M., et al., Tamoxifen-induced ER-alpha-SRC-3 interaction in HER2 positive human breast cancer; a possible mechanism for ER isoform specific recurrence. *Endocr. Relat. Cancer*, 2006. 13(4): p. 1135-45.
[18] Pandey, D.P., et al., Estrogenic GPR30 signalling induces proliferation and migration of breast cancer cells through *CTGF. EMBO J.*, 2009. 28(5): p. 523-32.
[19] Chong, Y.M., et al., The relationship between the insulin-like growth factor-1 system and the oestrogen metabolizing enzymes in breast cancer tissue and its adjacent non-cancerous tissue. *Breast Cancer Res. Treat*, 2006. 99(3): p. 275-88.
[20] Phaneuf, S., et al., Oxytocin signaling in human myometrium. *Adv. Exp. Med. Biol.,* 1995. 395: p. 453-67.
[21] Horner-Glister, E., et al., Influence of oestradiol and tamoxifen on estrogen receptors-alpha and -beta protein degradation and non-genomic signaling pathways in uterine and breast carcinoma cells. *J. Mol. Endocrinol.,* 2005. 35(3): p. 421-32.
[22] Britton, D.J., et al., Bidirectional cross-talk between ERalpha and EGFR signaling pathways regulates tamoxifen-resistant growth. *Breast Cancer Res. Treat,* 2006. 96(2): p. 131-46.
[23] Bjornstrom, L.,Sjoberg, M. Estrogen receptor-dependent activation of AP-1 via non-genomic signaling. *Nucl. Recept,* 2004. 2(1): p. 3.
[24] Kubarek, L., et al., Down-regulation of CXCR4 expression by tamoxifen is associated with DNA methyltransferase 3B up-regulation in MCF-7 breast cancer cells. *Biomed. Pharmacother.*, 2009. 63(8): p. 586-91.
[25] Kubarek, L., Jagodzinski, P.P. Epigenetic up-regulation of CXCR4 and CXCL12 expression by 17 beta-estradiol and tamoxifen is associated with formation of DNA methyltransferase 3B4 splice variant in Ishikawa endometrial adenocarcinoma cells. *FEBS Lett*, 2007. 581(7): p. 1441-8.

[26] Habauzit, D., et al., Development and validation of a test for environmental estrogens: Checking xeno-estrogen activity by CXCL12 secretion in BREAST CANCER CELL LINES (CXCL-test). *Environ. Toxicol.,* 2010. 25(5): p. 495-503.

[27] Wang, L., et al., Expression of monocyte chemotactic protein-1 in human endometrial cancer cells and the effect of treatment with tamoxifen or buserelin. *J. Int. Med. Res.*, 2006. 34(3): p. 284-90.

[28] Jiang, B., et al., Estrogen modulates bone marrow-derived DCs in SLE murine model-(NZB x NZW) F1 female mice. *Immunol. Invest.*, 2008. 37(3): p. 227-43.

[29] Bradshaw, L.N., et al., Estradiol stabilizes the 105-kDa phospho-form of the adhesion-docking protein NEDD9 and suppresses NEDD9-dependent cell spreading in breast cancer cells. *Biochim. Biophys. Acta.*, 2011. 1813(2): p. 340-5.

[30] Borley, A.C., et al., Anti-estrogens but not estrogen deprivation promote cellular invasion in intercellular adhesion-deficient breast cancer cells. *Breast Cancer Res.*, 2008. 10(6): p. R103.

[31] Tower, A.M., et al., AFPep, a novel drug for the prevention and treatment of breast cancer, does not disrupt the estrous cycle or fertility in rats. *Oncol. Rep.,* 2009. 22(1): p. 49-56.

[32] Tsujioka, S., et al., Collaborative work on evaluation of ovarian toxicity. 3) Effects of 2- or 4- week repeated-dose toxicity and fertility studies with tamoxifen in female rats. *J. Toxicol. Sci.*, 2009. 34 Suppl 1: p. SP43-51.

[33] Xu, S., et al., 17beta-estradiol activates estrogen receptor beta-signaling and inhibits transient receptor potential vanilloid receptor 1 activation by capsaicin in adult rat nociceptor neurons. *Endocrinology*, 2008. 149(11): p. 5540-8.

[34] Wang, Z., et al., Calmodulin antagonists induce platelet apoptosis. *Thromb. Res.*, 2010. 125(4): p. 340-50.

[35] Borras, C., et al., 17beta-oestradiol up-regulates longevity-related, antioxidant enzyme expression via the ERK1 and ERK2[MAPK]/NFkappaB cascade. *Aging Cell,* 2005. 4(3): p. 113-8.

[36] El-Beshbishy, H.A., et al., Amelioration of tamoxifen-induced liver injury in rats by grape seed extract, black seed extract and curcumin. *Indian J. Exp. Biol.*, 2010. 48(3): p. 280-8.

[37] Lee, M.H., et al., Gene expression profiling of murine hepatic steatosis induced by tamoxifen. *Toxicol Lett*, 2010. 199(3): p. 416-24.

[38] Shah, Y.M., Rowan, B.G. The Src kinase pathway promotes tamoxifen agonist action in Ishikawa endometrial cells through phosphorylation-dependent stabilization of estrogen receptor (alpha) promoter interaction and elevated steroid receptor co-activator 1 activity. *Mol. Endocrinol.,* 2005. 19(3): p. 732-48.

[39] Shao, C., et al., Estrogen enhanced cell-cell signaling in breast cancer cells exposed to targeted irradiation. *BMC Cancer*, 2008. 8: p. 184.

[40] Santen, R.J. Clinical review: Effect of endocrine therapies on bone in breast cancer patients. *J. Clin. Endocrinol. Metab.*, 2011. 96(2): p. 308-19.

[41] Henry, N.L., et al., Lack of association between estrogen receptor polymorphisms and change in bone mineral density with tamoxifen therapy. *Br. J. Cancer,* 2010. 102(2): p. 294-300.

[42] Tsai, K.S., Yang, R.S., Liu, S.H. Benzo[a]pyrene regulates osteoblast proliferation through an estrogen receptor-related cyclooxygenase-2 pathway. *Chem. Res. Toxicol.*, 2004. 17(5): p. 679-84.

[43] Ferrer-Lorente, R., et al., Tamoxifen does not prevent the mobilization of body lipids elicited by oleoyl-estrone. *Steroids,* 2004. 69(10): p. 661-5.

[44] Hutcheson, I.R., et al., Estrogen receptor-mediated modulation of the EGFR/MAPK pathway in tamoxifen-resistant MCF-7 cells. *Breast Cancer Res. Treat*, 2003. 81(1): p. 81-93.

[45] Dorssers, L.C., et al., Tamoxifen resistance in breast cancer: elucidating mechanisms. *Drugs,* 2001. 61(12): p. 1721-33.

[46] Tomlinson, D., Knowles,M.,, Speirs, V. Mechanisms of FGFR3 actions in endocrine resistant breast cancer. *Int. J. Cancer*, 2011.

[47] Hiscox, S., et al., Inhibition of focal adhesion kinase suppresses the adverse phenotype of endocrine-resistant breast cancer cells and improves endocrine response in endocrine-sensitive cells. *Breast Cancer Res. Treat,* 2011. 125(3): p. 659-69.

[48] Caiazza, F., et al., Cytosolic phospholipase A2-alpha expression in breast cancer is associated with EGFR expression and correlates with an adverse prognosis in luminal tumors. *Br. J. Cancer*, 2011. 104(2): p. 338-44.

[49] Watson, C., et al., High expression of sphingosine 1-phosphate receptors, S1P1 and S1P3, sphingosine kinase 1, and extracellular signal-regulated kinase-1/2 is associated with development of tamoxifen resistance in estrogen receptor-positive breast cancer patients. *Am. J. Pathol.*, 2010. 177(5): p. 2205-15.

[50] Chong, K., et al., Measuring IGF-1, ER-alpha and EGFR expression can predict tamoxifen-resistance in ER-positive breast cancer. *Anti-cancer Res.*, 2011. 31(1): p. 23-32.

[51] Ahnstrom, M., et al., Role of cyclin D1 in ErbB2-positive breast cancer and tamoxifen resistance. *Breast Cancer Res Treat,* 2005. 91(2): p. 145-51.

[52] Bates, N.P., Hurst, H.C. An intron 1 enhancer element mediates estrogen-induced suppression of ERBB2 expression. *Oncogene*, 1997. 15(4): p. 473-81.

[53] Martin, L.A., et al., The anti-estrogen ICI 182,780, but not tamoxifen, inhibits the growth of MCF-7 breast cancer cells refractory to long-term estrogen deprivation through down-regulation of estrogen receptor and IGF signaling. *Endocr. Relat. Cancer,* 2005. 12(4): p. 1017-36.

[54] Koutras, A.K., et al., The upgraded role of HER3 and HER4 receptors in breast cancer. *Crit. Rev. Oncol. Hematol.,* 2010. 74(2): p. 73-8.

[55] Godinho, M.F., et al., Relevance of BCAR4 in tamoxifen resistance and tumor aggressiveness of human breast cancer. *Br. J. Cancer*, 2010. 103(8): p. 1284-91.

[56] Svensson, S., et al., ERK phosphorylation is linked to VEGFR2 expression and Ets-2 phosphorylation in breast cancer and is associated with tamoxifen treatment resistance and small tumors with good prognosis. *Oncogene*, 2005. 24(27): p. 4370-9.

[57] Thomas, N.B., et al., Growth of hormone-dependent MCF-7 breast cancer cells is promoted by constitutive caveolin-1 whose expression is lost in an EGF-R-mediated manner during development of tamoxifen resistance. *Breast Cancer Res. Treat*, 2010. 119(3): p. 575-91.

[58] Nicholson, R.I., et al., Growth factor signaling and resistance to selective estrogen receptor modulators and pure anti-estrogens: the use of anti-growth factor therapies to treat or delay endocrine resistance in breast cancer. *Endocr. Relat. Cancer*, 2005. 12 Suppl 1: p. S29-36.

[59] Agrawal, A., et al., Overview of tyrosine kinase inhibitors in clinical breast cancer. *Endocr. Relat. Cancer,* 2005. 12 Suppl 1: p. S135-44.

[60] Gee, J.M., et al., Epidermal growth factor receptor/HER2/insulin-like growth factor receptor signaling and estrogen receptor activity in clinical breast cancer. *Endocr. Relat. Cancer*, 2005. 12 Suppl 1: p. S99-S111.

[61] Dowsett, M., et al., Growth factor signaling and response to endocrine therapy: the Royal Marsden Experience. *Endocr. Relat. Cancer,* 2005. 12 Suppl 1: p. S113-7.

[62] Jordan, N.J., et al., Increased constitutive activity of PKB/Akt in tamoxifen resistant breast cancer MCF-7 cells. *Breast Cancer Res. Treat*, 2004. 87(2): p. 167-80.

[63] Rayala, S.K., et al., P21-activated kinase 1 regulation of estrogen receptor-alpha activation involves serine 305 activation linked with serine 118 phosphorylation. *Cancer Res.*, 2006. 66(3): p. 1694-701.

[64] Wirtenberger, M., et al., The functional genetic variant Ile646Val located in the kinase binding domain of the A-kinase anchoring protein 10 is associated with familial breast cancer. *Carcinogenesis,* 2007. 28(2): p. 423-6.

[65] Tari, A.M., et al., Cyclooxygenase-2 protein reduces tamoxifen and N-(4-hydroxyphenyl)retinamide inhibitory effects in breast cancer cells. *Lab. Invest.,* 2005. 85(11): p. 1357-67.

[66] Cowell, L.N., et al., Tamoxifen treatment promotes phosphorylation of the adhesion molecules, p130Cas/BCAR1, FAK and Src, via an adhesion-dependent pathway. *Oncogene,* 2006. 25(58): p. 7597-607.

[67] Hiscox, S., et al., Elevated Src activity promotes cellular invasion and motility in tamoxifen-resistant breast cancer cells. *Breast Cancer Res. Treat,* 2006. 97(3): p. 263-74.

[68] Hiscox, S., et al., Src kinase promotes adhesion-independent activation of FAK and enhances cellular migration in tamoxifen-resistant breast cancer cells. *Clin. Exp. Metastasis.,* 2007. 24(3): p. 157-67.

[69] Hiscox, S., et al., Tamoxifen resistance in breast cancer cells is accompanied by an enhanced motile and invasive phenotype: inhibition by gefitinib ('Iressa', ZD1839). *Clin. Exp. Metastasis.*, 2004. 21(3): p. 201-12.

[70] Glaros, S., et al., Activation function-1 domain of estrogen receptor regulates the agonistic and antagonistic actions of tamoxifen. *Mol. Endocrinol.*, 2006. 20(5): p. 996-1008.

[71] Herrera, J.L., et al., Estradiol and tamoxifen differentially regulate a plasmalemmal voltage-dependent anion channel involved in amyloid-beta induced neurotoxicity. *Steroids,* 2011. 76(9): p. 840-4.

[72] Suuronen, T., et al., Anti-inflammatory effect of selective estrogen receptor modulators (SERMs) in microglial cells. *Inflamm. Res.*, 2005. 54(5): p. 194-203.

[73] Mitsukawa, K., X. Lu, and T. Bartfai, Galanin, galanin receptors and drug targets. *Cell Mol. Life Sci.*, 2008. 65(12): p. 1796-805.

[74] Hilke, S., et al., Estrogen induces a rapid increase in galanin levels in female rat hippocampal formation--possibly a non-genomic/indirect effect. *Eur. J. Neurosci.*, 2005. 21(8): p. 2089-99.

[75] Manji, H.K., Moore, G.J., Chen, G. Bipolar disorder: leads from the molecular and cellular mechanisms of action of mood stabilizers. *Br. J. Psychiatry,* 2001. 178(Suppl 41): p. S107-19.

[76] Zarate, C.A., Manji, H.K. Protein kinase C inhibitors: rationale for use and potential in the treatment of bipolar disorder. *CNS Drugs*, 2009. 23(7): p. 569-82.

[77] Trim, N., Holden-Dye, L.,. Walker, R.J. The inhibitory action of tamoxifen on the contraction of Ascaris suum somatic muscle in response to acetylcholine. *Parasitology,* 1999. 119 (Pt 6): p. 655-62.

[78] Younes, M., Honma, N. Estrogen receptor beta. *Arch. Pathol. Lab. Med.,* 2011. 135(1): p. 63-6.

[79] Badawy, A., Elnashar, A. Treatment options for polycystic ovary syndrome. *Int. J. Womens Health*, 2011. 3: p. 25-35.

[80] Kedia-Mokashi, N., et al., Chromosomal aberration in the post-implantation embryos sired by tamoxifen treated male rats. *Mutat. Res.*, 2010. 703(2): p. 169-73.

[81] Nobakht, M., Najafzadeh, N., Kordestani Shargh, B. Effects of tamoxifen on morphological and ultrastructural aspects of developing hippocampus of rat. *Iran Biomed. J.,* 2009. 13(4): p. 237-43.

[82] Seli, E., et al., Estradiol regulates monocyte chemotactic protein-1 in human coronary artery smooth muscle cells: a mechanism for its antiatherogenic effect. *Menopause*, 2001. 8(4): p. 296-301.

[83] Jaskelioff, M., et al., Telomerase reactivation reverses tissue degeneration in aged telomerase-deficient mice. *Nature,* 2011. 469(7328): p. 102-6.

[84] Hall, J.V., et al., The multifaceted role of estrogen in enhancing Chlamydia trachomatis infection in polarized human endometrial epithelial cells. *Cell Microbiol*, 2011. 13(8): p. 1183-99.

[85] Chumsri, S., et al., Aromatase, aromatase inhibitors, and breast cancer. *J. Steroid Biochem. Mol. Biol,* 2011. 125(1-2): p. 13-22.

[86] Henry, N.L., et al., Inflammatory cytokines and aromatase inhibitor-associated musculoskeletal syndrome: a case-control study. *Br. J. Cancer*, 2010. 103(3): p. 291-6.

[87] Miller, W.R., et al., Hormonal therapy for post-menopausal breast cancer: the science of sequencing. *Breast Cancer Res. Treat,* 2007. 103(2): p. 149-60.

[88] Mishra, R., et al., Glycine soya diet synergistically enhances the suppressive effect of tamoxifen and inhibits tamoxifen-promoted hepatocarcinogenesis in 7,12-dimethylbenz[alpha]anthracene-induced rat mammary tumor model. *Food Chem. Toxicol.*, 2011. 49(2): p. 434-40.

[89] Liu, B., et al., Low-dose dietary phytoestrogen abrogates tamoxifen-associated mammary tumor prevention. *Cancer Res.*, 2005. 65(3): p. 879-86.

[90] Albukhari, A.A., et al., Caffeic acid phenethyl ester protects against tamoxifen-induced hepatotoxicity in rats. *Food Chem. Toxicol.*, 2009. 47(7): p. 1689-95.

[91] Sacco, S.M., et al., Lignan-rich sesame seed negates the tumor-inhibitory effect of tamoxifen but maintains bone health in a post-menopausal athymic mouse model with estrogen-responsive breast tumors. *Menopause*, 2008. 15(1): p. 171-9.

[92] Chamras, H., et al., Novel interactions of vitamin E and estrogen in breast cancer. *Nutr. Cancer*, 2005. 52(1): p. 43-8.

[93] Yde, C.W., et al., The antipsychotic drug chlorpromazine enhances the cytotoxic effect of tamoxifen in tamoxifen-sensitive and tamoxifen-resistant human breast cancer cells. *Anticancer Drugs*, 2009. 20(8): p. 723-35.

[94] Hodges-Gallagher, L., et al., Inhibition of histone deacetylase enhances the anti-proliferative action of antiestrogens on breast cancer cells and blocks tamoxifen-induced proliferation of uterine cells. *Breast Cancer Res. Treat*, 2007. 105(3): p. 297-309.

[95] Bogush, T.A., et al., Estrogen receptors, antiestrogens, and non-small cell lung cancer. *Biochemistry* (Mosc), 2010. 75(12): p. 1421-7.

[96] Chatterjee, S.J., Pandey, S. Chemo-resistant melanoma sensitized by tamoxifen to low-dose curcumin treatment through induction of apoptosis and autophagy. *Cancer Biol. Ther.,* 2011. 11(2): p. 216-28.

[97] Lee, Y.S., Wurster, R.D. Dual effects of estrogen and anti-estrogens on the growth of SK-N-MC human neuroblastoma cells. *Cancer Lett*, 1994. 86(1): p. 119-25.

In: Tamoxifen Concepts and Cancer: New Paradigms
Editor: Ramon Andrade de Mello
ISBN: 978-1-62081-520-5

Chapter VIII

Tamoxifen: Biological Activities and Therapeutic Outcomes

Peter G. Bradford* and Atif B. Awad
State University of New York at Buffalo
Buffalo, NY, US

Abstract

Tamoxifen is the most widely used adjuvant endocrine therapy for breast cancer in pre- and postmenopausal women. Long-term studies have shown tamoxifen therapy to reduce the occurrence and reoccurrence of breast cancer and to prolong survival of patients with breast cancer and those predisposed to breast cancer. Early research with tamoxifen and other triphenylethylene compounds demonstrated their partial estrogenic activity but, perhaps more importantly, identified their antiestrogenic properties.

On the basis of this antiestrogenic activity, tamoxifen was approved in 1977 by the US Food and Drug Administration as adjuvant therapy in postmenopausal women with node positive breast cancer. Tamoxifen has also been approved to help reduce the risk for invasive breast cancer in women with ductal carcinoma *in situ* and to help reduce the incidence of breast cancer in women at high risk for such cancers. The demonstrated efficacy of tamoxifen in ER-positive breast cancers has led to the development and approval of aromatase inhibitor drugs, as well as to the conductance of large clinical trials comparing the two adjuvant hormonal therapies.

Clinical guidelines now recommend tamoxifen for premenopausal breast cancer patients and sequential aromatase inhibitor and tamoxifen therapies in postmenopausal patients especially those with high risk of recurrence. Long-term studies of tamoxifen have led to multiple discoveries: that to be optimally active tamoxifen must be metabolized to 4-hydroxytamoxifen and 4-hydroxy-N-desmethyltamoxifen (endoxifen) by cytochrome P450 systems, that CYP2D6 polymorphisms affect tamoxifen metabolism and may affect clinical outcomes, and that not all ER-positive breast cancer patients respond to tamoxifen.

* E-mail: pgb@buffalo.edu.

Tamoxifen, as a selective estrogen receptor modulator, has direct estrogenic activities in that it preserves bone mineral density and has favorable effects on serum lipids. However, concerns with the drug include the invariable acquired resistance, a small but significant risk of developing uterine cancer, and in patients who took the drug for at least five years, the increased risk of developing ER-negative and perhaps more difficult to treat contralateral breast cancers.

Tamoxifen continues to be studied in preclinical and clinical settings and further genetic marker studies may identify populations that benefit most from adjuvant tamoxifen treatment.

Historical Perspective

Tamoxifen is a nonsteroidal triphenylethylene antiestrogen that was developed following the initial studies with a similar compound, MER-25 (reviewed [1]). In studying the uterine stimulatory properties of estrogens in rodents, MER-25 was observed to completely inhibit the response to estradiol and the dose responsiveness of the effect of MER-25 established its competitive antagonism. Although MER-25 was antiestrogenic in every species tested, it was withdrawn from clinic development because of its relatively weak antiestrogenic activity, weak anti-gonadotropin activity, and CNS toxicity [2].

Tamoxifen became of subsequent interest because of its greater potency as well as its demonstrated antiestrogenic activity in the breast [1]. Pioneering studies gave promise that tamoxifen could cure animals of microscopic and palpable mammary tumors induced by the chemical carcinogens DMBA and N-methylnitrosourea [3]. These tumors were promoted by circulating estrogens and could be prevented by tamoxifen. The results demonstrated that tamoxifen inhibited the actions of estrogens at the level of the tumor and that this effect was fundamental to the antitumor effects of tamoxifen. The earliest clinical appraisal of tamoxifen, at that time ICI46474, showed certain potential [4]. In patients with recurrence of breast cancer or metastases of breast cancer and who were judged not suitable for further surgery or additional radiotherapy received 10 -20 mg ICI46474 for at least 3 months. The observed remission rate was 22% and, based upon the occurrence of hot flushes in responding patients, the basis of remission was deemed to be estrogen antagonism.

Tamoxifen was discovered to have estrogen-like effects in some tissues but to inhibit estrogen actions in other tissues, thus the term selective estrogen receptor modulator (SERM). Tamoxifen acts like estradiol in bone, maintaining bone density and reducing fractures in postmenopausal women [5]. Similarly, tamoxifen acts like estradiol in the uterus, stimulating proliferation of the endometrium in some patients and increasing the overall rate of fibroids, polyps, and endometrial carcinoma [6, 7]. Tamoxifen has estrogenic effects on blood coagulation, increasing the risks of thromboembolic events which are among the most serious complications associated with tamoxifen use.

As Factor V Leiden (FVL) is the most common genetic risk factor for venous thromboembolism (VTE), both large and small case control studies investigating FVL and women who experience VTE while on tamoxifen were conducted [8, 9].

Study outcomes showed that women on tamoxifen were five-to-twelve times more likely to carry FVL mutations compared to women receiving tamoxifen but who did not develop VTE. However, other retrospective studies of women on tamoxifen failed to show any relationship between the development of VTE and the presence of FVL [10].

Tamoxifen is antiestrogenic in breast and also seems to oppose the effects of estrogen in the pituitary, inhibiting the induction of the progesterone receptor by estradiol and increasing FSH secretion [11, 12]. Tamoxifen adjuvant therapy for breast cancer in premenopausal women dampens the normal negative feedback at the hypothalamus and pituitary, resulting in slightly increased FSH, stimulated ovarian steroidogenesis and elevated serum estradiol levels. These target site-specific actions of tamoxifen, both stimulatory and inhibitory, were of great potential and allowed it to be developed as a therapeutic agent to treat estrogen receptor (ER)-positive breast cancers.

Current Approvals

Medical Societal Recommendations

Tamoxifen has several approved indications (Table 1). Tamoxifenhas been approved by the U.S. Food and Drug Administration (FDA) initially in 1977 for use in treatment of patients with advanced breast cancer, in 1990 for node-negative breast cancer patients, and in 1998 as preventive therapy for breast cancer.

The long history of tamoxifen as being demonstrably safe and effective was considered by the American Society of Clinical Oncology (ASCO) when it published its clinical practice guidelines in 2002 and recommended a 5-year course of adjuvant tamoxifen as standard therapy for women with hormone receptor-positive breast cancer [13]. With the subsequent FDA approval in 2002 thru 2005 of three third-generation aromatase inhibitors for the treatment of early-stage breast cancer in postmenopausal women and with outcomes from several large scale comparative clinical trials of the two adjuvant therapies, updated ASCO guidelines have been published [14].

Table 1. U.S. Food and Drug Administration Approvals for Tamoxifen

Year of Approval	Indication
1977	Treatment of advanced breast cancer in postmenopausal women
1985	Adjuvant therapy in postmenopausal women with node positive breast cancer with chemotherapy
1986	Adjuvant therapy in postmenopausal women with node positive breast cancer alone
1989	Adjuvant therapy in premenopausal women with ER-positive advanced breast cancer
1990	Adjuvant therapy for pre- and postmenopausal women with node-negative ER-positive breast cancer
1998	Reduction of risk of breast cancer in high-risk pre- and postmenopausal women
2001	Adjuvant therapy of ductal carcinoma *in situ* after surgery and radiotherapy to reduce the incidence of invasive cancer
Based on references [108, 109].	

In 2010, the ASCO guidelines now recommend that postmenopausal women with hormone receptor positive breast cancer consider incorporating aromatase inhibitor therapy at some point during adjuvant treatment, either as upfront therapy or as sequential treatment after tamoxifen [14].

Tamoxifen is currently the only approved adjuvant endocrine therapy for premenopausal women with early stage hormone receptor-positive breast cancer. Adjuvant tamoxifen therapy is effective for these patients: systematic meta-analyses conducted by the Early Breast Cancer Trialists' Collaborative Group (EBCTCG) demonstrated that five years of tamoxifen adjuvant therapy for ER-positive disease reduced the recurrence rate by 41% and the annual breast cancer death rate by 31%, irrespective of age (<50, 50-59, or ≥ 70 years) [15, 16]. The current ASCO clinical practice guidelines include the recommendation that women who are pre- or perimenopausal at the time of breast cancer diagnosis be treated with 5 years of tamoxifen [14].

In 1998, at the recommendation of its Oncology Drugs Advisory Committee, the U.S. FDA approved tamoxifen as preventive therapy for breast cancer. The recommendation was based largely on the report of the National Surgical Adjuvant Breast and Bowel Project P-1 (NSABP-P1) which had an enrollment of 13,388 women at risk for breast cancer that showed tamoxifen reduced the overall occurrence of future invasive breast cancer by 49% [17]. Despite these and other consistent results showing tamoxifen to be an effective preventive therapy for breast cancer, its use by women for this indication has been less than might be expected, perhaps because of perceived concerns about side-effects or the poor ability to identify women at high risk [18, 19].

Adverse Effects, Precautions, and Side Effects

The known serious side effects of tamoxifen are blood clots, strokes, cataracts, and endometrial cancer. A comprehensive analysis of the four principal breast cancer prevention trials (Royal Marsden, NSABP-P1, Italian, and IBIS-I) showed that venous thromboembolic events were increased by tamoxifen in all studies with a relative risk of 1.9 (1.4-2.6) [20]. Subsequent data from the Breast Cancer Prevention Trial (BCPT) indicated a similar increase in blood clot frequency in women taking tamoxifen, particularly in women also on chemotherapy [21]. These same studies also identified an increased risk of endometrial cancers: a consensus relative risk of 2.4 (1.5-4.0) in the four principal breast cancer prevention trials and an increase from 1 to 2 cases per year per 1,000 women taking tamoxifen compared to placebo in the BCPT.

Results of a systematic literature review of adverse effects which included data from the Cochrane Central Register of Controlled Events, showed thatthe risk of adverse effects with tamoxifen therapy for women under 50 was lower than that for women on tamoxifen overall [22]. For women under 50, the relative risk for venous thrombosis while on tamoxifen was determined to be 2.30 (1.23-4.31) but decreased to 1.00 (0.38-2.67) in the follow-up phase, that is after stopping tamoxifen following five years of therapy. The same study identified the relative risk for endometrial cancer in women under 50 given tamoxifen to be 1.19 (0.53-2.65) and the relative risk for pulmonary embolism to be 1.16 (0.55-2.43) [22]. Tamoxifen therapy has been directly associated with noncancerous uterine effects including endometrial proliferation and thickening as assessed by ultrasonography as well as increased risks of polyps, leiomyoma, and irregular postmenopausal bleeding [23].

Common side effects of tamoxifen are similar to those experienced in menopause and include hot flashes, vaginal dryness and discharge, and fatigue. These effects are all consistent with the antagonism of estrogen actions. The occurrence of hot flashes in women receiving tamoxifen may be a good indicator of its pharmacological activation and its effectiveness [24].

Mechanism of Action

Selective Estrogen Receptor Modulator

Tamoxifen is classified as a selective estrogen receptor modulator (SERM) because it functions as an ER antagonist in some tissues but as an ER agonist in others. In the breast, tamoxifen acts at least initially like an ER antagonist, inhibiting the growth-stimulating activity of endogenous estrogens resulting in a highly significant reduction in breast cancer initiation and recurrence. However, in bone, tamoxifen has apparent ER agonistic effects more similar to estradiol, preserving or actually increasing bone mineral density in postmenopausal women who take the drug for as short a period as 2-5 years. In two controlled studies, therapy with 20 mg tamoxifen daily for 2 years increased the density of the lumbar spine by 0.6 – 0.7% per year [25, 26]. In the updated, 7-year follow-up of the large NSABP-P1, women who received tamoxifen for 5 years had significantly fewer fractures of the hip, spine, and radius compared to those receiving placebo [21]. Overall, in women over 50, the group in which most (89%) of the observed fractures occurred, tamoxifen reduced the incidence of fractures by 29%.

Tamoxifen and other SERMs are nonsteroidal, nonplanar triphenylethylene derivatives that bind with high affinity to ERs [27]. However, the mechanism by which tamoxifen and its more active metabolites selectively modulate ERs is not entirely understood. 4-Hydroxytamoxifen binds with high affinity and with approximately equal affinities to both ERα and ERβ [28]. The crystal structures of the ERα bound to estradiol or to 4-hydroxytamoxifen differ, suggesting that tamoxifen and its metabolites induce conformational changes in the ER distinct from those induced by endogenous estradiol [29]. These differences may account for the ability of the ER-tamoxifen complex to interact with select sets of coregulators and to function overall as a SERM.

The presence of tissue-specific coactivators and corepressors as well as differences in their relative expression within specific tissues along with the absolute concentrations of estradiol and tamoxifen will dictate the overall pharmacological outcomes of tamoxifen therapy in specific tissues. Even in the same tissue, for example the endometrium, the effects of tamoxifen have been observed to differ. In premenopausal women with high ambient estradiol levels, tamoxifen antagonizes the effects of ER activation; whereas, in postmenopausal women who have lower (<10%) endogenous estradiol levels, tamoxifen promotes ER activation and responses [30]. Endometrial gene-expression profiles from postmenopausal patients receiving tamoxifen or estradiol showed that tamoxifen-induced proliferation of endometrial tissue in postmenopausal women uses the same set of genes regulated by the ER agonist estradiol [31]. The latter observation may account for the observed 2- to 7-fold increase in the incidence of endometrial cancer in such a population.

SERMs, including tamoxifen, may therefore express an ER agonistic effect or an ER-antagonistic effect depending on the tissue targeted, on the ambient estradiol levels, and on the expression of other regulatory factors.

Production of Active Metabolites

Both basic research and clinical epidemiology suggest that the antiestrogenic and antiproliferative effects of tamoxifen in the breast are mediated by the tamoxifen metabolites 4-hydroxytamoxifen and 4-hydroxy-N-desmethyltamoxifen (endoxifen) (Figure 1).

Tamoxifen itself has only weak affinity for the ER, whereas 4-hydroxytamoxifen and endoxifen each have a hundred-fold higher affinities and are 30 – 100-fold more efficient in suppressing estrogenic responses including cell proliferation [32].

The metabolism of tamoxifen is complex as it involves the intestinal and hepatic cytochrome P450 drug-metabolizing enzyme systems, although the hepatic CYP3A4 and CYP2D6 mixed function oxidases are the predominant determinants [33]. Fundamental studies showed that the high first-pass metabolism of tamoxifen produced metabolites with increased ER binding affinities and more potent anti-estrogenic activity in vivo [34].

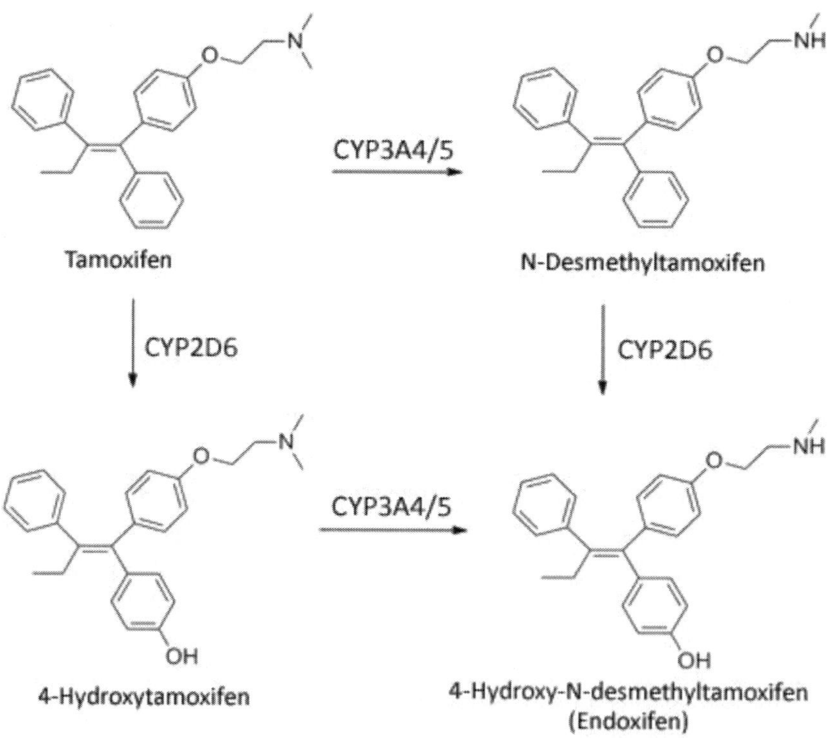

Figure 1. Metabolism of tamoxifen by cytochrome P450 enzymes. Phase I metabolism systems in the human liver convert tamoxifen primarily via CYP3A4 mixed function oxidase to N-desmethyltamoxifen and subsequently via CYP2D6 mixed function oxidase to 4-hydroxy-N-desmethyltamoxifen (endoxifen). As CYP2D6 is not inducible or regulated by known environmental agents, allelic variants of CYP2D6 largely determine the level of formation of the active metabolite endoxifen. Modified from [110].

Research revealed that endogenous metabolizing systems were promoting the conversion of tamoxifen as a prodrug to therapeutically active metabolites. Detailed studies identified these active metabolites as 4-hydroxytamoxifen and 4-hydroxy-N-desmethyltamoxifen (endoxifen) [35]. Endoxifen may be the more significant therapeutic metabolite as several studies have indicated higher circulating levels of endoxifen compared to 4-hydroxytamoxifen in patients receiving adjuvant tamoxifen therapy [36].

Potential Role of CYP2D6

Unlike other drug-metabolizing P450 enzymes, the CYP2D6 mixed function oxidase is not inducible and not regulated by many known environmental agents [37]. As such, variations in activity are largely attributable to genetic polymorphisms. There are over 100 allelic variants of the CYP2D6 gene, leading to differences in expressed CYP2D6 enzyme activity [38]. These phenotypic differences allow characterization of people into four basic metabolic classes: poor metabolizers (PM), intermediate metabolizers (IM), extensive metabolizers (EM), and ultrarapid metabolizers (UM) [39].

These patient genotypic characteristics may be significant to tamoxifen therapeutics. The basis of PM is the homozygous or compound heterozygous presence of *CYP2D6* null alleles. These null alleles of the *CYP2D6*gene encode nonfunctional proteins because of entire gene deletions, single base pair mutations, or small insertions/deletions that interrupt the correct reading frame or splice sites.

The most frequent null allele, *CYP2D6*4* (G1934-->A, splice site defect), occurs with estimated frequencies of 20-25% in Caucasians, 1-7% in Africans and African-Americans, and 0 - 1% in Oriental populations [33, 40]. These allelic frequencies are reflected in the measured occurrence of the PM phenotype: 9-10% Caucasian, 2-7% in African-Americans, and 0-1% in Chinese, Japanese, and Korean populations [37].

It is estimated that hepatic CYP2D6 metabolizes about one-quarter of currently used drugs including most antidepressants, class I antiarrhythmic drugs, antipsychotics, opioids, and anticancer drugs, and among them tamoxifen [37]. In one clinical study involving 1,370 women with early-stage breast cancer on tamoxifen endocrine therapy, the distribution of women in the PM, IM, EM, and UM phenotypes was determined to be 6%, 12%, 80%, and 2% [41].

Significantly, clinical studies suggest that women who have early stage breast cancer and who have null or reduced CYP2D6 activity have worse clinical outcomes when treated with tamoxifen, whereas women carrying two functional CYP2D6 alleles are associated with better clinical outcomes [42, 43]. Retrospective analyses with early stage breast cancer patients who had received 5 years adjuvant tamoxifen therapy indicated that at 9 year follow-up the recurrence rates were 14.9% for EM, 20.9% for heterozygous EM/IM, and 29% for PM [42]. Similarly, the predictive value of the CYP2D6*10 allele, which gives rise to CYP2D6 with significantly decreased enzymatic activity, was investigated in patients receiving adjuvant tamoxifen monotherapy [44].

Those homozygous for CYP2D6*10 alleles had significantly higher cancer recurrence within 10 years compared to those with wild-type CYP2D6*1 and the increased risk was proportional to the number of CYP2D6*10 alleles. Interestingly, the IM or EM patients had reduced tamoxifen compliance reportedly due to severe hot flushes as compared to PM patients, suggesting more efficient conversion to active antiestrogenic metabolites [45].

Overall, these observations are consistent with the hypothesis that CYP2D6 polymorphisms associated with reduced CYP2D6 enzymatic activity promote lower plasma endoxifen levels which manifest as adversely affecting tamoxifen efficacy. Significantly, those women with low capacity to convert tamoxifen to endoxifen are overrepresented among those women who have a high breast cancer recurrence rate [41]. A recent clinical study identified median baseline endoxifen concentrations in the EM, IM, and PM metabolizer groups as 34.3, 18.5, and 4.2 ng/mL [46].

As part of the study, when the IM or PM patients had their tamoxifen dose increased from 20 to 40mg, endoxifen levels in the IM group were no longer different from those of the EM patients; however, the PM endoxifen concentrations were still significantly lower than those in EM patients despite an average rise of 6.1 ng/mL [46].

Not all analyses support an influential role of variations in CYP2D6 activity in affecting breast cancer outcomes in patients receiving tamoxifen.A comprehensive review of ten epidemiologic studies investigating the association of CYP2D6 genotype and breast cancer recurrence rates reported heterogeneous results and determined relative risks outside of reasonable bounds [47].

A separate meta-analysis of published data also noted heterogeneity in outcomes although there was a non-significant trend toward improved disease-free survival for women with normal versus reduced CYP2D6 function [48].

This trend was also seen when comparing nonusers versus women who were using CYP2D6 inhibitor drugs such as SSRIs [48]. In one large case-controlled study involving over 11,000 women diagnosed with breast cancer between ages 35-69, there was only minimal association between reduced functioning CYP2D6 alleles (*4), use of CYP2D6 inhibitor drugs, and recurrence of cancer in tamoxifen-treated patients [49].

Significantly, in retrospective analyses of two large clinical trials, the Breast International Group BIG 1-98 trial and the Arimidex, Tamoxifen Alone or in Combination (ATAC) trail, no association was found between CYP2D6 genotype and control of breast cancer recurrence[50, 51].These analyses have been further extended through a straight forward model of ER ligand binding, using reported tamoxifen metabolite serum concentrations in CYP2D6 genotypic groups and calculated ER binding activities [47].

The model suggests that the serum concentrations of tamoxifen and of its metabolites under normal tamoxifen dosing should be sufficient to overwhelm the ER (>99% binding) and therefore all patients should have serum concentrations of tamoxifen and its metabolites sufficient to manifest full antitumorigenic effect regardless of genotype. Perhaps one limitation of this analysis is that plasma tamoxifen metabolite concentrations for the homozygous CYP2D6 *4/*4 PM group was based on measurements from few subjects [36].

In other analyses of retrospective clinical data, 10-of-14 studies reported poorer clinical outcomes for patients taking tamoxifen who were determined to be of the PM genotypes (CYP2D6*4,*5,*10,*41) [52].

Another study examined the potential correlation among breast cancer outcomes, measured serum endoxifen levels, and CYP2D6 metabolizer phenotype. [41]. This study, engaging 1,370 women with ER-positive breast cancer who were participating in the Women's Healthy Eating and Living (WHEL) study, identified a predictive concentration threshold for the active metabolite endoxifen.

Eighty percent of the women were identified by CYP2D6 allelic determination to be extensive metabolizers (EM) whereas 6% were identified as poor metabolizers (PM). The PM had approximately one-third the endoxifen levels as the EM and one-quarter the level as the ultrarapid (UM) metabolizers. The women in the lowest quintile of serum endoxifen levels had a 26% higher breast cancer recurrence rate compared to those women in the upper four quintiles. The identified associated predictors of this higher-risk, bottom quintile were poor and intermediate CYP2D6 metabolizer phenotype.

Tamoxifen Resistance

In advanced disease, only half of the patients with ER-positive primary tumors respond to tamoxifen. Often resistance is considered to be either intrinsic, in which ER-positive tumors intrinsically express enhanced growth factor pathways, or acquired, in which tumors initially responsive to tamoxifen become unresponsive or even stimulated by the antiestrogen [53].

Many tumor-associated mechanisms of tamoxifen resistance have been identified which can be considered as forms of acquired resistance and can be broadly classified into three categories: changes or deregulation in ER and its coregulators, alterations in expression of cell cycle signaling molecules (including MYC, cyclins E1 and D1), and enhancements in signaling of growth factor receptor pathways (including HER2 and EGFR) [54]. One identified example of dysregulated ER signaling is the observed activation of ER by tamoxifen through nongenomic means driven by hyperactivation of HER2 signaling [55].

Breast cancer antiestrogen resistance genes have been identified through in vitro functional screening with subsequent evaluation for relevance through mRNA expression screening of patients receiving tamoxifen as first-line therapy and determining association with tumor aggressiveness [56].

High tumor mRNA levels of *GRB7* and *ERBB2* were significantly associated with a short progression-free survival after first line tamoxifen treatment with ER-positive primary breast tumors. *GRB7* and *ERBB2* encode growth-promoting receptors or adaptor proteins.

Global gene expression analysis has been used to subcategorize breast tumors into risk groups and to help understand of the cancer biology associated with poor outcome on adjuvant tamoxifen therapy [57, 58].

Such a study using genome-wide mRNA expression and based on a limited number of primary tumors treated with tamoxifen that did not recur and along with tumors from patient that while on tamoxifen did progress identified the signaling gene product, Rho GDIα [59]. RhoGDIα is a negative regulator of the Rho family of GTP-binding proteins and had been identified to be associated with DNA-bound ERα in breast cancer cells and to regulate ER-driven gene transcription [60].

Tamoxifen-resistant tumors had lower levels of Rho GDIα gene expression compared with responsive tumors [59].

Of note, is that loss of Rho GDIα increased the growth rate of tumors while inhibiting ER expression and thus preventing tamoxifen from acting as an ER antagonist in breast tissue. Identifying the mechanisms of tamoxifen resistance will aid in the classification of breast cancer patients into different prognostic groups and identify individualized treatment approaches.

Tamoxifen Use in Preventive Therapy for Breast Cancer

Strategies have been identified to prevent breast cancer in high risk women. These strategies involve both lifestyle changes as well as medical therapies [19, 61, 62]. Lifestyle strategies that have been positively identified as reducing the risk of breast cancer include the adoption of low-fat diet, weight loss, exercise, and reduced alcohol intake [61, 63]. The one medical therapy currently approved by the U.S. Food and Drug Administration for preventive therapy of breast cancer is the use of the SERMs tamoxifen and raloxifene. Clinical prevention trials are currently underway using aromatase inhibitors to determine whether they also can be used successfully for the prevention of breast cancer. Of the SERMs, tamoxifen may be advantageous since it has greater efficacy than raloxifene and it can be used in premenopausal women.

Identifying Women at High Risk

Essential to using tamoxifen as breast cancer preventive medical therapy is to identify those women at high risk for breast cancer who would benefit most from treatment. Means of risk assessment to identify such women include an determination of family history such as prior precancerous breast biopsies, the existence of two or more first- or second-degree relatives with breast cancer, specific genetic testing, and evaluation of mammographic density [64].

Precancerous breast biopsies include proliferative lesions such as atypical ductal hyperplasia and atypical lobular hyperplasia, both of which raise the risk of subsequent cancer 4-5 fold [65]. Atypical hyperplasias are generally treated surgically but tamoxifen is often recommended as preventative therapy for these women. In such studies, tamoxifen as preventive therapy reduced the occurrence of breast cancer by 86% in women with a history of atypical hyperplasia [66].

The presence of an affected first-degree relative increases a woman's risk for breast cancer, a conclusion clearly supported by a large meta-analysis from 52 epidemiological studies [67].

The risk ratios for breast cancer increased with increasing numbers of affected first-degree relatives: compared with women who had no affected relatives, the risk ratios were 1:80 (99% CI, 1·69–1·91), 2:93 (2·36–3·64), and 3:90 (2·03–7·49), respectively, for one, two, and three or more affected first-degree relatives. It is clear, however, that although these women are at increased risk, most will never develop breast cancer and those that do will most likely be over age 50 when the cancer is first detected [67].

Genetic Predisposition

Five-to-ten percent of breast cancer cases are thought to be hereditary, resulting directly from gene mutations. Mutations in the high penetrance genes BRCA1 and BRCA2 were identified early through linkage studies in families with multiple cases of breast and ovarian cancers [68]. Genome-wide studies have more recently identified variants in other genes (includingTP53, PTEN, CHEK2, ATM, NBN) each with strong evidence of association with breast cancer, although these are all with more modest odds ratios compared to BRCA1 and BRCA2 and of only intermediate penetrance [69-71]. Post-randomization analyses show that tamoxifen was up to 50% effective in preventing breast cancer in these patients and, in patients already diagnosed with cancer, tamoxifen was associated with prevention of contralateral breast cancers, particularly in carriers of BRCA1 mutations [72].

Role of Breast Density

High mammographic density is a clear phenotypic marker of breast cancer. Large nested case-control studies and meta-analyses have shown extensive mammographic density to be strongly and reproducibly associated with increased risk of breast cancer [61, 73, 74]. Specific data show that women with density in 75% of the mammogram have a four-to-five fold increased risk of breast cancer. Of significance, tamoxifen therapy has been observed in numerous investigations to decrease breast density, this effect occurring primarily during the first 18 months of treatment [75, 76].

In a nested case-control study within the first International Breast Cancer Intervention Study (IBIS-1) and involving over a thousand women, baseline mammograms and mammograms that took place 12-18 months after treatment with tamoxifen were examined and quantified according to density [77, 78]. Forty-six percent of the women in the tamoxifen group were observed to have a reduction of breast density of 10% or more. Those women in the tamoxifen group experiencing a reduction in breast density of at least 10% had a 63% reduction in the risk of breast cancer, whereas women who took tamoxifen but experienced less than a 10% reduction in mammographic density had no risk reduction [77, 78]. The results suggest that changes in mammographic breast density might be a strong predictor of tamoxifen response. It is not certain whether those women who did not experience response to tamoxifen or a reduction in mammographic density were of the CYP2D6 genotypes that do not efficiently metabolize tamoxifen to more active products; thus, more closely associating the efficacy of tamoxifen with changes in breast density.

Despite the success in identifying several factors predisposing a woman to breast cancer, extensive review of risk assessment models show them currently to be of only moderate discriminatory accuracy [62]. Their limitations are cited to be their reliance on known risk factors and advances are predicted to come from more refined information on genotypes and better understanding of the mechanisms of gene regulation in cancer types [79].

Breast Cancer Preventive Clinical Trials

Clinical trial data clearly show that tamoxifen therapy is associated with breast cancer prevention. This effect is most definitive in preventing ER-positive breast cancers. Data on tamoxifen therapy from four large breast cancer preventive clinical trials with long-term follow-up are available (Table 2).

Table 2. Tamoxifen Breast Cancer Prevention Trials: Relative Risk for Primary ER-Positive Tumors

Randomized Trial	Patient Enrollment	Follow-Up (Years)*	Relative Risk ER-Positive Tumors
Royal Marsden	2471	13.2	0.61 (0.43-0.86)
NSABP P-1	13388	7.0	0.38 (0.28-0.50)
Italian Prevention	5408	11.0	0.77 (0.51-1.16)
IBIS-I	7139	8.0	0.66 (0.50-0.87)

NSABP P-1, National Surgical Breast and Bowel Project; IBIS-I, International Breast Cancer Intervention Study-I; *median follow-up; relative risk and 95% confidence interval are shown; data from [19].

The first study, the National Surgical Adjuvant Breast and Bowel Project (NSABP P-1) Breast Cancer Prevention Trial began in 1992 enrolling more than 13,000 women aged 35 and older who were at high risk for developing breast cancer. Initial results from NSABP P-1 showed that women taking tamoxifen had an overall 49% reduction in developing breast cancer when tamoxifen was taken for 5-years [17].

In the follow-up study, the NSABP protocol P-2, the Study of Tamoxifen and Raloxifene (STAR), both drugs were shown to be similar in reducing the risk of invasive breast cancer in postmenopausal women at high risk; however, tamoxifen seemed more effective in preventing noninvasive disease [80]. Updated, more recent analysis of the STAR trial with median follow-up of 81-months showed that tamoxifen had increased efficacy relative to raloxifene with longer term benefits in preventing invasive disease [81].

The second trial, the International Breast Cancer Intervention Study (IBIS-I) which enrolled over 7,000 women aged 35 to 70 showed that after 4 years, women on tamoxifen therapy had a 32% reduction in the incidence of breast cancer compared to placebo [82]. Importantly again, long-term observation with median follow-up of 96 months showed that the relative risk for breast cancer was 0.73 for women taking tamoxifen. Moreover, this preventive effect was constant in the entire follow-up period,after tamoxifen therapy had ceased, without diminution of benefit for up to 10 years [82].

The Royal Marsden Hospital Tamoxifen Trial is a third significant study. The Royal Marsden trial included more than 2,500 women and has data from extensive follow-up [83, 84]. Despite a null effect of tamoxifen in the early years, significant breast cancer risk reduction was observed after the 8-year treatment period; and after median follow-up of 13years, the incidence of ER-positive invasive cancer in the tamoxifen arm was reduced by 39%.

Finally, in the Italian Tamoxifen Prevention Study, which enrolled women with hysterectomy, the rates of breast cancer were no different among the groups. However, the calculated rates were much lower (relative risk 0.24) in the tamoxifen group for women who were stratified to be at high risk of developing breast cancer [85].

In summary, overall data from these four large preventive clinical trials showed a 43% reduction in ER-positive invasive breast cancer but no effect on ER-negative cancers [19]. Each of the four trials included tamoxifen therapy for five years. As these are all long-term studies with extended observation after the tamoxifen period, a significant finding to arise is that in years 6-10 and beyond, after tamoxifen therapy had ceased and when adverse effect profiles were minimal, the incidence of breast cancer was reduced an additional 38% in women who took tamoxifen [19]. These studies identify an apparent durable preventative effect of tamoxifen on ER-positive breast cancer extending beyond the period of treatment. Based upon these analyses and a broader systematic review of MEDLINE and Cochrane databases, the American Society of Clinical Oncology made the recommendation that for women at increased risk for breast cancer tamoxifen (20 mg/d for 5 years) be offered to reduce the risk of invasive ER-positive breast cancer, with benefits for at least 10 years [86].

Tamoxifen Use as Adjuvant Therapy for Breast Cancer

Use in Breast Cancers Diagnosed in Pre- and Perimenopausal Women

Approximately 12% of women diagnosed with breast cancer are diagnosed under the age of 45 and about 25% of women receiving such a diagnosis do so before menopause [87-89]. Optimal adjuvant therapy includes chemotherapy, ovarian suppression, and tamoxifen. Aromatase inhibitors are not recommended in the absence of direct ovarian suppression. Thus, in premenopausal patients tamoxifen alone (20 mg/daily for 5 years) or the combination of ovarian function ablation and tamoxifen are standard therapies [14, 87]. Through comprehensive meta-analysis of the Early Breast Cancer Trialists' Collaborative Group (EBCTCG), allocation to adjuvant tamoxifen therapy was associated with a 41% reduction in breast cancer recurrence and a 34% reduction in mortality in premenopausal women with ER-positive cancers [15]. Significantly, the risk reductions produced by tamoxifen were little affected by age, with the risk reductions for women younger than 40 similar to those for women who were older. These beneficial effects of tamoxifen for premenopausal women were shown to be remarkably persistent for 15-years despite receiving active therapy for only 5-years, with an absolute gain through treatment generally twice as great observed at 15-years compared to 5-years [15].

Outcomes from the randomized placebo control study of tamoxifen following chemotherapy in premenopausal women with early breast cancer conducted by the NCI of Canada showed that tamoxifen improved 5-year disease free survival, although with only non-significant improvement in overall survival [90]. The study included 672 women and detailed comparative data on compliance showed that nearly one-third of the women stopped medication prematurely, most of those stopped within 24 months.

Adjuvant chemotherapy has indirect benefit in ER-positive breast cancers in premenopausal women through induction of partial or complete ovarian suppression [91]. However, chemotherapy-induced amenorrhea may be only temporary and when menopausal status is uncertain the current recommendation is that endocrine adjuvant therapy should be with tamoxifen rather than an aromatase inhibitor. Long-term efficacy of the addition of zoledronic acid to adjuvant endocrine therapy in premenopausal women has been demonstrated in a 62-month follow-up from the ABCSG-12 randomized trial [92]. In the course of this study, which included direct ovarian suppression, disease-free survival was unchanged but overall survival was better for women treated with tamoxifen compared to women treated with the aromatase inhibitor anastrazole [92].

Use in Breast Cancers Diagnosed in Postmenopausal Women

Tamoxifen has been the standard adjuvant hormonal therapy for many years for postmenopausal women diagnosed with breast cancer. The overview of randomized trails reported by the EBCTCG showed a reduction in the reoccurrence of breast cancer of 40% and in death by 26% after five years tamoxifen therapy [15]. With the introduction of aromatase inhibitors, many comparative studies have shown superior efficacy with lower recurrence rates of breast cancer in women treated with the one of the aromatase inhibitors anastrazole, exemestane, or letrozole versus tamoxifen (Table 3) [93-96]. Comprehensive meta-analysis of all trials of aromatase inhibitors versus tamoxifen indicated their superiority to tamoxifen when the outcome was disease-free survival [97]. However, the studies did not show an advantage in terms of improvement in overall survival.

Trials Comparing Tamoxifen and Aromatase Inhibitors in Early Breast Cancer

The ATAC trial is one of the principal comparative studies of 5-year treatment of early-stage breast cancer with aromatase inhibitors versus tamoxifen. The most recent analysis of long-term outcomes after median follow-up of 120-month reflects 24,522 women-years of follow-up for the anastrozole group and 23,950 women-years in the tamoxifen group [98]. For hormone-receptor-positive patients, the recent results significantly favor the anastrozole group in terms of disease-free survival (0.86, 0.78-0.95), time to recurrence (0.79, 0.70-0.89), and time to distant recurrence (0.85, 0.73-0.98)[98]. However, there was little difference in overall mortality (0.95, 0.84-1.0-6) and there was a significant increase in bone fractures during active period of treatment with anastrozole (1.33, 1.15-1.55).

Despite the long-term follow-up and relatively recent reporting of the 10-year analysis, there has been published controversy regarding the interpretation of these results [99, 100].

Citing evidence that anastrozole failed to show improvement in overall survival and that tamoxifen may be a safer drug, some published opinions state that tamoxifen should still be the preferred drug for most postmenopausal women with hormone-receptor positive breast cancer [99].

The Breast International Group BIG 1-98 trail is a randomized, double-blinded trial involving postmenopausal women with hormone-receptor-positive early breast cancer. In the study, disease-free survival is compared in women receiving 5-year monotherapies with either tamoxifen or the aromatase inhibitor letrozole. Also included in the study are women receiving sequential therapies of tamoxifen for 2 years followed by letrozole for 3 years or letrozole for 2 years followed by tamoxifen for 3 years. At median follow-up of 51-months, letrozole monotherapy had longer disease-free survival compared to tamoxifen monotherapy (0.83, 0.71-0.96) [101]. Patients on tamoxifen experienced more thromboembolic events, endometrial pathology, hot flashes, night sweats, and vaginal bleeding.

Table 3. Studies Comparing Tamoxifen and Aromatase Inhibitors as Adjuvant Therapy for Postmenopausal Women with Breast Cancer

Randomized Trial	Treatments	Patient Number	Disease-Free Survival Events (%)		HR	95% CI	*P*
Primary Adjuvant							
ATAC	ANA x TAM	6,241	26.1	28.5	0.90	0.82 - 0.99	.025
BIG 1-98	LET x TAM	4,922	20.7	23.0	0.88	0.78 - 0.99	.03
ABCSG-12	ANA x TAM	1,803	8.0	7.2	1.10	0.78 - 1.53	.59
Sequential Therapy							
BIG 1-98	TAM/LET x LET	3,094	16.7	16.0	1.05	0.84 - 1.32	--
BIG 1-98	LET/TAM x LET	3,086	15.3	16.0	0.96	0.76 - 1.21	--
ABCSG-8	TAM/ANA x TAM	3,714	12.2	14.1	0.85	0.71 - 1.01	.067
TEAM	TAM/EXE x EXE	9,766	14.5	14.7	0.97	0.88 - 1.08	.604
ARNO	TAM x TAM/ANA	979	11.4	7.8	0.66	0.44 - 1.00	.049

ATAC, Arimidex, Tamoxifen, Alone or in Combination trial; BIG, Breast International Group; ABCSG, Austrian Breast and Colorectal Cancer Study Group; TEAM, Tamoxifen Exemestane Adjuvant Multinational trial; ARNO, Arimidex-Nolvadex trial; HR, hazard ratio; data from [14] ASCO Clinical Practice Guideline.

Patients on letrozole experienced more bone fractures, arthralgia, hypercholesterolemia, cardiovascular events, and cardiac failure [101]. Neither sequential treatment improved disease-free survival as compared to letrozole monotherapy and after initial analysis, there was no significant difference between letrozole monotherapy and tamoxifen monotherapy with respect to overall survival[94]. Despite the initial analysis showing that letrozole therapy did not provide a significant overall survival advantage compared to tamoxifen, more recent analysis adjusting for selective crossover effects did reveal a significant survival advantage with letrozole [94, 102].

The Tamoxifen Exemestane Adjuvant Multinational (TEAM) phase 3 trial is a third important large randomized trial comparing tamoxifen with an aromatase inhibitor in the treatment of postmenopausal women with early breast cancer [95]. The TEAM trial compared 5 years of treatment with the aromatase inhibitor exemestane with sequential strategy of tamoxifen for 2.5 years followed by exemestane for 2.5 years. At median follow-up of 5.1 years, there was no difference between therapy arms in terms of disease-free survival or overall survival. Review of the outcomes showed serious adverse effects to be rare, although the exemestane-alone arm was associated with increased joint disorders, bone fractures, and diagnoses of osteoporosis, as well as hypertension and cardiac failure [95, 103].

A recent meta-analysis designed to examine the toxicities of tamoxifen and aromatase inhibitors identified seven trials with 30,023 patients that met inclusion criteria [104]. Longer duration of aromatase inhibitor therapy was associated with increased risk of bone fractures (1.47, 1.34-1.61), and cardiovascular disease (1.26, 1.10 – 1.43) but lower risks for uterine cancer (0.34, 0.22 – 0.53) and blood clots (0.55, 0.46 – 0.64) [104].

Although these large clinical trials have shown adjuvant aromatase inhibitor therapy to be consistently more beneficial to tamoxifen in terms of disease-free survival, debate continues as to whether tamoxifen should continue to be the preferred therapy particularly for women with node-negative disease [105]. Overall survival advantage with aromatase inhibitor therapy has not been consistently demonstrated. It has been suggested that the statistical impact of CYP2D6 poor metabolizers in studies may have created the small but significant advantage in clinical trials of aromatase inhibitors versus tamoxifen in disease-free survival of postmenopausal women with early, hormone receptor-positive breast cancer [33].

Based on current evidence it has been suggested that women at high risk of recurrence, especially those with node-positive disease, should receive an aromatase inhibitor as part of their treatment but routine prescription of such drugs to postmenopausal patients with low-risk disease may not appropriate [106]. Moreover, some clinicians have questioned whether the toxicity of adjuvant aromatase inhibitor therapy has not been underestimated and they have noted that there is a demonstrated overall poorer tolerance of women for aromatase inhibitors versus tamoxifen [106, 107]. The difference in financial costs of tamoxifen and aromatase inhibitor therapies is also a factor. Without clear meaningful overall survival advantage or improvements in the quality of life, are more expensive medicines justified [33, 105]

Conclusion

Tamoxifen has been approved for the treatment of breast cancer for over 35 years. Many women have taken tamoxifen and as a result of carefully conducted clinical trials both as a preventative medicine and as a cancer therapeutic agent, extensive data exist on its effectiveness. The adverse effects of tamoxifen are also well known and are generally mild but in rare instances may be more severe. The balance of risk versus benefit should be an individual decision. With advancing knowledge about drug metabolism and breast tumor biology, those women who would benefit most from tamoxifen therapy can be determined. For these women, the benefit tamoxifen therapy is that it can reduce the risk of breast cancer recurrence and breast cancer related death and provide a high health-related quality of life.

The positive effects of 5 years of tamoxifen therapy are long-term with effects on diminishing cancer recurrence continuing for up to 10 years and on reducing the incidence of breast cancer death extending beyond 10 years. Despite tamoxifen being an old drug, these data have prompted the American Society of Clinical Oncology in its clinical practice guidelines to recommend that most postmenopausal women receive an aromatase inhibitor regimen either as sole therapy or after 2 to 3 years of tamoxifen [14].

References

[1] MacGregor, J.I. and V.C. Jordan, Basic guide to the mechanisms of antiestrogen action. *Pharmacol. Rev.,* 1998. 50(2): p. 151-96.

[2] Lerner, L.J. and V.C. Jordan, Development of antiestrogens and their use in breast cancer: eighth Cain memorial award lecture. *Cancer Res.*, 1990. 50(14): p. 4177-89.

[3] Jordan, V.C., Antiestrogenic and antitumor properties of tamoxifen in laboratory animals. *Cancer Treatment Reports*, 1976. 60: p. 1409-1419.

[4] Cole, M.P., C.T. Jones, and I.D. Todd, A new anti-oestrogenic agent in late breast cancer. An early clinical appraisal of ICI46474. *Br. J. Cancer*, 1971. 25(2): p. 270-5.

[5] Santen, R.J., Clinical review: Effect of endocrine therapies on bone in breast cancer patients. *J. Clin. Endocrinol. Metab.*, 2011. 96(2): p. 308-19.

[6] Assikis, V.J. and V.C. Jordan, Gynecologic effects of tamoxifen and the association with endometrial carcinoma. *Int. J. Gynaecol. Obstet.*, 1995. 49(3): p. 241-57.

[7] Ali, S., L. Buluwela, and R.C. Coombes, Antiestrogens and their therapeutic applications in breast cancer and other diseases. *Annu. Rev. Med.*, 2011. 62: p. 217-32.

[8] Garber, J.E., et al., Factor V Leiden mutation and thromboembolism risk in women receiving adjuvant tamoxifen for breast cancer. *J. Natl. Cancer Inst*, 2010. 102(13): p. 942-9.

[9] Eroglu, A. and N. Akar, Factor V Leiden, prothrombin G20210A and methylenetetrahydrofolate reductase (MTHFR) C677T polymorphisms and the risk of tamoxifen-associated thromboembolism in breast cancer patients. *Thromb. Res.*, 2011. 127(4): p. 384-5.

[10] Cuzick, J., Tamoxifen and the factor V Leiden mutation. *J. Natl. Cancer Inst*, 2010. 102(13): p. 918-9.

[11] Bellido, C., et al., Tamoxifen induces gonadotropin-releasing hormone self-priming through an estrogen-dependent progesterone receptor expression in the gonadotrope of the rat. *Neuroendocrinology*, 2003. 77(6): p. 425-35.

[12] Gjerde, J., et al., Associations between tamoxifen, estrogens, and FSH serum levels during steady state tamoxifen treatment of postmenopausal women with breast cancer. *BMC Cancer,* 2010. 10: p. 313.

[13] Winer, E.P., et al., American Society of Clinical Oncology technology assessment on the use of aromatase inhibitors as adjuvant therapy for women with hormone receptor-positive breast cancer: status report 2002. *J. Clin. Oncol.*, 2002. 20(15): p. 3317-27.

[14] Burstein, H.J., et al., American Society of Clinical Oncology clinical practice guideline: update on adjuvant endocrine therapy for women with hormone receptor-positive breast cancer. *J. Clin. Oncol.*, 2010. 28(23): p. 3784-96.

[15] Effects of chemotherapy and hormonal therapy for early breast cancer on recurrence and 15-year survival: an overview of the randomised trials. *Lancet,* 2005. 365(9472): p. 1687-717.

[16] Pritchard, K.I. Adjuvant endocrine therapy for premenopausal women with early stage breast cancer. 2011 [cited 2011 August 5]; Available from: http://www.uptodate.com/contents/adjuvant-endocrine-therapy-for-premenopausal-women-with-early-stage-breast-cancer.

[17] Fisher, B., et al., Tamoxifen for prevention of breast cancer: report of the National Surgical Adjuvant Breast and Bowel Project P-1 Study. *J. Natl. Cancer Inst.*, 1998. 90(18): p. 1371-88.

[18] Waters, E.A., et al., Prevalence of tamoxifen use for breast cancer chemoprevention among U.S. women. *Cancer Epidemiol. Biomarkers Prev*, 2010. 19(2): p. 443-6.

[19] Cuzick, J., et al., Preventive therapy for breast cancer: a consensus statement. *Lancet Oncol.*, 2011. 12(5): p. 496-503.

[20] Cuzick, J., et al., Overview of the main outcomes in breast-cancer prevention trials. *Lancet,* 2003. 361(9354): p. 296-300.

[21] Fisher, B., et al., Tamoxifen for the prevention of breast cancer: current status of the National Surgical Adjuvant Breast and Bowel Project P-1 study. *J. Natl. Cancer Inst.*, 2005. 97(22): p. 1652-62.

[22] Iqbal, J., et al., Endometrial cancer and venous thromboembolism in women under age 50 who take tamoxifen for prevention of breast cancer: A systematic review. *Cancer Treat Rev.,* 2011.

[23] Haskell, S.G., Selective estrogen receptor modulators. *South Med. J., 2003. 96(5): p. 469-76.*

[24] Bevers, T.B., et al., Breast cancer risk reduction. *J. Natl. Compr. Canc.* Netw., 2010. 8(10): p. 1112-46.

[25] Love, R.R., et al., Effects of tamoxifen on bone mineral density in postmenopausal women with breast cancer. *N. Engl. J. Med.*, 1992. 326(13): p. 852-6.

[26] Gray, S., Breast cancer. Role of the research nurse. *Nurs. Times*, 1995. 91(5): p. 33-5.

[27] Maximov, P.Y., et al., Structure-function relationships of estrogenic triphenylethylenes related to endoxifen and 4-hydroxytamoxifen. *J. Med. Chem.*, 2010. 53(8): p. 3273-83.

[28] Kuiper, G.G., et al., Comparison of the ligand binding specificity and transcript tissue distribution of estrogen receptors alpha and beta. *Endocrinology*, 1997. 138(3): p. 863-70.

[29] Wu, Y.-L., et al., Structural Basis for an Unexpected Mode of SERM-Mediated ER Antagonism. *Molecular Cell*, 2005. 18(4): p. 413-424.

[30] Mourits, M.J., et al., Tamoxifen treatment and gynecologic side effects: a review. *Obstet. Gynecol,* 2001. 97(5 Pt 2): p. 855-66.

[31] Gielen, S.C.J.P., et al., Signaling by estrogens and tamoxifen in the human endometrium. *The Journal of Steroid Biochemistry and Molecular Biology*, 2008. 109(3-5): p. 219-223.

[32] Lim, Y.C., et al., Endoxifen, a secondary metabolite of tamoxifen, and 4-OH-tamoxifen induce similar changes in global gene expression patterns in MCF-7 breast cancer cells. *J. Pharmacol. Exp. Ther.*, 2006. 318(2): p. 503-12.

[33] Jordan, V.C., New insights into the metabolism of tamoxifen and its role in the treatment and prevention of breast cancer. *Steroids*, 2007. 72(13): p. 829-42.

[34] Jordan, V.C., Metabolites of tamoxifen in animals and man: identification, pharmacology, and significance. *Breast Cancer Res. Treat*, 1982. 2(2): p. 123-38.

[35] Desta, Z., et al., Comprehensive evaluation of tamoxifen sequential biotransformation by the human cytochrome P450 system in vitro: prominent roles for CYP3A and CYP2D6. *J. Pharmacol. Exp. Ther.*, 2004. 310(3): p. 1062-75.

[36] Jin, Y., et al., CYP2D6 genotype, antidepressant use, and tamoxifen metabolism during adjuvant breast cancer treatment. *J. Natl. Cancer* Inst., 2005. 97(1): p. 30-9.

[37] Zhou, S.F., Polymorphism of human cytochrome P450 2D6 and its clinical significance: part II. *Clin Pharmacokinet,* 2009. 48(12): p. 761-804.

[38] CYP2D6 allele nomenclature. 2011; Available from: http://www.cypalleles.ki.se/cyp2d6.htm.

[39] Zanger, U.M., S. Raimundo, and M. Eichelbaum, Cytochrome P450 2D6: overview and update on pharmacology, genetics, biochemistry. Naunyn Schmiedebergs *Arch. Pharmacol.*, 2004. 369(1): p. 23-37.

[40] Bradford, L.D., CYP2D6 allele frequency in European Caucasians, Asians, Africans and their descendants. *Pharmacogenomics*, 2002. 3(2): p. 229-43.

[41] Madlensky, L., et al., Tamoxifen metabolite concentrations, CYP2D6 genotype, and breast cancer outcomes. *Clin. Pharmacol. Ther.*, 2011. 89(5): p. 718-25.

[42] Schroth, W., et al., Association between CYP2D6 polymorphisms and outcomes among women with early stage breast cancer treated with tamoxifen. *JAMA,* 2009. 302(13): p. 1429-36.

[43] Higgins, M.J. and V. Stearns, Pharmacogenetics of endocrine therapy for breast cancer. *Annu. Rev. Med.,* 2011. 62: p. 281-93.

[44] Kiyotani, K., et al., Impact of CYP2D6*10 on recurrence-free survival in breast cancer patients receiving adjuvant tamoxifen therapy. *Cancer Sci.*, 2008. 99(5): p. 995-9.

[45] Rae, J.M., et al., Cytochrome P450 2D6 activity predicts discontinuation of tamoxifen therapy in breast cancer patients. *Pharmacogenomics J.,* 2009. 9(4): p. 258-64.

[46] Irvin, W.J., et al., Genotype-Guided Tamoxifen Dosing Increases Active Metabolite Exposure in Women With Reduced CYP2D6 Metabolism: A Multicenter Study. *Journal of Clinical Oncology*, 2011.

[47] Lash, T.L., et al., Genotype-guided tamoxifen therapy: time to pause for reflection? *Lancet Oncol.,* 2009. 10(8): p. 825-33.

[48] Seruga, B. and E. Amir, Cytochrome P450 2D6 and outcomes of adjuvant tamoxifen therapy: results of a meta-analysis. *Breast Cancer Res. Treat,* 2010. 122(3): p. 609-17.

[49] Lash, T.L., et al., CYP2D6 inhibition and breast cancer recurrence in a population-based study in Denmark. *J. Natl. Cancer Inst.,* 2011. 103(6): p. 489-500.

[50] Rae JM, D.S., Hayes DF, et al, Lack of correlation between gene variants in tamoxifen metabolizing enzymes with primary endpoints in the ATAC trial., in Program and abstracts of the 33rd *Annual San Antonio Breast Cancer Symposium.* 2010.

[51] Leyland-Jones B, R.M., Bouzyk M, et al., Outcome according to CYP2D6 genotype among postmenopausal women with endocrine-responsive early invasive breast cancer randomized in the BIG 1-98 trial. Program and abstracts of the 33rd *Annual San Antonio Breast Cancer Symposium*, 2010. Abstract S1-8.

[52] Singh, M.S., P.A. Francis, and M. Michael, Tamoxifen, cytochrome P450 genes and breast cancer clinical outcomes. *The Breast*, 2011. 20(2): p. 111-118.

[53] Orlando, L., et al., Molecularly targeted endocrine therapies for breast cancer. *Cancer Treatment Reviews*, 2010. 36(Supplement 3): p. S67-S71.

[54] Osborne, C.K. and R. Schiff, Mechanisms of Endocrine Resistance in Breast Cancer. *Annual Review of Medicine,* 2011. 62(1): p. 233-247.

[55] Shou, J., et al., Mechanisms of Tamoxifen Resistance: Increased Estrogen Receptor-HER2/neu Cross-Talk in ER/HER2–Positive Breast Cancer. *Journal of the National Cancer Institute*, 2004. 96(12): p. 926-935.

[56] van Agthoven, T., et al., Relevance of Breast Cancer Antiestrogen Resistance Genes in Human Breast Cancer Progression and Tamoxifen Resistance. *Journal of Clinical Oncology*, 2009. 27(4): p. 542-549.

[57] Van Tine, B.A. and M.J. Ellis, Understanding the Estrogen Receptor–Positive Breast Cancer Genome: Not Even the End of the Beginning. *Journal of the National Cancer Institute*, 2011. 103(7): p. 526-527.

[58] van 't Veer, L.J., et al., Gene expression profiling predicts clinical outcome of breast cancer. *Nature*, 2002. 415(6871): p. 530-536.

[59] Barone, I., et al., Loss of Rho GDIα and Resistance to Tamoxifen via Effects on Estrogen Receptor α. *Journal of the National Cancer Institute*, 2011. 103(7): p. 538-552.

[60] El Marzouk, S., et al., Rho GDP dissociation inhibitor α interacts with estrogen receptor α and influences estrogen responsiveness. *Journal of Molecular Endocrinology*, 2007. 39(4): p. 249-259.
[61] Cummings, S.R., et al., Prevention of breast cancer in postmenopausal women: approaches to estimating and reducing risk. *J. Natl. Cancer Inst.*, 2009. 101(6): p. 384-98.
[62] Amir, E., et al., Assessing women at high risk of breast cancer: a review of risk assessment models. *J. Natl. Cancer Inst.*, 2010. 102(10): p. 680-91.
[63] Tirona, M.T., R. Sehgal, and O. Ballester, Prevention of breast cancer (Part II): risk reduction strategies. *Cancer Invest.,* 2010. 28(10): p. 1070-7.
[64] Afonso, N., Women at high risk for breast cancer--what the primary care provider needs to know. *J. Am. Board Fam. Med.,* 2009. 22(1): p. 43-50.
[65] Arpino, G., R. Laucirica, and R.M. Elledge, Premalignant and in situ breast disease: biology and clinical implications. *Annals Of Internal Medicine*, 2005. 143(6): p. 446-457.
[66] Venkitaraman, R., Lobular Neoplasia of the Breast. *The Breast Journal*, 2010. 16(5): p. 519-528.
[67] Familial breast cancer: collaborative reanalysis of individual data from 52 epidemiological studies including 58[punctuation space]209 women with breast cancer and 101[punctuation space]986 women without the disease. *The Lancet,* 2001. 358(9291): p. 1389-1399.
[68] Nathanson, K.L. and S.M. Domchek, Therapeutic approaches for women predisposed to breast cancer. *Annu. Rev. Med.*, 2011. 62: p. 295-306.
[69] Turnbull, C. and N. Rahman, Genetic predisposition to breast cancer: past, present, and future. *Annu. Rev. Genomics. Hum. Genet.,* 2008. 9: p. 321-45.
[70] Narod, S.A., Genetic variants associated with breast-cancer risk. *Lancet Oncol.,* 2011. 12(5): p. 415-6.
[71] Zhang, B., et al., Genetic variants associated with breast-cancer risk: comprehensive research synopsis, meta-analysis, and epidemiological evidence. *Lancet Oncol.*, 2011. 12(5): p. 477-88.
[72] Calderon-Margalit, R. and O. Paltiel, Prevention of breast cancer in women who carry BRCA1 or BRCA2 mutations: a critical review of the literature. *Int. J. Cancer,* 2004. 112(3): p. 357-64.
[73] Boyd, N.F., et al., Mammographic density and the risk and detection of breast cancer. N. Engl. J. Med., 2007. 356(3): p. 227-36.
[74] Kerlikowske, K., et al., Breast cancer risk by breast density, menopause, and postmenopausal hormone therapy use. *J. Clin. Oncol.*, 2010. 28(24): p. 3830-7.
[75] Chow, C.K., et al., Effect of tamoxifen on mammographic density. *Cancer Epidemiol Biomarkers Prev*, 2000. 9(9): p. 917-21.
[76] Cuzick, J., et al., Tamoxifen and breast density in women at increased risk of breast cancer. *J. Natl. Cancer Inst.,* 2004. 96(8): p. 621-8.
[77] Boyd, N.F., Tamoxifen, mammographic density, and breast cancer prevention. *J. Natl. Cancer Inst.,* 2011. 103(9): p. 704-5.
[78] Cuzick, J., et al., Tamoxifen-induced reduction in mammographic density and breast cancer risk reduction: a nested case-control study. *J. Natl. Cancer Inst.*, 2011. 103(9): p. 744-52.

[79] Gail, M.H. and P.L. Mai, Comparing breast cancer risk assessment models. J. Natl. Cancer Inst., 2010. 102(10): p. 665-8.
[80] Vogel, V.G., et al., Effects of tamoxifen vs raloxifene on the risk of developing invasive breast cancer and other disease outcomes: the NSABP Study of Tamoxifen and Raloxifene (STAR) P-2 trial. *JAMA*, 2006. 295(23): p. 2727-41.
[81] Vogel, V.G., et al., Update of the National Surgical Adjuvant Breast and Bowel Project Study of Tamoxifen and Raloxifene (STAR) P-2 Trial: Preventing breast cancer. *Cancer Prev Res.* (Phila), 2010. 3(6): p. 696-706.
[82] Cuzick, J., et al., Long-term results of tamoxifen prophylaxis for breast cancer--96-month follow-up of the randomized IBIS-I trial. *J. Natl. Cancer Inst.*, 2007. 99(4): p. 272-82.
[83] Powles, T., et al., Interim analysis of the incidence of breast cancer in the Royal Marsden Hospital tamoxifen randomised chemoprevention trial. *Lancet*, 1998. 352(9122): p. 98-101.
[84] Powles, T.J., et al., Twenty-year follow-up of the Royal Marsden randomized, double-blinded tamoxifen breast cancer prevention trial. *J. Natl. Cancer Inst.*, 2007. 99(4): p. 283-90.
[85] Veronesi, U., et al., Tamoxifen for the prevention of breast cancer: late results of the Italian Randomized Tamoxifen Prevention Trial among women with hysterectomy. *J. Natl. Cancer Inst.*, 2007. 99(9): p. 727-37.
[86] Visvanathan, K., et al., American society of clinical oncology clinical practice guideline update on the use of pharmacologic interventions including tamoxifen, raloxifene, and aromatase inhibition for breast cancer risk reduction. *J. Clin. Oncol.*, 2009. 27(19): p. 3235-58.
[87] Aebi, S., et al., Primary breast cancer: ESMO Clinical Practice Guidelines for diagnosis, treatment and follow-up. *Ann. Oncol.*, 2010. 21 Suppl 5: p. v9-14.
[88] Siegel, R., et al., Cancer statistics, 2011. CA: *A Cancer Journal for Clinicians*, 2011. 61(4): p. 212-236.
[89] National Cancer Institute SEER 2011; Available from: http://seer.cancer.gov/statfacts/html/breast.html.
[90] Bramwell, V.H., et al., A randomized placebo-controlled study of tamoxifen after adjuvant chemotherapy in premenopausal women with early breast cancer (National Cancer Institute of Canada--Clinical Trials Group Trial, MA.12). *Ann. Oncol.*, 2010. 21(2): p. 283-90.
[91] Ortmann, O., et al., Which factors should be taken into account in perimenopausal women with early breast cancer who may become eligible for an aromatase inhibitor? Recommendations of an expert panel. *Cancer Treat Rev.*, 2011. 37(2): p. 97-104.
[92] Gnant, M., et al., Adjuvant endocrine therapy plus zoledronic acid in premenopausal women with early-stage breast cancer: 62-month follow-up from the ABCSG-12 randomised trial. *Lancet Oncol*, 2011. 12(7): p. 631-641.
[93] Comprehensive side-effect profile of anastrozole and tamoxifen as adjuvant treatment for early-stage breast cancer: long-term safety analysis of the ATAC trial. *The Lancet Oncology*, 2006. 7(8): p. 633-643.
[94] Letrozole Therapy Alone or in Sequence with Tamoxifen in Women with Breast Cancer. *New England Journal of Medicine*, 2009. 361(8): p. 766-776.

[95] van de Velde, C.J., et al., Adjuvant tamoxifen and exemestane in early breast cancer (TEAM): a randomised phase 3 trial. *Lancet,* 2011. 377(9762): p. 321-31.

[96] Cuzick, J., et al., Effect of anastrozole and tamoxifen as adjuvant treatment for early-stage breast cancer: 10-year analysis of the ATAC trial. *The Lancet Oncology*, 2010. 11(12): p. 1135-1141.

[97] Dowsett, M., et al., Meta-analysis of breast cancer outcomes in adjuvant trials of aromatase inhibitors versus tamoxifen. *J. Clin. Oncol*., 2010. 28(3): p. 509-18.

[98] Effect of anastrozole and tamoxifen as adjuvant treatment for early-stage breast cancer: 100-month analysis of the ATAC trial. *The Lancet Oncology*, 2008. 9(1): p. 45-53.

[99] Tannock, I.F., 10-year analysis of the ATAC trial: wrong conclusion? *The Lancet Oncology*, 2011. 12(3): p. 216-217.

[100] Cuzick, J., et al., 10-year analysis of the ATAC trial: wrong conclusion? - Authors' reply. *The Lancet Oncology,* 2011. 12(3): p. 217-217.

[101] Coates, A.S., et al., Five Years of Letrozole Compared With Tamoxifen As Initial Adjuvant Therapy for Postmenopausal Women With Endocrine-Responsive Early Breast Cancer: Update of Study BIG 1-98. *Journal of Clinical Oncology*, 2007. 25(5): p. 486-492.

[102] Colleoni, M., et al., Analyses Adjusting for Selective Crossover Show Improved Overall Survival With Adjuvant Letrozole Compared With Tamoxifen in the BIG 1-98 Study. *Journal of Clinical Oncology,* 2011. 29(9): p. 1117-1124.

[103] Coombes, R.C. and L.S. Kilburn, Time to TEAM: exemestane, or tamoxifen then exemestane? *The Lancet,* 2011. 377(9762): p. 280-281.

[104] Amir, E., et al., Toxicity of Adjuvant Endocrine Therapy in Postmenopausal Breast Cancer Patients: A Systematic Review and Meta-analysis. *Journal of the National Cancer Institute*, 2011.

[105] Houston, K.E. and D.B. Thomson, Aromatase inhibitors: what is the true cost? *Internal Medicine Journal,* 2011. 41(2): p. 139-140.

[106] Petit, T., P. Dufour, and I. Tannock, A critical evaluation of the role of aromatase inhibitors as adjuvant therapy for postmenopausal women with breast cancer. *Endocrine-Related Cancer,* 2011. 18(3): p. R79-R89.

[107] Oberguggenberger, A., et al., Is the toxicity of adjuvant aromatase inhibitor therapy underestimated? Complementary information from patient-reported outcomes (PROs). *Breast Cancer Research and Treatment*, 2011. 128(2): p. 553-561.

[108] Friedman, M.A. Tamoxifen. 1998; Available from: http://www.fda.gov/NewsEvents/Testimony/ucm115118.htm.

[109] Miller, R.W. TAmoxifen as a Breast Cancer Treament. 2011; Available from: http://ezinearticles.com/?Tamoxifen-As-A-Breast-Cancer-Treatmentandid=5706893.

[110] Huttunen, K.M., H. Raunio, and J. Rautio, Prodrugs—from Serendipity to Rational Design. *Pharmacological Reviews,* 2011. 63(3): p. 750-771.

In: Tamoxifen Concepts and Cancer: New Paradigms
Editor: Ramon Andrade de Mello
ISBN: 978-1-62081-520-5

Chapter IX

The Role of Pharmacogenomics in Personalising the Use of Tamoxifen in Breast Cancer

***S. J. Johnston*[1], *L. C. Chen*[2] *and K. L. Cheung*[1*]**

[1]Division of Breast Surgery and [2]School of Pharmacy,
University of Nottingham, UK

Abstract

Tamoxifen is a well-established endocrine therapy used in the treatment of hormone-receptor positive breast cancer. In recent years, its role in adjuvant and advanced breast cancer settings has been superseded by aromatase inhibitors. The prodrug tamoxifen is metabolised in the liver into several primary and secondary metabolites via cytochrome P450 enzymes. The main active forms are endoxifen and 4-hydroxytamoxifen, with CYP2D6 being a key enzyme in the production of both.

There is evidence that tamoxifen-associated hot flushes are an indicator of clinical efficacy of tamoxifen. Co-prescription of CYP2D6 inhibitors, including selective serotonin re-uptake inhibitors (SSRIs) commonly used to treat hot flushes, may decrease the clinical efficacy of tamoxifen and should be used with caution. Moreover, there is evidence that patients with poor CYP2D6-mediated tamoxifen metaboliser phenotype have worse clinical outcomes, and fewer hot flushes, than those with other phenotypes.

Further research is necessary to clarify whether extensive metabolisers have the best clinical outcomes on tamoxifen.

Preliminary data suggest that in individuals of certain CYP2D6 phenotype, tamoxifen may have equivalent efficacy, and be considered as an alternative to aromatase inhibitors if there were concerns over the side effect profile and cost of the latter. Thus the role of tamoxifen may be redefined in a new era of personalised breast cancer treatment.

[*] E-mail address: kl.cheung@nottingham.ac.uk.

Introduction

With the introduction of tamoxifen in 1973 [1] it became possible to personalise breast cancer treatment according to oestrogen receptor (ER) status, as determined by an immunocytological or histochemical technique. Selection of individual patients according to ER status for 5 years treatment with tamoxifen following surgery for early breast cancer is made in the light of data from worldwide randomised trials. Meta-analysis of these data indicates a reduction of around 50% in recurrence and 40% in breast cancer mortality in patients with ER positive tumours, but no effect in patients with ER negative tumours [2]. For several decades, tamoxifen has been the first line endocrine agent for adjuvant treatment and for post-menopausal women with hormone receptor-positive advanced breast cancer. Tamoxifen is an effective and well-tolerated endocrine treatment in these settings, but has side effects which are potentially serious, e.g. endometrial proliferation and deep vein thrombosis, and more common side effects such as hot flushes, which may impact adversely on quality of life and affect compliance to treatment. Moreover, between 30% and 50% of those taking adjuvant tamoxifen will eventually relapse or die of breast cancer, which may in part be explained by tumour-dependent ER activation [3]. In recent years, tamoxifen has been superseded by the third-generation aromatase inhibitors (AIs), anastrozole [4,5,6], letrozole [7,8] and exemestane [9], with evidence demonstrating a significant efficacy advantage for AIs over tamoxifen. However, the magnitude of this benefit is not large: for example, long-term follow-up of the Arimidex (anastrozole), Tamoxifen, Alone or in Combination (ATAC) trial [10] demonstrated an absolute difference in disease-free survival of 4% at 100 months in favour of anastrozole. The wide inter-individual variation in clinical effectiveness of tamoxifen may be due to intrinsic host factors including phenotypic variation of tamoxifen metabolism into its active components. This chapter outlines key developments over the last decade that have increased knowledge of the metabolism of tamoxifen via cytochrome P450 enzymes and explored links between pharmacogenetic factors and response to tamoxifen. The implications for the role of pharmocogenetics in personalising the use of tamoxifen therapy in breast cancer are then discussed, including the potential to enable clinicians to predict the benefits and risks of tamoxifen therapy through testing for individual genes, and hence tailor the choice of hormone treatment to the individual patient.

Tamoxifen Metabolism

Irrespective of selection for hormone receptor positivity, there remains wide inter-individual variation in clinical response to tamoxifen, both in terms of efficacy and in relation to side effects, which may be caused by variation in the metabolism of the prodrug, tamoxifen, into its active components.

Tamoxifen is metabolised extensively in the liver into several primary and secondary metabolites (Figure 1) via cytochrome P450 (CYP) enzymes. Studies on tamoxifen metabolites have established that 4-hydroxytamoxifen and 4-hydroxy-N-desmethyltamoxifen (endoxifen) are the main active therapeutic components, being of similar potency, with at least 100-fold greater affinity to the ER, and 30- to 100-fold greater potency in the suppression of oestrogen-dependent proliferation of breast cancer cells compared with the prodrug [1].

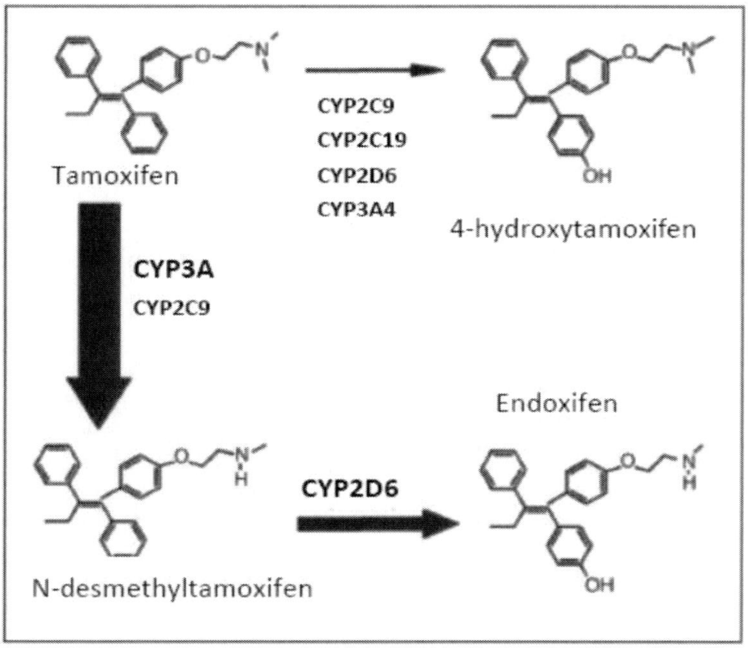

Figure 1. Metabolic pathway of tamoxifen. The width of the arrow represents the relative contribution of each pathway. [Adapted from Goetz et al, *J. Clin. Oncol.* 2005;23(36)9312-8].

CYP2D6 Activity and Effect on Plasma Endoxifen Levels

Factors affecting CYP2D6 activity and thus tamoxifen metabolism in individuals on tamoxifen may include genetic polymorphism of the enzyme, and concomitant drug interactions via competitive inhibition (acting as substrate to the enzyme) and direct inhibition of enzyme function.

The influence of the enzyme CYP2D6 on plasma endoxifen levels during tamoxifen treatment was demonstrated in three prospective clinical trials. In the first of these, Stearns et al. [13] measured the plasma concentration of tamoxifen and its metabolites (N-desmethyl-tamoxifen, 4-hydroxytamoxifen and endoxifen) in the plasma of 12 women of known CYP2D6 genotype with breast cancer who were taking adjuvant tamoxifen before and after 4 weeks of coadministered paroxetine.

The trial found that the mean plasma concentration of endoxifen decreased by 56% (p=0.02), whilst none of the other metabolites underwent statistically significant changes in concentration. Analysis by CYP2D6 genotype indicated that baseline plasma endoxifen concentration in those with variant genotype were lower, and that the reduction in endoxifen concentration was evident primarily in women with wild-type compared to variant genotype

(64% versus 24%, p=0.03). Indeed, there was no statistical reduction in endoxifen concentration for those with variant genotype.

Although this was a small preliminary study, the results raised the possibility that pharmacogenetic variation in CYP2D6 activity may influence therapeutic outcomes from tamoxifen treatment, with potential implications for CYP2D6 variant allele carriers, having lower plasma endoxifen, and those with wild-type genotype, whose plasma endoxifen concentrations may be reduced by concomitant enzyme inhibiting drugs.

Further evidence of the importance of CYP2D6 genotype and concomitant use of SSRIs was subsequently presented in a larger prospective clinical trial [14] of 80 patients with newly diagnosed breast cancer beginning adjuvant tamoxifen therapy. Of these patients, 24 were taking CYP2D6 inhibiting drugs (SSRIs paroxetine (n=10), sertraline (n=4), citalopram (n=4), fluoxetine (n=2) or the SNRI venlafaxine (n=3)).

Patients were genotyped for common CYP2D6 and other tamoxifen-metabolising enzyme (CYP2C9, CYP3A5 and sulfotransferase 1A1) alleles. The primary outcome measure was plasma concentration of tamoxifen and its metabolites, after one and four months of tamoxifen therapy.

The study found that those with a CYP2D6 homozygous wild-type genotype had statistically higher levels of plasma endoxifen after four months of tamoxifen therapy compared to those with homozygous variant or heterozygous genotypes, and that for homozygous wild-type genotype, plasma endoxifen concentration was reduced substantially when co-administered with paroxetine. Of the other CYP2D6 inhibiting drugs, venlafaxine was the weakest inhibitor and the effect of sertraline was intermediate between paroxetine and venlafaxine, which is consistent with in vitro data (although data for the two patients taking fluoxetine was not reported).

The largest of these prospective trials was conducted by Borges et al [15], in which 158 breast cancer patients taking tamoxifen were genotyped for 33 CYP2D6 alleles and had medication history taken. The outcome measure was plasma concentration of tamoxifen and its metabolites at the fourth month of tamoxifen treatment. The study used a mixture model approach to define phenotypic groups according to endoxifen/N-desmethyltamoxifen plasma concentration ratio, identifying three distinct genotype groups in the distribution of this ratio (Table 1).

Table 1. Mixture model in Borges et al, (Clin. Pharmacol. Ther. 2006;80(1):61-74). "NDM" = N-desmethyltamoxifen

Phenotypic group	Mean ratio endoxifen/NDM	p-value
No functional CYP2D6 allele	0.04	<0.001
1 active CYP2D6 allele	0.08	
2 or more active CYP2D6 allele	0.15	

The study also identified two phenotypic groups by plasma endoxifen concentration, and showed that those with CYP2D6 extensive metaboliser phenotype taking potent CYP2D6 inhibitors had significantly lower mean endoxifen plasma concentration than those who were not taking CYP2D6 inhibitors (23.5 +/- 9.5 nmol/L versus 84.1 +/- 39.4 nmol/L, p<0.001). Together, these three prospective clinical trials provided evidence that steady-state endoxifen plasma concentrations during tamoxifen treatment were reduced in women that carry certain

CYP2D6 genetic variants, or who carry wild-type alleles and are co-prescribed CYP2D6 inhibitors, while the concentration of tamoxifen or other metabolites remained unaffected by CYP2D6 metabolic status.

Moreover, the plasma concentrations of endoxifen were on average ten-fold higher than those of 4-hydroxytamoxifen, with a large degree of interpatient variability: up to one hundred-fold greater endoxifen exposure relative to 4-hydroxytamoxifen in some patients [13, 15, 16].

Endoxifen and Potential Indicators of Tamoxifen Response CYP2D6 Phenotype

In order to determine whether changes in active metabolite concentration resulting from genetic polymorphisms affect clinical outcomes of women receiving adjuvant tamoxifen, a prospective adjuvant tamoxifen trial [17] was used to explore the association between variation of tamoxifen metabolising genes and disease outcomes and toxicity in the form of hot flushes [18]. The study determined the genotype of CYP2D6 (based on aforementioned preliminary study findings) and CYP3A5 (selected because it has been shown to be the principal enzyme catalysing the elimination of tamoxifen) from 223 patients in the adjuvant tamoxifen trial.

Primary outcome measures were relapse-free (RF) time, disease-free survival (DFS) and overall survival (OS), and a secondary outcome measure was incidence of hot flushes. At 12 years of follow-up, for CYP3A5 there was no difference in RF-time, DFS or OS between genotypes, whilst for CYP2D6, unadjusted data indicated an advantage in RF-time and DFS, but not OS, for those with CYP2D6*4*4 (homozygous variant) genotype compared to patients with one or no variant alleles (Figure 2).

However, Cox proportional hazards modelling found a significant association between both nodal status and tumour size with RF-time, DFS and OS. Once adjustment had been made for these associations, there was no statistically significant difference in hazard ratios – so it may have been more forthright for the article to display the Kaplan-Meier curves for the adjusted rather than unadjusted data.

Similarly for the secondary outcome measure, the incidence of hot flushes did not vary by CYP3A5 genotype, but there was a non-significant lower incidence of hot flushes in the homozygous variant CYP2D6 group compared to those with wild-type alleles (Table 2).

Table 2. Incidence of moderate or severe hot flushes by CYP2D6 genotype

CYP2D6 genotype	Total patients	Patients with moderate or severe hot flushes	
		Number	%
Homozygous variant	13	0	0
Heterozygous wild-type	40	9	23
Homozygous wild-type	137	27	20

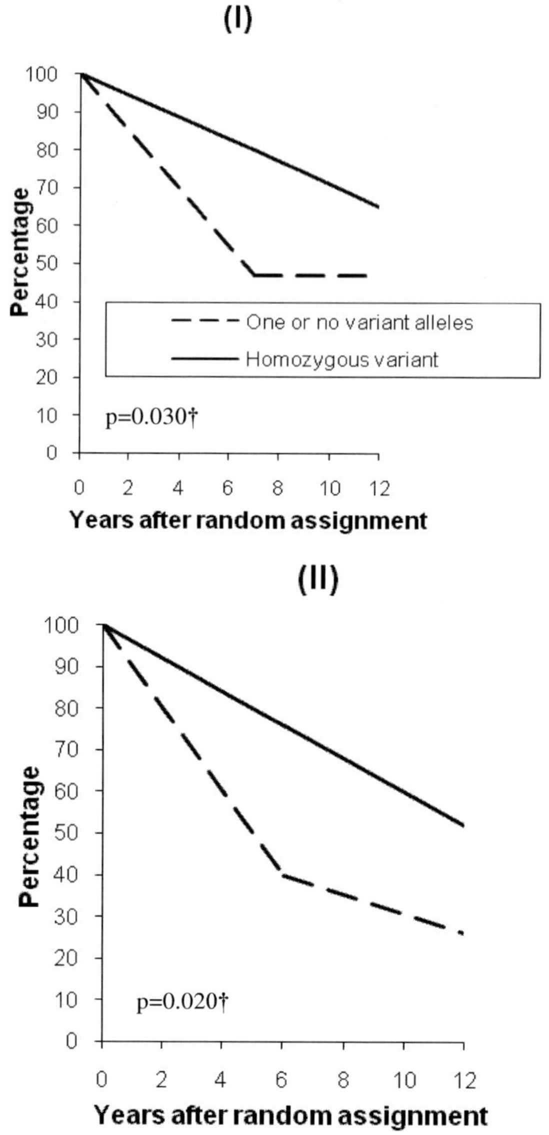

Figure 2. Kaplan-Meier estimates (approximate representation) of (I) relapse-free time; (II) disease-free survival for unadjusted† data, Wt (wild-type)/*4 or Wt/Wt vs. *4/*4 (adjusted data hazard ratios not significant: p=0.176 and 0.089 respectively). [Adapted from Goetz et al, 2005;23(36):9312-8].

Co-Prescription of SSRIs

Goetz et al [19] then undertook a retrospective review of the medical records of the patients in the North Central Cancer Treatment Group adjuvant tamoxifen trial [17], from which they defined metaboliser status based on a combination of CYP2D6 genotype and inhibition via co-prescribed medications (classified as moderate or potent inhibitors). From this information, they classified patients into extensive metabolisers (homozygous wild-type genotype not co-prescribed a CYP2D6 inhibitor) or decreased metabolisers, further classified into intermediate or poor metabolisers based on the presence of one or two CYP2D6 variant (*4) alleles or the co-prescription of a moderate or potent CYP2D6 inhibitor. Outcome measures were breast cancer recurrence and death.

By defining the patients in this manner, the study found that those with decreased metabolism (n=65) had significantly shorter time to recurrence (HR=1.91, p=0.034) and worse relapse-free survival (HR=1.74, p=0.017) relative to patients with extensive metabolism (n=115), and that compared to extensive metabolisers, poor metabolisers had the most significant risk of breast cancer relapse (HR 3.12, p=0.007).

Thus the study concludes that CYP2D6 metabolism as measured by genetic variation and enzyme inhibition is an independent predictor of breast cancer outcome in post-menopausal women receiving tamoxifen for early breast cancer – although the "measurement" of CYP2D6 metabolism in this study is based on several layers of classification of retrospective data, with the effect of moderate and potent enzyme inhibitors (co-prescribed in 13 patients) being somewhat indeterminate.

Hot Flushes

The evidence of increased risk of disease relapse and fewer hot flushes with those with decreased CYP2D6 mediated metabolism, along with poorer outcome with co-administration of SSRIs in patients receiving adjuvant tamoxifen therapy, was presented as an "*a priori*" hypothesis [20] at the Annual Scientific Meeting of the American Society of Clinical Oncology in 2007: that hot flushes themselves are an indicator of tamoxifen efficacy, and that the absence of hot flushes may be an indication of poor prognosis.

The evidence for this was taken from the Women's Healthy Eating and Living (WHEL) study [21], a large randomised trial of the effect of a major increase in vegetable consumption on future breast cancer events among breast cancer survivors. Between 1995 and 2000, the WHEL study recruited 3088 women aged 18-70 years, diagnosed (within 2-48 months) with stage I (T1c) to III breast cancer, and randomly assigned subjects to a WHEL healthy cancer prevention diet or control arm (National Cancer Institute based diet).

Baseline information included dietary intake, menopause status and anti-oestrogen use, and the study recorded information about cancer pathology and treatment, along with patient questionnaire data on symptoms. Retrospective analysis was then performed on the control arm (n=1551) to explore links between tamoxifen use, hot flushes and breast cancer events. Unadjusted cancer event proportions for hot flushes were compared to those without. The average time after study entry was 7.3 years, and there were 864 patients on tamoxifen in the analysis. At 7.3 years of follow-up, the study found that women with hot flushes had fewer breast cancer specific events (locoregional or contralateral recurrence, or metastatic disease) than those without hot flushes (12.9% vs. 21%, p=0.01), and that recurrence-free survival was better for those who reported hot flushes (figure 3).

The study also found that hot flushes were more predictive of breast cancer specific outcomes than age, hormone receptor status or stage I vs. II disease. Thus a relationship between hot flushes and efficacy of adjuvant tamoxifen was suggested.

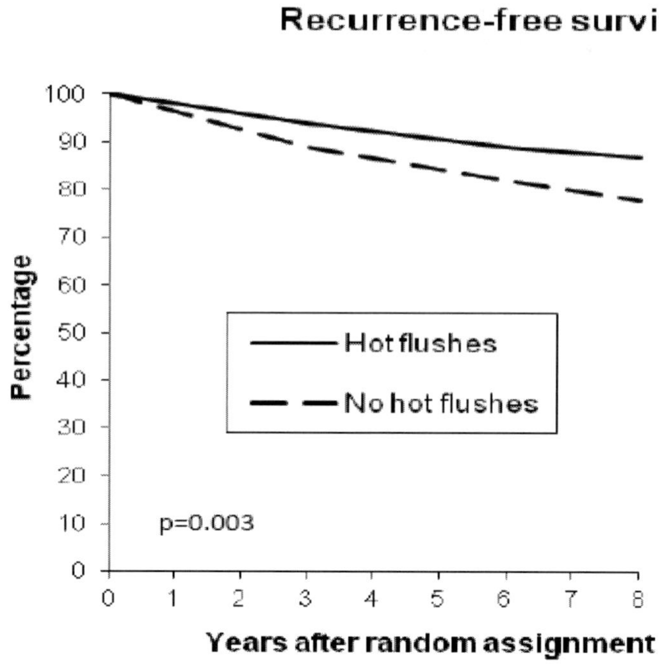

Figure 3. Kaplan-Meier recurrence-free survival (approximate representation) as a function of reported hot flashes in patients on tamoxifen (n=864) [Adapted from ASCO Proceedings, Chicago, 1-5 June 2007].

In summary, the evidence from trials looking at clinical outcomes according to variously defined metaboliser phenotypic status has identified CYP2D6 genotype, individually and in conjunction with SSRI co-prescription, as a potential predictive factor of tamoxifen response. The proposed mechanism, as suggested by prior clinical trials, is CYP2D6-mediated metabolism of the prodrug tamoxifen to endoxifen. Furthermore, there is evidence that hot flushes themselves might indicate an efficacious, endoxifen-mediated response to tamoxifen therapy.

Association Between CYP2D6 Genetic Variation and Tamoxifen Response

A further study attempted to define the predictive value of genetic variants of CYP enzymes including CYP2D6 for tamoxifen treatment outcome [22]. The study was a non-randomised, retrospective analysis of 486 ER-positive postmenopausal breast cancer patients, with 206 patients taking adjuvant tamoxifen compared to a control population of 280 patients not taking tamoxifen, using archival material. Patients receiving adjuvant tamoxifen and concomitant chemotherapy or patients with an unclear ER status (n=135) were excluded from the analysis. Information on co-prescription of SSRIs was incomplete and also excluded from analysis. Outcome measures were relapse-free time (time from surgery to locoregional recurrence or contralateral disease), event-free survival (time to relapse or death from any cause) and overall survival.

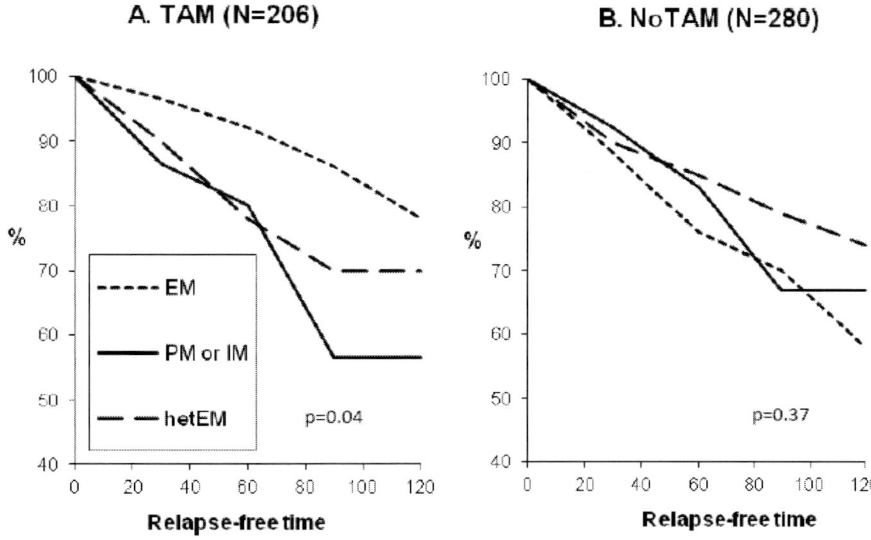

Figure 4. Kaplan-Meier probabilities (approximate representation) of relapse-free time (RFT) of breast cancer patients on adjuvant tamoxifen for CYP2D6-metaboliser phenotypes. [Adapted from Scroth et al *J. Clin. Oncol.* 2007;25(33):5187-93]. TAM=patients on tamoxifen, NoTAM= patients not on tamoxifen, EM=extensive metabolisers, hetEM=heterozygous EM, IM=intermediate metabolisers, PM=poor metabolisers.

At a median follow-up of 71 months, carriers of CYP2D6*4, *5, *10 and *41 alleles, with phenotypes defined as poor and intermediate metabolisers, had significantly more breast cancer recurrences, shorter relapse-free times, and worse event-free survival than carriers of functional alleles (Figure 4). No such association was found for the control population.

The authors concluded by suggesting that genetic testing for CYP2D6 status could be used to refine the choice and / or sequencing of hormonal therapy in prospective clinical trials, and identified a potential role for pharmacogenetics, with upfront genetic testing of CYP2D6 genotype, to predicting response to tamoxifen.

Implications

Research into pharmacogenetics of tamoxifen therapy has identified CYP2D6 as a key enzyme in the metabolism of tamoxifen, with a critical role in the formation of endoxifen. Along with 4-hydroxytamoxifen, endoxifen is a major active metabolite of the prodrug. In women treated with tamoxifen, plasma endoxifen levels are on average five to ten times higher than those of 4-hydroxytamoxifen, with wide inter-individual variation, suggesting a dominant active role for endoxifen determined via genetic variation in CYP2D6. By defining CYP2D6 phenotypes such as extensive and poor tamoxifen metabolisers based on genotype and the co-prescription of known CYP2D6 inhibitors such as SSRIs that are commonly used to treat hot flushes, evidence is presented of an association between pharmacogenetic factors and clinical response to tamoxifen. This implies that CYP2D6 genotype could be used in upfront genetic testing to help clinicians weigh up the potential benefits versus the risks of tamoxifen therapy for the individual patient.

Research has also asked questions about the practice of prescribing SSRIs to treat tamoxifen-associated hot flushes, and found evidence that SSRIs, which are both competitive and direct inhibitors of CYP2D6, contribute to decreased tamoxifen metaboliser status with an associated diminished clinical response to tamoxifen. Alongside evidence that hot flushes are associated with fewer breast cancer events, the implication is that hot flushes indicate an efficacious clinical response to tamoxifen, via CYP2D6-mediated metabolism into endoxifen and SSRIs should therefore be avoided, or at least used with caution, in patients treated with tamoxifen. Given that hot flushes may be interpreted as a surrogate of adequate endoxifen levels in the body, patients could be reassured that with the development of hot flushes, they are likely to be deriving clinical benefit from tamoxifen.

Whilst aromatase inhibitors have replaced tamoxifen as the first line endocrine therapy in the adjuvant breast cancer setting for postmenopausal women, the absolute DFS advantage is small; thus the subgroup of patients who are extensive CYP2D6 metabolisers (e.g. homozygous wild type alleles) may benefit more from tamoxifen therapy. Whether or not pharmacogenomics could be used to tailor therapy to the individual would require prospective clinical trials to test whether individual genes such as CYP2D6 can be used to predict outcomes. In the meantime, genetic testing could be applied on an individual basis, for example if there are concerns over toxicities of aromatase inhibitors such as osteoporotic risk, in which case tamoxifen may be preferable and of similar efficacy for individuals with CYP2D6 homozygous wild-type genotype. With improved knowledge of global and ethnic variation in CYP2D6 genotype, the application of pharmacogenomics could be targeted to certain groups in order to make more informed decisions in tailoring endocrine therapy. Thus a new role for tamoxifen may emerge in a new era of personalised medicine.

References

[1] Cole M, Jones C, Todd I: A new antioestrogenic agent in late breast cancer. An early appraisal of ICI 46,474. *Br J Cancer* 1971;25:270-5.

[2] Early Breast Cancer Trialists' Collaborative Group: Effects of chemotherapy and hormonal therapy for early breast cancer on recurrence and 15-year survival: an overview of the randomised trials. *Lancet.* 2005 May 14-20;365(9472):1687-717.

[3] Ring A and Dowsett M: Mechanisms of tamoxifen resistance. *Endocr. Rel. Cancer.* 11:643-58.

[4] Bonneterre J, Thurlimann D, Robertson J, et al. Anastrozole versus tamoxifen as first-line therapy for advanced breast cancer in 668 postmenopausal women: results of the Tamoxifen or Arimidex randomised group efficacy and tolerability study. *J. Clin. Oncol.* 2003;39:2310-7.

[5] Nabholtz J, Buzdar A, Pollak M, et al. Anastrozole is superior to tamoxifen as first-line therapy for advanced breast cancer in postmenopausal women: results of a North American multicenter randomised trial. *J. Clin. Oncol.* 2000;18:3758-67.

[6] Milla-Santos A, Milla L, Portella J, et al. Anastrozole versus tamoxifen as first-line therapy in postmenopausal patients with hormone-dependent advanced breast cancer: a prospective, randomised, phase III study. *Am. J. Clin. Oncol.* 2003;26:317-22.

[7] Mourisden H, Gershanovich M, Sun Y, et al. Superior efficacy of letrozole versus tamoxifen as first-line therapy for post-menopausal women with advanced breast cancer: results of a phase III study of the International Letrozole Breast Cancer Group. *J. Clin. Oncol.* 2001;19:2596-606.

[8] Eirmann W, Paepke S, Appfelstaedt J, et al. Letrozole Neo-Adjuvant Breast Cancer Study Group: Preoperative treatment of postmenopausal breast cancer patients with letrozole: a randomised double-blind multicenter study. *Ann Oncol.* 2001;12:1527-32.

[9] Paridaens R, Dirix L, Lohrisch C, et al. European Organsiation for the Research and Treatment of Cancer (EORTC) – Investigational Drug Branch for Breast Cancer (IDBBC). Mature results of a randomised phase II multicenter study of exemestane versus tamoxifen as first-line hormone therapy for post-menopausal women with metastatic breast cancer. *Ann. Oncol.* 2003;14:1391-8.

[10] Forbes JF, Cuzick J, Buzdar A, et al. Effect of anastrozole and tamoxifen as adjuvant treatment for early-stage breast cancer: 100-month analysis of the atac trial. *Lancet Oncol.* 2008;9:45-53.

[11] Lee KH, Ward BA, Desta Z, et al: Quantification of tamoxifen and three metabolites in plasma by high-performance liquid chromatography with fluorescence detection: application to a clinical trial. *J. Chromatogr. B. Analyt. Technol. Biomed. Life Sci.* 2003;791:245-53.

[12] Desta Z, Ward BA, Soukhova NV, et al: Comprehensive evaluation of tamoxifen sequential biotransformation by the human cytochrome P450 system in vitro: prominent roles for CYP3A and CYP2D6. *J. Pharmacol. Exp. Ther.* 2004;310:1062-75.

[13] Stearns V, Johnson MD, Rae JM, et al: Active tamoxifen metabolite plasma concentrations after coadministration of tamoxifen and the selective serotonin reuptake inhibitor paroxetine. *J. Natl. Cancer Inst.* 2003;95(23):1758-64.

[14] Jin Y, Desta Z, Stearns V, et al: CYP2D6 genotype, antidepressant use, and tamoxifen metabolism during adjuvant breast cancer treatment. *J. Natl. Cancer Inst.* 2005;97(1):30-9.

[15] Borges S, Desta Z, Li L, et al: Quantitative effect of CYP2D6 genotype and inhibitors on tamoxifen metabolism: implication for optimization of breast cancer treatment. *Clin. Pharmacol. Ther.* 2006;80(1):61-74.

[16] Desta Z, Flockhart DA: Germline pharmacogenetics of tamoxifen response: have we learned enough? *J. Clin. Oncol.* 2007;25(33):5147-9 (editorial).

[17] Ingle J, Suman V, Mailliard J, et al: Randomized trial of tamoxifen alone or combined with fluoxymesterone as adjuvant therapy in postmenopausal women with resected primary breast cancer: A North Central Cancer Treatment Group Study. *Proc. Am. Soc. Clin. Oncol.* 2000;19:86a (abstract).

[18] Goetz MP, Rae JM, Suman VJ, et al: Pharmacogenetics of tamoxifen biotransformation is associated with clinical outcomes of efficacy and hot flashes. *J. Clin. Oncol.* 2005;23(36):9312-8.

[19] Goetz MP, Knox SK, Suman VJ, et al: The impact of cytochrome P450 2D6 metabolism in women receiving adjuvant tamoxifen. *Breast Cancer Res. Treat.* 2007;101(1):113-21. Epub 2006 Nov 18.

[20] Mortimer JE, Flatt SW, Parker BA, et al: Tamoxifen, hot flashes and recurrence in breast cancer: Support for pharmacogenetics. *J. Clin. Oncol.* 2007;25(18S):500 (abstract).

[21] Pierce JP, Natarajan L, Caan BJ, et al: Influence of a diet very high in vegetables, fruit, and fiber and low in fat on prognosis following treatment for breast cancer: the Women's Healthy Eating and Living (WHEL) randomized trial. *JAMA*. 2007;298(3):289-98.

[22] Scroth W, Antoniadou L, Fritz P, et al: Breast cancer treatment outcome with adjuvant tamoxifen relative to patient CYP2D6 and CYP2C19 genotypes. *J. Clin. Oncol.* 2007;25(33):5187-93.

In: Tamoxifen Concepts and Cancer: New Paradigms
Editor: Ramon Andrade de Mello
ISBN: 978-1-62081-520-5

Chapter X

Tamoxifen and Antidepressants in the Breast Cancer Setting

Álber Morais Dias [*]
Service of Psychiatry - Sao Paulo State Court of Justice,
São Paulo, Brazil

Abstract

Breast cancer is the most commonly diagnosed cancer in women worldwide, and many patients experience clinically significant depression that require psychiatric intervention. Tamoxifen is a selective oestrogen receptor modulator that reduces the risk of recurrence in early-stage patients whose tumour cells express the oestrogen receptor. To be effective, it depends on metabolic activation via cytochrome P450 2D6 (CYP2D6). Many medications, including antidepressants used for hot flashes, pain or depression in breast cancer patients, may compromise CYP2D6 activity and interfere with plasma concentration of endoxifen (tamoxifen active metabolic), affecting survival in those patients. With so many treatment options, many questions arise about which antidepressant to choose in those patients. The data suggest that strong CYP2D6 inhibitors, such as fluoxetine and paroxetine, should probably be avoided, and weak inhibitors (venlafaxine, mirtazapine and citalopram) are safer choices, with less potential to decrease the clinical efficacy of tamoxifen. Studies with long follow-up periods and with greater power to look at individual antidepressants are necessary.

Abbreviations

SSRI - Selective serotonin reuptake inhibitor
SNRI - Serotonin–norepinephrine reuptake inhibitor

[*] E-mail: albermorais@bol.com.br.

1. Introduction

Breast cancer remains a life-threatening and life-altering experience than can be associated with significant psychological distress[1] While many women experience "normal" distress, there is a subset that experience clinically significant depression that may benefit from specialized psychiatric intervention[2].

Newer antidepressants are widely used in women with breast cancer for treatment of depression and are prescribed for pain[3], tamoxifen related hot flashes and various other indications; this practice is particularly relevant in the context of tamoxifen therapy because selective serotonin reuptake inhibitor (SSRI) antidepressants inhibit CYP2D6 to varying degrees[4], as the selective estrogen-receptor modulator tamoxifen. Because of this, tamoxifen´s prevention of breast cancer recurrence could be reduced[5].

This chapter will summarize information about coadministration of antidepressants and tamoxifen in the breast cancer setting.

2. Depression in Breast Cancer

The estimated point prevalence of major depressive disorder in all women ranges from 3.5 to 7% [6];the rate of depression disorder in women with breast cancer is estimated to be 10-25%, depending on the method of assessment.It appears that depression is more common in the first year following diagnosis (especially in younger women), and that systemic therapies likely influence the development of symptoms [1]. The effects of chemotherapy on fertility, sexuality and menopause-associated health problems (e.g., osteoporosis and cardiovascular disease) can lead to high levels of distress [7]. Besides, after primary cancer therapy, patients are often fearful of cancer recurrence and face the loss of support and frequent visits with medical professionals, contributing to high rates of anxiety, which is often comorbid with depression [8,9]. Depression is often associated with decreased acceptance of and compliance with adjuvant therapy in women with breast cancer, which may, in turn, affect disease outcome [10]. Despite the mean level of adherence to tamoxifen is high compared with other chronic medications, nearly one fourth of patients may be at risk for inadequate clinical response because of poor adherence [11].

3. Tamoxifen

Because breast cancer is estrogen-dependent, reducing estrogen secretion by oophorectomy, hypophysectomy,or adrenalectomy can cause the cancer to regress.The need for these surgical procedures was reduced by the introduction of tamoxifen, which acts as an antiestrogen by inhibiting the binding of estrogen to estrogen receptors [12].It reduces by half the risk of breast cancer recurrence in early-stage patients whose tumour cells express the oestrogen receptor [13]. Tamoxifen is converted to endoxifen (active metabolic) principally by a noninducible P450 enzyme that is coded for by the most polymorphic, and most studied, gene in the cytochrome P450 system: CYP2D6. There are more than 80 different major alleles of the CYP2D6 identified, many of which confer decreased or absent CYP2D6 activity and patients can be divided into poor, intermediate, extensive and ultrarapid metabolizers on the basis of their genotype [14]. Interactions between CYP2D6 polymorphisms and other drugs that are CYP2D6 inhibitors (antidepressants, for example) may be associated with altered tamoxifen activity [15], even if they have the homozygous active genotype, in a manner similar to the poor metabolizer genotype [14].

4. Coadministration of SSRIs/SNRIs and Tamoxifen

Anti-estrogen therapy for patients with breast cancer, which may induce or exacerbate depression and anxiety and which frequently causes hot flashes, has led to an intersection between clinical oncology and clinical psychiatry [14]. The links between vasomotor symptoms and depression are both clinical and neurobiological. The clinical link is demonstrated by the high degree of overlap between the symptoms of depression and the symptoms of perimenopause and menopause. The neurobiological link between vasomotor symptoms and depression is that both are regulated by the trimonoamine neurotransmitter system. Estrogen affects the trimonoamine system by regulating the expression of genes for numerous neurotransmitter receptors, synthesizing enzymes, and metabolizing enzymes. Given the clinical and neurobiological link between vasomotor symptoms and the symptoms of depression, it was logical to look at antidepressants that target the trimonoaminergic neurotransmitter system to find a treatment for vasomotor symptoms, but the most promising results to date seem to be with SNRIs (serotonin–norepinephrine reuptake inhibitors), especially the SNRI desvenlafaxine. Perhaps it is necessary to target both the profound hypothalamic regulation of temperature by norepinephrine as well as serotonin to achieve optimal efficacy in the treatment of vasomotor symptoms, rather than targeting just serotonin regulation of temperature with an SSRI [16].

Since SSRIs and SNRIs have been demonstrated to decrease hot flashes in otherwise healthy postmenopausal women who are not taking tamoxifen, and since citalopram, venlafaxine and gabapentin are as effective in reducing hot flashes as strong CYP2D6 inhibitors in women taking tamoxifen, the mechanism by which these antidepressants reduce hot flashes is likely not due to blockade of endoxifen production. These data suggest that concomitant use of potent CYP2D6 inhibitors should be avoided in women taking tamoxifen, unless the patient is committed to one of these drugs as an effective antidepressant where other medications have been ineffective, or a patient requiring antidepressant therapy cannot tolerate alternative agents [14].

Table 1 lists the antidepressants that are considered"strong""moderate"' or "weak" inhibitors of CYP2D6, or "noninhibitors" [17].

The choice of antidepressant can significantly affect survival in women receiving tamoxifen for breast cancer. According to one study, use of paroxetine during tamoxifen treatment is associated with an increased subsequent risk of death due to breast cancer in a fashion that correlates with the duration of combined use. This study found no association between fluoxetine (another strong CYP2D6 inhibitor) and death from breast cancer among women taking tamoxifen, which might reflect the relatively small number of women in the sample [4].

Table 1. Antidepressants classified by potency of CYP2D6 inhibition

Strong CYP2D6 Inhibitors
Fluoxetine
Paroxetine
Sertraline
Bupropion
Moderate CYP2D6 Inhibitors
Duloxetine
Mild CYP2D6 Inhibitors
Citalopram
Escitalopram
Noninhibitors of CYP2D6
Venlafaxine
Desvenlafaxine
Mirtazapine

However, in a 2009 review of the literature, the authors found consistent evidence that paroxetine and fluoxetine have large effect on the metabolism of tamoxifen and recommended that these drugs should not be used in conjunction with tamoxifen treatment in breast cancer.

Indirect evidence suggests that bupropion also has considerable effects on the metabolism of tamoxifen. Safer choices, according to the authors, given a lack of CYP2D6 inhibition, include venlafaxine, desvenlafaxine and mirtazapine. The question remains as to whether these inhibitory effects on tamoxifen metabolism translate into poorer clinical outcomes [17,18]. Lash and colleagues found no reduction in tamoxifen´s protection against breast cancer in patients using citalopram [19].

Conclusion

It appears to be an emerging consensus that antidepressants that are potent inhibitors of CYP2D6 (ie, fluoxetine, paroxetine and sertraline) used concurrently with tamoxifen therapy for women with breast cancer may reduce the clinical efficacy of tamoxifen.

Furthermore, evidence suggests that antidepressants that are either milder or CYP2D6 or noninhibitors are in fact safer choices, with less potential to decrease the clinical efficacy of tamoxifen [17]. However, it will be important to confirm these results in results in studies with long follow-up periods and with greater power to look at individual antidepressants [20].

References

[1] Coyne JC,Palmer SC,Shapiro PJ, et al. Distress, psychiatric morbidity, and prescriptions for psychotropic medication in a breast cancer waiting room sample.*General Hospital Psychiatry* 2004;26(2):121-128.

[2] Fann JR,Thomas-Rich AM,Katon WJ, et al. Major depression after breast cancer: a review of epidemiology and treatment.*General Hospital Psychiatry* 2008;30(2):112-126.

[3] MacDonald RN, Hugi MR, Graydon JE, et al.The management of chronic pain in patients with breast cancer. The steering committee on clinical practice guidelines for the care and treatment of breast cancer. *CMAJ* 1998;158(3):s71-S81.

[4] Kelly, CM, Juurlink DN, Gomes T, et al. Selective serotonin reuptake inhibitors and breast cancer mortality in women receiving tamoxifen: a population based cohort study. BMJ 2010;340:c693.

[5] Lash TL, Cronin-Fenton D, Ahern TP, et al. Breast cancer recurrence risk related to concurrent use of SSRI antidepressants and tamoxifen. *Acta Oncologica* 2010;49(3): 305-312.

[6] Murphy JM, Laird NM, Monson RRet al. A 40-year perspective on the prevalence of depression: the Stirling County Study. *Arch. Gen. Psychiatry* 2000;57(3):209-15.

[7] Couzi RJ, Helzlsouer KJ, Fetting JH. Prevalence of menopausal symptoms among women with a history of breast cancer and attitudes toward estrogen replacement therapy. *Journal of Clinical Oncology* 1995; 13(11): 2737-2744.

[8] Sarenmalm EK, Ohlen J, Jonsson T, et al. Coping with Recurrent Breast Cancer: Predictors of Distressing Symptoms and Health-Related Quality of Life. Journal of Pain and Symptom Management 2007;34(1):24-39.

[9] Rowland JH. Anxiety and the blues after breast cancer: how common are they? *CNS Spectr* 1999;4(10):40-54.

[10] Pasacreta JV. Depressive phenomena, physical symptom distress, and functional status among women with breast cancer. *Nurs. Res.* 1997;46:214-21.

[11] Partridge AH, Wang PS, Winer EP, et al. Nonadherence to adjuvant tamoxifen therapy in women with primary breast cancer. *Journal of Clinical Oncology* 2003;21(4): 602-606.

[12] Osborne, CK. Tamoxifen in the Treatment of Breast Cancer. *N. Engl. J. Med.* 1998; 339:1609-1618.

[13] Early Breast Cancer Trialists' Collaborative Group. Effects of chemotherapy and hormonal therapy for early breast cancer on recurrence and 15-year survival: an overview of the randomised trials. *Lancet* 2005;365:1687-1717.

[14] Henry NL, Stearns V, Flockhar DA, et al. Drug Interactions and Pharmacogenomics in the Treatment of Breast Cancer and Depression. *Am. J. Psychiatry* 2008;165:1251-1255.

[15] Jin Y, Desta Z, Stearns V, et al. CYP2D6 Genotype, Antidepressant Use, and Tamoxifen Metabolism During Adjuvant Breast Cancer Treatment *JNCI J. Natl. Cancer Inst.* 2005;97(1):30-39.

[16] Stahl, SM. Stahl´s Essential Psychopharmacology – Neuroscientific Basis and Practical Applications. 3rded. New York: Cambridge University Press, 2008.

[17] Breitbart, W. Do antidepressants reduce the effectiveness of tamoxifen?. *Psycho-Oncology* 2011;20:1–4.
[18] Desmarais JE, Looper KJ. Interactions between tamoxifen and antidepressants via cytochrome P450 2D6. *The Journal of Clinical Psychiatry* 2009;70(12):1688-97.
[19] Lash TL, Pedersen L, Cronin-Fenton D. Tamoxifen's protection against breast cancer recurrence is not reduced by concurrent use of the SSRI citalopram. *British Journal of Cancer* 2008; 99:616–621.
[20] Chubak J, Buist DSM, Boudreau DM, et al. Breast cancer recurrence risk in relation to antidepressant use after diagnosis. *Breast Cancer Res. Treat* 2008; 112:123-132.

In: Tamoxifen Concepts and Cancer: New Paradigms
Editor: Ramon Andrade de Mello
ISBN: 978-1-62081-520-5

Chapter XI

Obesity in Breast Cancer Treated with Tamoxifen

Karla Sánchez-Lara[1*] and Jenny G. Turcott[2]
[1]Oncology Center, Médica Sur
[2]Thoracic Oncology Clinic,
Instituto Nacional de Cancerología de México (INCan)
Mexico City, Mexico

Abstract

Background. Breast cancer is the most frequent type of cancer in women. Epidemiological studies suggest that lifestyle factors including dietary patterns and physical activity play a significant role in the development and survival of breast cancer. In particular, there is convincing evidence that obesity is a potent risk factor for both cancer development and prognosis.

The pathophysiological link is not fully elucidated, but may include an increased estrogen production by adipose-tissue stromal cells, elevated levels of insulin and insulin-like growth factor (IGF)-1, increased adipose tissue-derived factors (adipokines), and possibly other mechanisms related to an expanded fat mass.

In addition, the pharmacological therapy in estrogen-positive breast cancer is a hormonal therapy focused in diminishing the estrogen levels, Tamoxifen. Thus, if high fat volume is associated with elevated levels of serum estrogen, an important question is whether obesity affects treatment efficacy, and if modifiable risk factors related to lifestyle and obesity could be an important and necessary part of the breast cancer treatment.

Conclusion. There is convincing evidence of the association between obesity and breast cancer risk and prognosis, consequently more studies of the effect of lifestyle factors such as diet patterns, physical activity and body mass index in breast cancer hormonal treatment as Tamoxifen are needed. Integral treatment including additional strategies that target other potential mediators of obesity-related prognostics effects are also necessary to improve prognosis in these patients.

* E-mail: ksanchez@medicasur.org.mx and kpao82@hotmail.com.

Abbreviations

BMI - Body mass index
ER - Estrogen receptor
PR - Progesteron receptor
NASH - Non alcoholic steatohepatitis
HR - Hazard ratio
CI - Confidence Interval

1. Introduction

Breast cancer is a worldwide problem affecting more than 1 million women annually [1]. Knowledge of preventable risk factors and recognition of epidemiologic, prognostic and predictive factors, are essentially to risk-reduction strategies.

There are well known risk factors for breast cancer, included advanced age, a first-degree relative with history of breast cancer, genes mutations and hormonal factors that increase exposure to estrogen like early menses or late pregnancy. Besides, a direct correlation between obesity, estrogen levels and higher breast cancer risk has been evidenced in both development and prognosis.

One of the most important pharmacological treatments are anti-estrogen therapies, like Tamoxifen; since adipose tissue are a main estrogen producer, an integral treatment including weight control, healthy diet and physical activity must be considered [2]. This chapter will summarize information on potential nutritional and behavioral approaches to reducing breast cancer risk.

2. Obesity and Breast Cancer

Obesity is considered as a risk factor for developed and less favorable disease features at diagnosis, larger tumors and prognosis in breast cancer before and after menopause [3-4], the relationship between obesity and worst prognosis in breast cancer has been investigated extensively, and it is generally accepted that women with a greater body mass index (BMI) have less favorable outcomes than lean women, in both premenopausal and postmenopausal patients [5].

The predominant hypothesis relating obesity to prognosis concerns the influence of adipose tissue volume on hormone levels; higher fat tissue is associated with elevated serum estrogen levels [6], a major contributor to the growth of hormone receptor-positive breast cancer [7-8]. Before menopause, obesity may interfere with normal menstrual cycling, potentially leading to reductions in estrogen levels; after menopause, increased production of estrogen in excess adipose tissue is associated with obesity, secondary to the aromatization of adrenal androgens which translates to obese women having a higher risk of developing breast cancer.

There are many studies that confirm this association [9], one interesting study found that women who gained 55 pounds or more after age of 18 had an approximately 55% greater risk of breast cancer compared with those who maintained their weight. A gain of 22 pounds or more after menopause was associated with 82% greater risk of breast cancer, whereas losing at least 22 pounds after menopause and maintaining the weight loss was associated with a trend toward decreased breast cancer risk [10]. The complexity of the relationship between obesity and breast cancer also reflects important contributions of obesity-related factors other than estrogen to breast cancer risk and prognosis. These factors include insulin resistance, adiponectin as well as inflammatory markers such as C-reactive protein, interleukins and adipocytokines [7], like leptin, a hormone that is produced mainly by the fat tissue, but it can also be synthesized by breast cancer cells in response to obesity-related stimuli [11-13]. Leptin induces breast cancer cell growth, transformation, and survival and reduces the efficacy of breast cancer treatments [14].

Both leptin and its receptor (ObR) are over expressed in breast cancer, especially in higher grade tumors, but are absent in normal epithelial breast tissues [15-16].

3. Diet and Physical Activity

Links between adult diet and risk of breast cancer have been extensively investigated, but many topics remain controversial because the diet of an individual or of a specific group/population represents a complex phenomenon that may vary day by day, and may change markedly over longer periods. Another limitation is the instruments to measure dietary intake. In addition, it is difficult to randomize large numbers of women to specific diets and maintain good long-term compliance. In view of these limitations, it may be more reasonable and reliable to consider data on dietary patterns rather than focusing on single food components or ingredients [17-18]. However, there are some dietetic factors in these patients that had been investigated: fat, carbohydrates, soy and alcohol consumption.

Dietary fat has been a topic of extensive investigation in breast cancer development; potential mechanisms of action includes an influence on steroid hormone levels or higher energy density affecting other established risk factors, such as weight gain or age at menarche; in a large prospective study of 188,736 postmenopausal women with 3,501 cases of invasive breast cancer, a small increase in risk was seen among women with the highest intake of dietary fat [19]. However, there are several studies including meta analysis that found no association between dietary fat and breast cancer [20-22]. The World Cancer Research Fund/American Institute for Cancer Research panel concluded that there is only limited or suggestive evidence that total fat may increase the risk of breast cancer after menopause [23].

Higher carbohydrates consumption could influence breast cancer risk by affecting circulating insulin levels, insulin resistance, insulin-like growth factors, and sex hormone bioavailability. Conversely, prospective cohort studies have not shown consistent associations between total carbohydrate, glycemic index and breast cancer risk [24, 25]. NHS-II study [26], which used a validated food-frequency questionnaire to assess the diet of 45,947 nurses, showed a positive association between the consumption of foods with a high glycemic index and the incidence of breast cancer.

About specific diet consumption, red meat, soy and alcohol has been investigated; some hypothesis proposed that red meat could induce carcinogenesis by growth-promoting hormones used in animal production, carcinogenic heterocyclic amines formed in cooking and its specific fatty acid content. In a sub-analysis of the NHS II (n =1,021), red meat intake was strongly related to an elevated risk of breast cancers that were estrogen- and progesterone receptor-positive (n = 512) but not to those that were estrogen- and progesterone receptor-negative (n = 167).

Compared with those eating 3 or fewer servings per week of red meat, the multivariate relative risks (95% confidence intervals) for ER+/PR+ breast cancer with increasing servings of red meat intake were 1.14 (0.90-1.45) for more than 3 to 5 or fewer servings per week, 1.42 (1.06-1.90) for more than 5 per week to 1 or fewer servings per day, 1.20 (0.89-1.63) for more than 1 to 1.5 or fewer servings per day, and 1.97 (1.35-2.88) for more than 1.5 servings per day (test for trend, P = .001) [27].

Phytoestrogens present in soy are structurally and functionally similar to estrogen and have hence received significant attention as potential dietary modifiers of breast cancer risk. High soy and phytoestrogen consumption in adolescence are related to lower breast cancer rates in several case-control studies [28,29]. Asian studies showed that an increased intake of isoflavones (range of 5–20 mg per day) reduced the risk of breast cancer [30]; a meta analysis of published studies on soy consumption and breast cancer noted a significant protective effect of high soy intake on risk of breast cancer [31].

Several studies show a positive association between alcohol consumption and breast cancer, especially for estrogen- and progesterone receptor-positive cancers, such as study of Nurses' Health Study II, that shows a statically difference comparing more than 1.5/d servings to $\leq$ 3/wk. Alcohol represents a risk factor possibly mediated by the direct effect of metabolites such as acetaldehyde or oxygen radicals, estimating a 10% increased risk per every 10 gr of alcohol consumed [32,33].

Physical activity and obesity are closely related through many factors that may independently or jointly influence breast cancer risk (eg, estrogen levels, body-fat distribution, insulin levels, insulin-like growth hormone, and mammographic density). Although observational studies provide evidence that higher levels of physical activity result in lower rates of breast cancer [34], some researchers have argued that intervention trials are needed to better define this relationship [35], even though the feasibility of maintaining compliance for a sufficiently long time is doubtful. Moreover, diets with low fat and glycemic index and regular physical activity are an important weight-control strategy, and synergism between dietary patterns and exercise could diminish breast cancer incidence and improve the prognosis of the patients, as proved in a recent prospective observational cohort studies.

The first study included 670 women with breast cancer diagnosis, patients consuming better-quality diets (defined by higher healthy eating index- 2005 scores) had a 88% reduced risk of death from breast cancer (HR(Q4:Q1) = 0.12, 95% CI: 0.02, 0.99) compared with inactive survivors consuming poor-quality diets. Survivors engaging in any recreational physical activity and consuming better-quality diets had a 91% reduced risk of death from breast cancer (HR: 0.09, 95% CI: 0.01, 0.89) [36]. The second study including 65,374 women with 2381 postmenopausal invasive breast cancer cases, 2 relevant dietary patterns related to breast cancer risk were identified. An alcohol/Western dietary pattern was positively associated with breast cancer risk (HR = 1.20; 95% CI: 1.03–1.38, p = 0.007), whereas the healthy/Mediterranean dietary pattern was negatively associated with breast cancer risk (HR, 0.85; 95% CI: 0.75–0.95, p = 0.003), especially when tumors were estrogen-receptor (ER) positive [37].

4. Tamoxifen Treatment and Obesity

For more than 30 years, Tamoxifen has been used to reduce the risk of both recurrence and contralateral breast cancers. Studies show that this hormone therapy reduces the incidence of recurrent breast cancer by 42%, and the incidence of contralateral breast cancer by 47% [38]. This anti-estrogen treatment is the standard of care in patients with ER-positive breast cancer [39.40].

Thus, if the pharmacological therapy is focused on diminishing the estrogen levels, and at the same time, high fat volume is associated with elevated levels of serum estrogen, an important question concerning obesity and breast cancer is whether obesity affects treatment efficacy; an integral treatment of these patients including nutritional strategies must be considerate, in order to avoid overweight and insulin resistance.

Consistent with studies; in a large cohort study (n=3,385) evaluating Tamoxifen for lymph node-negative, ER-positive breast cancer [41], results shows that contralateral breast cancer HR was higher in obese women than in underweight/normal-weight women (HR 1.58, 95% CI=1.10-2.25) and higher risk of other primary cancers (HR= 1.62, 95%CI= 1.16-2.24) Figure 1.

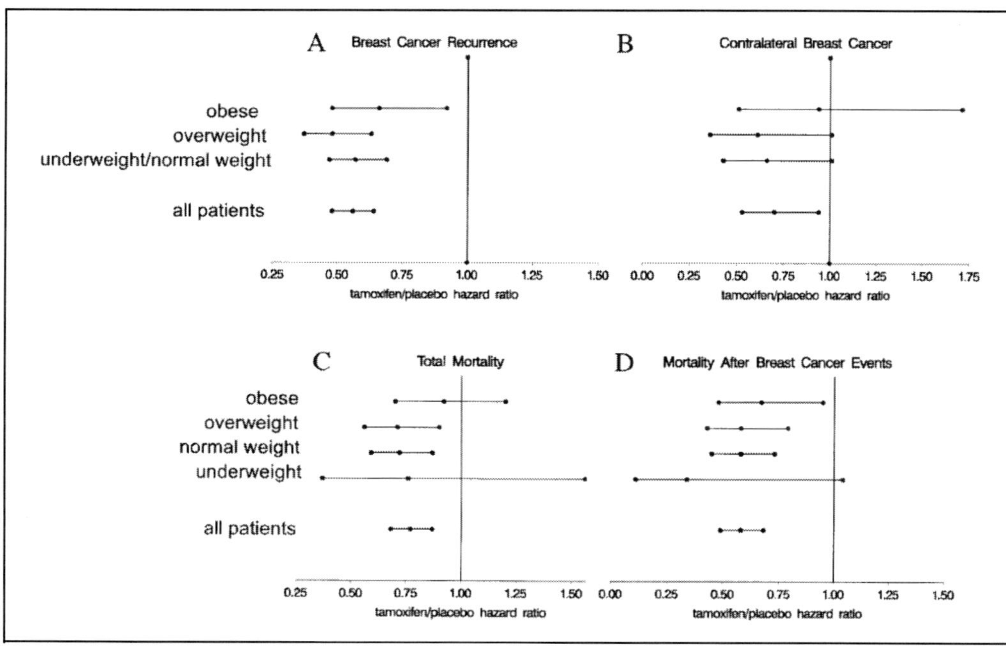

Figure 1. [41]. Tamoxifen/placebo HR according to BMI. HR with 95% CI was computed within BMI categories for breast cancer recurrence (A) and contralateral breast cancer (B). HR with 95% CI were computed within BMI categories (obese, overweight, normal weight, underweight) for all deaths (c) and deaths preceded by breast cancer recurrence or occurrence of contralateral breast tumor (D). for all panels, HR of less than 1.0 indicate a more favorable outcome for women receiving Tamoxifen.

Another important point is Tamoxifen dosage (ie, whether the standard dose of 20 mg daily is sufficient across the full range of BMIs). Although Sestak et al [42] reported that BMI was not significantly associated with risk of recurrence in those receiving tamoxifen, there was a modest increase of risk in those with BMIs greater than 35 kg/m2 (HR=1.18; 95%CI, 0.90 to 1.84).

Given these findings suggest that a 1-mg daily dose of anastrozole may be insufficient to adequately reduce estrogen levels in heavier patients, rigorous examination of BMI-related efficacy in other randomized trials in both the adjuvant and metastatic settings is critically important [7].

5. Tamoxifen and Steatosis

Non-alcoholic steatohepatitis (NASH) is associated with some medications, possibly including Tamoxifen, albeit the exact mechanism is not known, this therapy has been shown to increase hepatic fat content by blocking the role of estrogen in maintaining hepatic lipid homeostasis by supporting the expression of genes involved in lipid β-oxidation [43]. Other reports in which hypertriglceridemia was recognized as a risk factor for inducing NASH in patients using Tamoxifen, authors conclude that this hormone therapy may induce hypertriglyceridemia and, via this mechanism, also may produce fatty changes in the liver [1-44].

Imaging studies documented the development of fatty liver in approximately 33% of patients treated with Tamoxifen [45-51]; Saphner et al [52] evaluated 1,105 patients and found a NASH prevalence of 2.2%, seven patients had NASH before their diagnosis of breast cancer and 17 patients developed NASH after their diagnosis of breast cancer. In multivariate analysis, the factors associated with NASH in these patients were Tamoxifen, BMI >25 kg/m^2, and age; the median time to development of NASH was 22 months; Transaminase levels tended to return to normal after Tamoxifen was discontinued. Authors concluded that routine liver function testing is not required even in patients who have other risk factors for NASH as obesity, diabetes and alcohol intake. If a patient does develop NASH while on Tamoxifen, it is reasonable to stop Tamoxifen and consider other therapy. Cirrhosis is a rare complication, Bruno et al documented a prevalence: 0 of 2540 patients who took Tamoxifen [53].

Conclusion

Due to the high incidence of breast cancer, risk-reduction strategies are essential. While there is no clear evidence that specific dietary components can effectively reduce breast cancer risk, weight gain and obesity in adulthood are important factors in the development of postmenopausal breast cancer.

Additional research will be required to determine whether more complete pharmaceutical estrogen suppression is sufficient to improve breast cancer outcomes, or if additional strategies that target other potential mediators of obesity-related prognostics effects like diet patterns and physical activity will also be necessary to improve prognosis in these patients. Besides, women with this pathology should be encouraged to maintain a healthy lifestyle for their overall well-being and to remain up-to-date with recommendations for screening and surveillance.

References

[1] Akhondi-Meybodi, M., Mortazavy-Zadah, M.R., Hashemian, Z., Moaiedi, M. Incidence and risk factors for non-alcoholic steatohepatitis in females treated with tamoxifen for breast cancer. *Arab. J. Gastroenterol.* 2011;12:34-6.

[2] Stuckey, A. Breast cancer: epidemiology and risk factors. *Clin Obstet Gynecol* 2011;54:96-102.

[3] Moorman, P.G., Jones, B.A., Millikan, R.C., Hall, I.J., Newman, B. Race, anthropometric factors, and stage at diagnosis of breast cancer. *Am. J. Epidemiol.* 2001;153:284-91.

[4] Cui, Y., Whiteman, M.K., Flaws, J.A., Langenberg, P., Tkaczuk, K.H., Bush, T.L. Body mass and stage of breast cancer at diagnosis. *Int. J. Cancer* 2002;98:279-83.

[5] Zhang, S., Folsom, A.R., Sellers, T.A., Kushi, L.H., Potter, J.D. Better breast cancer survival for postmenopausal women who are less overweight and eat less fat. The Iowa Women's Health Study. *Cancer* 1995;76:275-83.

[6] Bernstein, L., Ross, R.K. Endogenous hormones and breast cancer risk. *Epidemiol. Rev.* 1993;15:48-65.

[7] Goodwin, P.J., Pritchard, K.I. Obesity and hormone therapy in breast cancer: an unfinished puzzle. *J. Clin. Oncol.* 2010;28:3405-7.

[8] Cleary, M.P., Grossmann, M.E., Ray, A. Effect of obesity on breast cancer development. Vet Pathol 2010;47:202-13.

[9] McTiernan, A., Irwin, M., Vongruenigen, V. Weight, physical activity, diet and prognosis in breast and gynecologic cancers. *J. Clin. Oncol.* 2010;28:4074-80.

[10] Eliassen, A.H., Colditz, G.A., Rosner, B., Willett, W.C., Hankinson, S.E. Adult weight change and risk of postmenopausal breast cancer. *JAMA* 2006;296:193-201.

[11] Garofalo, C., Koda, M., Cascio, S., et al. Increased expression of leptin and the leptin receptor as a marker of breast cancer progression: possible role of obesity-related stimuli. *Clin. Cancer Res.* 2006;12:1447-53.

[12] Bartella, V., Cascio, S., Fiorio, E., Auriemma, A., Russo, A., Surmacz, E. Insulin-dependent leptin expression in breast cancer cells. *Cancer Res.* 2008;68:4919-27.

[13] Cascio, S., Bartella, V., Auriemma, A., et al. Mechanism of leptin expression in breast cancer cells: role of hypoxia-inducible factor-1alpha. *Oncogene* 2008;27:540-7.

[14] Garofalo, C., Surmacz, E. Leptin and cancer. J Cell Physiol 2006;207: 12-22.

[15] Surmacz, E. Obesity hormone leptin: a new target in breast cancer? *Breast Cancer Res.* 2007;9:301.

[16] Ishikawa, M., Kitayama, J., Nagawa, H. Enhanced expression of leptin and leptin receptor (OB-R) in human breast cancer. *Clin. Cancer Res.* 2004;10:4325-31.

[17] Hauner, H., Hauner, D. The Impact of Nutrition on the Development and Prognosis of Breast Cancer. *Breast Care* (Basel) 2010;5:377-81.

[18] Singletary, S.E. Rating the risk factors for breast cancer. *Ann. Surg.* 2003;237:474-82.

[19] Thiebaut, A.C., Kipnis, V., Chang, S.C., et al. Dietary fat and postmenopausal invasive breast cancer in the National Institutes of Health-AARP Diet and Health Study cohort. *J. Natl. Cancer Inst.* 2007;99:451-62.

[20] Boyd, N.F., Stone, J., Vogt, K.N., Connelly, B.S., Martin, L.J., Minkin, S. Dietary fat and breast cancer risk revisited: a meta-analysis of the published literature. *Br. J. Cancer* 2003;89:1672-85.

[21] Prentice, R.L., Caan, B., Chlebowski, R.T., et al. Low-fat dietary pattern and risk of invasive breast cancer: the Women's Health Initiative Randomized Controlled Dietary Modification Trial. *JAMA* 2006;295:629-42.

[22] Smith-Warner, S.A., Spiegelman, D., Adami, H.O., et al. Types of dietary fat and breast cancer: a pooled analysis of cohort studies. *Int. J. Cancer* 2001;92:767-74.

[23] Mahoney, M.C., Bevers, T., Linos, E., Willett, W.C. Opportunities and strategies for breast cancer prevention through risk reduction. *CA Cancer J. Clin* 2008;58:347-71.

[24] Sieri, S., Pala, V., Brighenti, F., et al. Dietary glycemic index, glycemic load, and the risk of breast cancer in an Italian prospective cohort study. *Am. J. Clin. Nutr.* 2007;86: 1160-6.

[25] Michels, K.B., Mohllajee, A.P., Roset-Bahmanyar, E., Beehler, G.P., Moysich, K.B. Diet and breast cancer: a review of the prospective observational studies. *Cancer* 2007;109:2712-49.

[26] Frazier, A.L., Li, L., Cho, E., Willett, W.C., Colditz, G.A. Adolescent diet and risk of breast cancer. *Cancer Causes Control* 2004;15:73-82.

[27] Cho, E., Chen, W.Y., Hunter, D.J., et al. Red meat intake and risk of breast cancer among premenopausal women. *Arch. Intern. Med.* 2006;166:2253-9.

[28] Wu, A.H., Wan, P., Hankin, J., Tseng, C.C., Yu, M.C., Pike, M.C. Adolescent and adult soy intake and risk of breast cancer in Asian-Americans. *Carcinogenesis* 2002;23:1491-6.

[29] Thanos, J.C.M., Boucher, B.A., et al. Adolescent dietary phytoestrogen intake and breast cancer risk (Canada). . *Cancer Causes Control* 2006:1253-61.

[30] Wu, A.H., Yu, M.C., Tseng, C.C., Pike, M.C. Epidemiology of soy exposures and breast cancer risk. *Br. J. Cancer* 2008;98:9-14.

[31] Trock, B.J. H-CL, Clarke, R. . Metaanalysis of soy intake and breast cancer risk. *J. Nat. Cancer Inst.* 2006;98:459-71.

[32] Hamajima, N., Hirose, K., Tajima, K., et al. Alcohol, tobacco and breast cancer--collaborative reanalysis of individual data from 53 epidemiological studies, including 58,515 women with breast cancer and 95,067 women without the disease. *Br. J. Cancer* 2002;87:1234-45.

[33] Zhang, S.M., Lee, I.M., Manson, J.E., Cook, N.R., Willett, W.C., Buring, J.E. Alcohol consumption and breast cancer risk in the Women's Health Study. *Am. J. Epidemiol.* 2007;165:667-76.

[34] Friedenreich, C.M., Orenstein, M.R. Physical activity and cancer prevention: etiologic evidence and biological mechanisms. J. Nutr. 2002;132:3456S-64S.

[35] Irwin, M.L. Randomized controlled trials of physical activity and breast cancer prevention. *Exerc. Sport. Sci. Rev.* 2006;34:182-93.

[36] George, S.M., Irwin, M.L., Smith, A.W., et al. Postdiagnosis diet quality, the combination of diet quality and recreational physical activity, and prognosis after early-stage breast cancer. *Cancer Causes Control* 2011;22:589-98.

[37] Cottet, V., Touvier, M., Fournier, A., et al. Postmenopausal breast cancer risk and dietary patterns in the E3N-EPIC prospective cohort study. *Am. J. Epidemiol.* 2009;170: 1257-67.

[38] Tamoxifen for early breast cancer: an overview of the randomised trials. Early Breast Cancer Trialists' Collaborative Group. *Lancet* 1998;351:1451-67.

[39] Fleeman, N., Martin, Saborido C., Payne, K., et al. The clinical effectiveness and cost-effectiveness of genotyping for CYP2D6 for the management of women with breast cancer treated with tamoxifen: a systematic review. *Health Technol. Assess.* 2011;15: 1-102.

[40] Thurlimann, B., Keshaviah, A., Coates, A.S., et al. A comparison of letrozole and tamoxifen in postmenopausal women with early breast cancer. *N. Engl. J. Med.* 2005;353:
2747-57.

[41] Dignam, J., Wieand, K., Johnson, K.A., Fisher, B., Xu L. Obesity, Tamoxifen Use and outcomes in Women With Estrogen Receptor-Positive Early-Stage Breast Cancer. *J. Nat. Cancer Inst.* 2003;95:1467-76.

[42] Sestak, I., Distler, W., Forbes, J.F., Dowsett, M., Howell, A., Cuzick, J. Effect of body mass index on recurrences in tamoxifen and anastrozole treated women: an exploratory analysis from the ATAC trial. *J. Clin. Oncol.* 2010;28:3411-5.

[43] Osman, K.A. O.M., Ahmed, M.H. Tamoxifen-induced non-alcoholic steatohepatitis: where are we now and where are we going*? Expert Opin. Drug Saf.* 2007;6:1-4.

[44] Gudbrandsen, O.A., Rost, T.H., Berge, R.K. Causes and prevention of tamoxifen-induced accumulation of triacylglycerol in rat liver. *J. Lipid Res.* 2006;47:2223-32.

[45] Ogawa, Y., Murata, Y., Nishioka, A., Inomata, T., Yoshida, S. Tamoxifen-induced fatty liver in patients with breast cancer. *Lancet* 1998;351:725.

[46] Murata, Y., Ogawa, Y., Saibara, T., et al. Unrecognized hepatic steatosis and non-alcoholic steatohepatitis in adjuvant tamoxifen for breast cancer patients. *Oncol. Rep.* 2000;7:1299-304.

[47] Nguyen, M.C., Stewart, R.B., Banerji, M.A., Gordon, D.H., Kral, J.G. Relationships between tamoxifen use, liver fat and body fat distribution in women with breast cancer. *Int. J. Obes. Relat. Metab. Disord.* 2001;25:296-8.

[48] Nemoto, Y., Saibara, T., Ogawa, Y., et al. Tamoxifen-induced non-alcoholic steatohepatitis in breast cancer patients treated with adjuvant tamoxifen. *Intern. Med.* 2002;41:345-50.

[49] Murata, Y., Ogawa, Y., Saibara, T., et al. Tamoxifen-induced non-alcoholic steatohepatitis in patients with breast cancer: determination of a suitable biopsy site for diagnosis. *Oncol. Rep.* 2003;10:97-100.

[50] Ogawa, Y., Murata, Y., Saibara, T., Nishioka, A., Kariya, S., Yoshida, S. Follow-up CT findings of tamoxifen-induced non-alcoholic steatohepatitis (NASH) of breast cancer patients treated with bezafibrate. *Oncol. Rep.* 2003;10:1473-8.

[51] Gunel, N., Coskun, U., Toruner, F.B., et al. Serum leptin levels are associated with tamoxifen-induced hepatic steatosis. *Curr. Med. Res. Opin.* 2003;19:47-50.

[52] Saphner, T., Triest-Robertson, S., Li, H., Holzman, P. The association of non-alcoholic steatohepatitis and tamoxifen in patients with breast cancer. *Cancer* 2009;115:3189-95.

[53] Bruno, S., Maisonneuve, P., Castellana, P., et al. Incidence and risk factors for non-alcoholic steatohepatitis: prospective study of 5408 women enrolled in Italian tamoxifen chemoprevention trial. *BMJ* 2005;330:932.

In: Tamoxifen Concepts and Cancer: New Paradigms
Editor: Ramon Andrade de Mello
ISBN: 978-1-62081-520-5

Chapter XII

Electrically Enhanced Tamoxifen Delivery for Breast Cancer Treatments

Ignacio G. Camarillo[1], Maxine Nichols[1], Funian Xiao[1], Therese Salameh[1], Arutselvan Natarajan[2], Ganesh Venkatraman[3] and Raji Sundararajan[1*]

[1]Purdue University, West Lafayette, IN, US
[2]Stanford Medical School, Stanford, CA, US
[3]Sri Ramachandra University, Chennai, India

Abstract

Tamoxifen is one of the most effective anti-hormonal agents for the treatment of estrogen receptor-positive breast cancer, for both pre- and post-menopausal patients. However, with its poor response rate of 21% to 41%, it is not benefitting all the estrogen receptor-positive (ER+) patients. This necessitates its delivery using other means, whose attributes include less-invasive, physical and lower dosages. Electrical pulse-mediated drug delivery is gaining momentum as a promising alternate technique. This involves the application of high intensity, short pulses that open up the normally impermeable cell plasma membranes allowing the external drug molecules in. This chapter presents the findings of the in vitro study of electrical pulse-mediated Tamoxifen delivery on MCF-7 breast cancer cells at low and high voltages and at various durations, from milli to micro to nanoseconds, and their efficacies. Our results indicate the proliferation control of breast cancer cells using as low as one to five μM dosages of Tamoxifen at an electric field strenth of 200V/cm and the potential of transferring this technique for clinical use for treating those patients who do not respond well to current Tamoxifen therapy.

* E-mail: raji@purdue.edu 765 494 6912.

Introduction

Once a disease of the industrialized, affluent western world, today, breast cancer is everywhere, including Asia, Africa, and Eastern Europe [1]. It is the second most common cancer among women, estimated at 719,000 cases worldwide, with thousands of deaths, as conventional treatments, such as surgery, radiation therapy and chemotherapy do not work for all patients as indicated by the above deaths and the poor response rate of most commonly used breast cancer drugs (Table 1 [2]).

Thus, there is a compelling need for the development of alternate, affordable therapies, that are less costly and have fewer side effects. In addition, there is a lack of safe and efficient delivery systems that allow a drug to easily enter the cell through the plasma membrane. Medicines administered orally must circulate throughout the entire body before taking effect. This poses a potential threat to the patient, as the drug could take action in any part of the body causing adverse effects, as well as creating an opportunity for the drug to be broken down through enzymatic degradation. An improved delivery system, such as electroporation, which will provide a more targeted pathway into the cell, will increase the cell's receptiveness to the drug and enhance the drug's capabilities while reducing systemic effects.

Table 1. Response rate of metastatic breast cancer to single drug systemic therapy [2]

Drug	Response Rate
Tamoxifen	21% to 41%
Doxorubicin	25% to 40%
Paclitaxel	17% to 54%
Trastuzumab	10% to 20%

The goal of our research is to develop safe and efficient novel therapies to treat breast tumors using electrical pulses to enhance drug uptake for breast cancer treatment as it is less costly, has fewer side effects, and is simple (could be performed as an outpatient treatment [3]), requiring no costly outfits, like a radiation facility. The attractiveness of this technique is that it is applicable to all types of histologies of cancers at any stage, due to its very physical nature. Since charge distribution contributes to the cytotoxicity of membranes and cells, it is possible to reap enormous benefits from applications of electrical pulses for targeted macromolecular delivery where they redistribute the charges and the synergy of the drug and pulses results in an improved outcome compared to drug alone, and thus the reduction in the dosage and the associated side effects and cost. This physical technique, known as electroporation or electropermeabilization (EP) utilizes precisely controlled electric fields of short duration (microseconds) and high intensities to open up transient pores (aqueous pathways) through semi-permeable membranes and tissues allowing targeted delivery of therapeutic materials including drugs, antibodies and genes (DNA) [3-5].

EP has been shown to offer a 100-1000 fold improved therapeutic benefit compared to using a drug alone, and is gaining acceptance as a viable technique to enhance the efficacy of drug delivery for cancer treatment, gene transfer and similar applications in biology, biotechnology and medicine [6-8].

Electroporation-mediated chemotherapy-electrochemotherapy (ECT) is a viable alternative to conventional cancer treatments as evidenced by successful Phase I and II clinical trials for various skin cancers, such as lymphomas, squamous cell carcinomas, testicular carcinomas, and malignant pleural effusions [3, 7, 8]. When surgery, radiotherapy, and/or chemotherapy did not work, ECT was found to be effective for the treatment of chest wall breast carcinoma [9, 10].

Typically, eight 1200 or 1300V/cm, 100μs pulses at one second intervals are used for the clinical trials [3-10]. Recently, ultra-short pulses of nanosecond (ns) durations such as 10-300ns and 10 to 300kV/cm have been used for electroporation [11-14]. For example, three 60ns, 60kV/cm pulses at one second intervals [14] applied in a nanosecond pulse study on Jurkat cells induced apoptosis.

In addition, nano pulses of 300ns, 26kV/cm and 10ns, 150kV/cm strengths were also studied. In the present study, we have investigated the effects of milli, micro, and nanosecond pulses at low (200V/cm), high (1200V/cm) and medium (400V/cm) voltages using low doses of Tamoxifen.

Tamoxifen Characteristics

Pharmacology

Tamoxifen is a pro-drug which has less affinity for its target protein, the estrogen receptor. It is metabolized in the liver by the cytochrome P450 isoform CYP2D6 and CYP3A4 into active metabolites such as 4-hydroxytamoxifen and N-desmethyl-4-hydroxytamoxifen which have 30-100 times more affinity with the estrogen receptor than Tamoxifen itself. Figure 1 shows the biotransformation and mechanism of action of Tamoxifen. These active metabolites compete with estrogen in the body for binding to the estrogen receptor. In breast tissue, 4-hydroxytamoxifen acts as an estrogen receptor antagonist so that transcription of estrogen-responsive genes is inhibited [15].

Mechanism of Action

Tamoxifen binds to ER, inducing a conformational change in the receptor. The ER/Tamoxifen complex recruits co-repressors - NCoR (nuclear receptor co-repressor 1) and SMRT (nuclear receptor co-repressor 2) which results in a blockage or change in the expression of estrogen dependent genes. In the presence of high PAX2 expression (Paired box gene 2), the Tamoxifen/estrogen receptor complex is able to suppress the expression of the pro-proliferative ERBB2 protein [16, 17]. The prolonged binding of Tamoxifen to the nuclear chromatin of these complexes results in reduced DNA polymerase activity, impaired thymidine utilization, blockade of estradiol uptake, and decreased estrogen response thus inhibiting the cell cycle in G_0 and G_1 phase.

It is likely that Tamoxifen interacts with other coactivators or corepressors in the tissue and binds with different estrogen receptors, ER-α or ER-β, producing both estrogenic and antiestrogenic effects.

Pharmacodynamics

Following a single oral dose of 20 mg Tamoxifen, an average peak plasma concentration of 40 ng/mL occurs approximately 5 hours after dosing. The decline in plasma concentrations of Tamoxifen is biphasic with a terminal elimination half-life of about 5 to 7 days. Women receiving 20mg of Tamoxifen have shown approximately 65% of the administered dose excreted from the body over a period of 2 weeks with fecal excretion as the primary route of elimination.

Side effects

The common side effects of Tamoxifen include

- Hot flashes
- Vaginal discharge
- Water retention
- Irregular menstrual periods
- Weight loss
- Vaginal bleeding

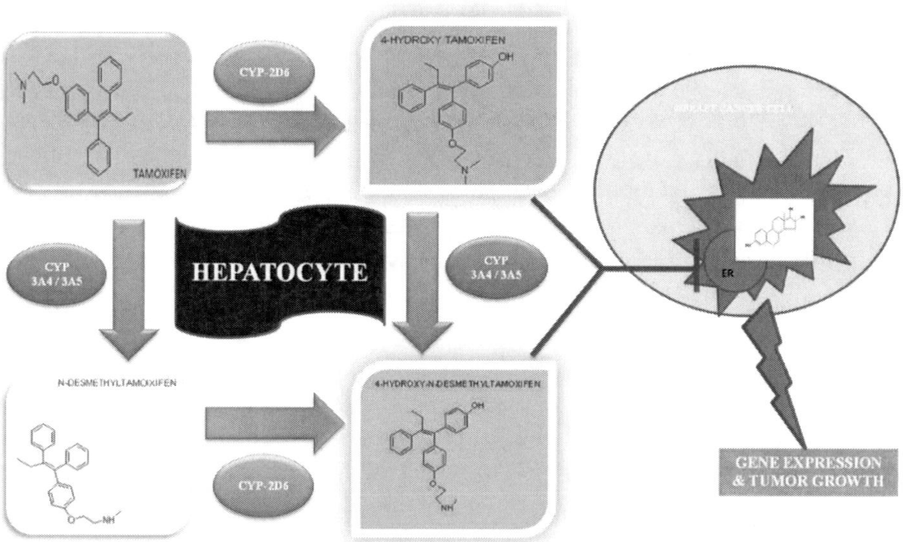

Figure 1. Biotransformation and mechanism of action of Tamoxifen.
Tamoxifen, a selective estrogen receptor modulator (SERM) used in the treatment of ER(+) breast cancer is hydroxylated by CYP2D6 and demethylated by CYP3A4 and CYP3A5, producing the active metabolites 4-hydroxytamoxifen and endoxifen (4-hydroxy-N-Desmethyl Tamoxifen), which possess anti-estrogen activity. These metabolites inhibit estrogen binding to ER in breast cancer cells, which, in turn, inhibit tumor growth.

Usage

The first clinical trial demonstrated that Tamoxifen given in addition to chemotherapy improved survival for patients with early breast cancer [18]. Since then, Tamoxifen has been used for the treatment of both early and advanced estrogen receptor-positive (ER+) breast cancer in pre- and post-menopausal women [19].

Additionally, it is also the most common hormone treatment for male breast cancer [20]. It is also approved by the FDA for the prevention of breast cancer in women at high risk of developing the disease [21]. It has been further approved for the reduction of contralateral (in the opposite breast) cancer.

The detailed study by Cuzick et al reported the long term biological effects of Tamoxifen in 153 breast cancer patients who participated in two trials of adjuvant Tamoxifen and who had not recurred were recruited into a study of the long term effects of Tamoxifen [22]. This study report confirmed that there were no potential biological negative side-effects.

Resistance to Tamoxifen

The estrogen antagonist, Tamoxifen is a commonly used anti-tumor agent for the treatment of ER-positive breast cancer. Although many patients benefit from Tamoxifen in the adjuvant and metastatic settings, resistance is an important clinical problem. The resistance to treatment can be attributed to changes in the expression of ERα or ERβ, alterations in co-regulatory proteins, and the influences of cellular kinase signal transduction pathways [23].

Thus, electrical-pulse-mediated Tamoxifen delivery is a viable option.

Materials and Methods

The Cells - MCF-7 Breast Cancer Cells

In this research, MCF-7, estrogen receptor-positive breast cancer cells were used (Figure 2). They were cultured in a mixture media of 90% RPMI 1640, 10% FBS serum (ATTC, Manassas, VA), and 1% Penicillin/Streptomysin (Invitrogen, Carlsbad, CA.). Cells grow in an incubator at $37^{o}C$ with 5% CO_2. After 24 hours, cells were washed twice with warm 7.4pH 1x PBS. Then they are left in a culture cell plate with serum-free-199 medium (Invitrogen) in the incubator for 24 hours before the electroporation.

For electroporation, the cells are transferred from the plate into a 750μL cuvette with a mixed medium made of 90% RPMI 1640 and 10% charcoal stripped fetal bovine serum. The density of the cells was $1x10^6$/mL.

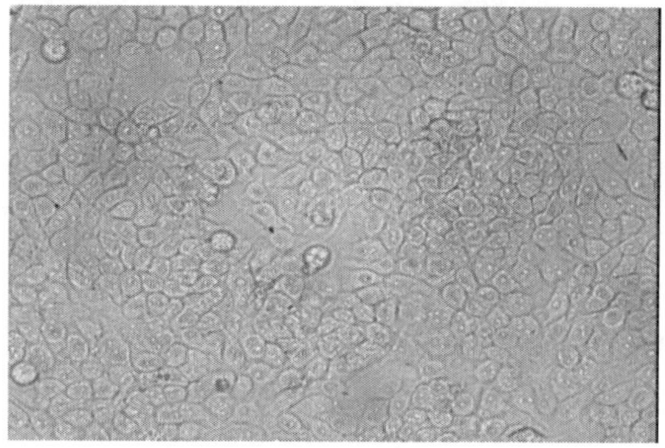

Figure 2. MCF-7 breast cancer cells under microscope.

The Drug - Tamoxifen

Tamoxifen (Figure 3) is a SERM with tissue-specific activity. It acts as an anti-estrogen (inhibiting agent) in the mammary tissue, but as an estrogen (stimulating agent) in cholesterol metabolism, bone density, and cell proliferation in the endometrium. The anti-estrogenic activity of Tamoxifen is attributed to an additional side chain - the *trans* isomer [24].

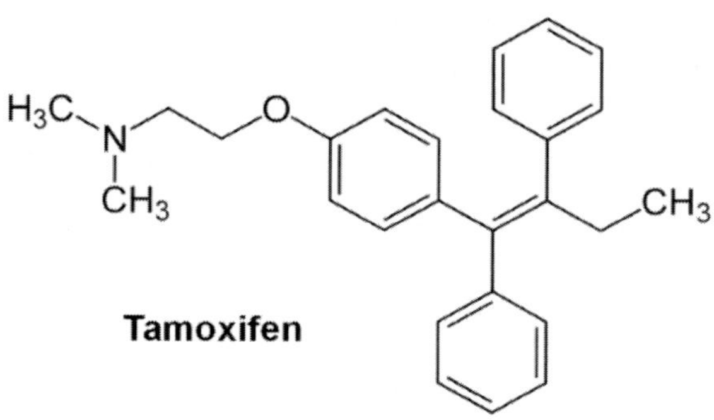

Figure 3. Chemical structure of Tamoxifen.

Under SERM categories, Tamoxifen belongs to the non-steroidal triphenylethylene family which exhibits steroid mimicking characteristics, and therefore adopts a structural conformation which resembles the steroid nucleus and effectively blocks the ER sites and hinders binding of estrogen thereby inhibiting tumor cell proliferation [25].

The Technique - Electroporation

Typically two conditions have to be met for efficient ECT. First, sufficient amounts of a chemotherapeutic drug must be present in the targeted tissue/tumor when the pulses are applied. Second, electric pulses have to be of appropriate magnitude to create reversible (transient) pores in the cell plasma membranes. Thus, it is critical to choose appropriate electrical parameters to achieve pore formation in the cell membrane without cell death. Typically, 1200 or 1300V/cm, 100μs pulses were applied in the skin cancer trials [3-10].

Most studies have used 6 or 8 pulses with an interval of 1s (1Hz) [3, 4, 7]. In our study, we investigated the efficacies of milli, micro and nanosecond pulses.

Using Milli and Microsecond Pulses

Both high intensity, short duration pulses (1200V/cm, 100 and 200μs, used in the clinical electrochemotherapy trials [8-10]) and low intensity, long duration pulses (200V/cm, 10-40ms, 100V/cm, 1ms) were investigated in this study. In order to study the effects of intermediate values, 400V/cm, 20ms, and 500V/cm, 260μs pulses were also studied. Each trial with the above parameters used 8 pulses at a frequency of 1Hz, unless otherwise mentioned.

A BTX ECM 830 (Genetronics, Inc, San Diego, CA), square wave electroporator with 0.4cm (electrode gap) cuvette was used in this study. The electroporation buffer used was DMEM.

The sample to be electroporated is taken in the cuvette and is generally fixed at a volume of 200μL. For those experiments requiring electroporation without any drug, 100μL of the cell suspension with 100μL of media is electroporated. For electroporation in the presence of the drug, 100μL of cell suspension was made up to 200μL with DMEM, after the addition of an appropriate volume of the drug. The micro and millisecond pulses were applied using BTX ECM830 commercial, square wave electroporator (Figure 4).

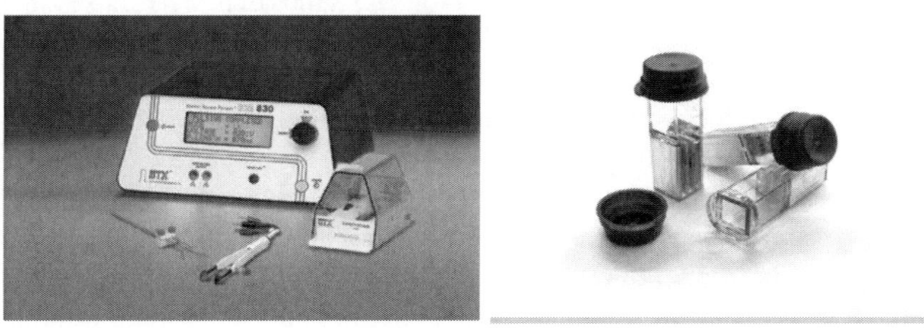

(a) (b)

Figure 4. a) BTX ECM 830 Square Wave Electroporator with the Cuvette Holder (that holds the cells), b) Cuvettes used for Electroporation Study.

Using Nanosecond Pulses

20ns pulses voltages were applied at 200V/cm for 10minutes; 500V/cm for 5minutes and 1200V/cm for 5minutes.

For this purpose, the pulse generator designed and developed in our lab, a 0 to 1000V, compact (just 4" x 4" x 2"), MOSFET-based nanosecond pulser was used that could operate using a 9.6VDC rechargeable battery, with variable pulse durations of 20ns to 20μs and with variable pulse repetition rate (PRF) of 1 kHz to 6 kHz.

The Assay -Cell Viability and Growth Assay

A cytometer, auto-T4 Cellometer Auto (Nexcelom Bioscience LLC., MA) along with software that works similar to a hemacytometer was used to study the viability of the various samples. It includes three components, an automatic microscope, a disposable counting slide and a computer. A mixture of 10μl of the cancer cells and equal volume trypan blue is made and 10μl of this is injected into the disposable slide, in each side. The disposable slide was loaded into the automatic microscope, which separates the slide into eight areas and then scans the number of live and dead cells in each area. The software in the computer contains various cell type profiles. Users can also customize any new cell profile. After scanning eight areas, the software calculates the viability of the cells based on the cell's profile.

Preparation of cells: after electroporation and incubation, cells suspended in media were stained with a 1:1 concentration of Trypan Blue. The dead cells are stained blue so they could be distinguished from the clear, live cells and were counted using the Cellometer.

Results and Discussion

Using Millisecond Pulses

Figure 5a shows the live cell numbers (Y-axis) and hence the viability of the MCF-7 cells due to the electroporation using 1μM concentration of Tamoxifen. The pulses applied were 200V/cm, at 10, 20, 30 and 40ms, denoted by LP1, LP2, LP3, and LP4, respectively. None is the control sample which had no treatment.

These results illustrate the reduction in the viability with an increase in the pulse duration for the same drug dose, indicating more cell death at longer pulse durations due to the increased energy applied. A comparison of these results with electroporation only cells (Figure 5b) indicate an increase in the cell viability using pulses only (without the drug). The reduction with pulses and Tamoxifen is about 39% compared to 28% using drug only. This illustrates the effectiveness of the combination therapy in controlling the proliferation of the cancer cells leading to effective curing of the cancer.

Using Micro and Millisecond Pulses

Figure 6 shows the viabilities at another set of various conditions of pulse parameters. Table 1 shows the micro- and millisecond electrical pulses used to deliver Tamoxifen in the MCF-7 cells. The control has no treatment. The next four samples were treated with electroporation only and the 6th sample is with drug only. The last four samples illustrate the synergy of the combination therapy investigated using both electrical pulses and the drug.

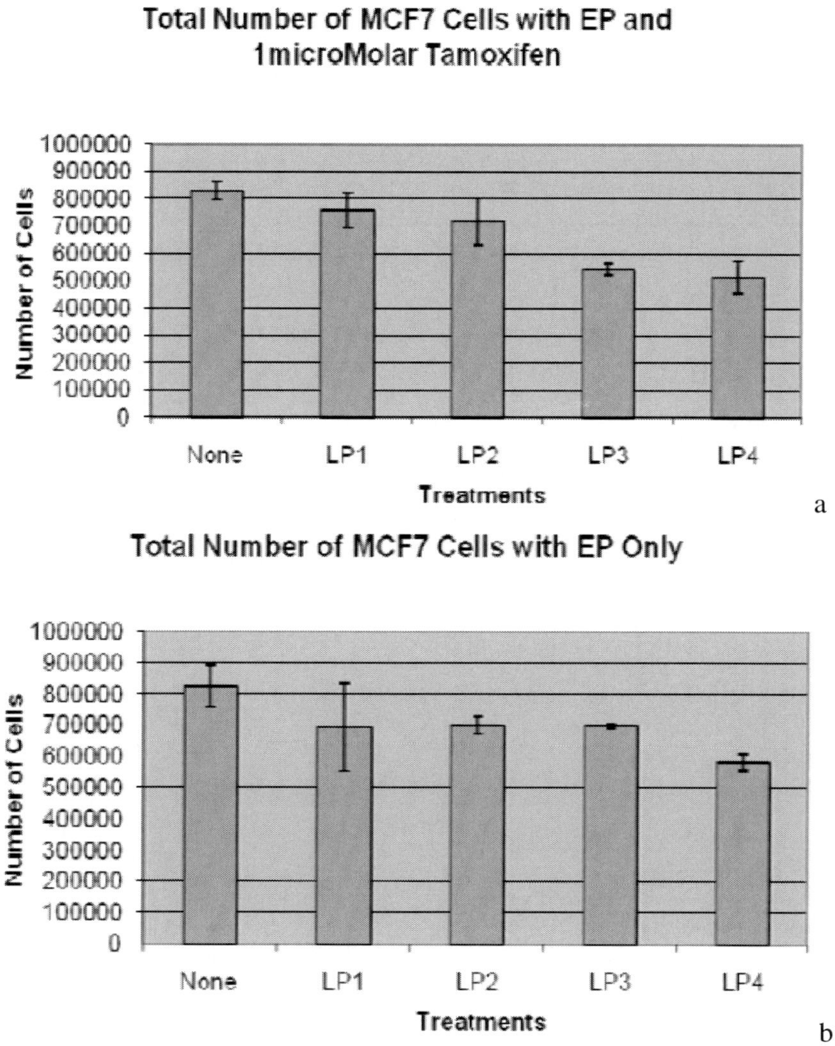

Figure 5. Viability using electroporation and 1μM Tamoxifen (a) and viability with electroporation only of MCF-7 cells. LP1, 2, 3, and 4 are 200V/cm, 10, 20, 30, and 40ms, respectively – 8 pulses at one second interval. None is the control sample that was not treated.

The four samples, after the control indicates that the viabilities of the two samples treated with the microsecond electrical pulse durations were reduced almost 15% compared with control, while the others with millisecond electrical pulse durations were reduced 20% compared with the control. The viability of the MCF-7 cancer cells treated with 5μM Tamoxifen only was reduced almost 20% compared with the control and was similar to the viability of samples treated with only electroporation.

The last four samples on the right depict the viabilities of electroporated samples with 5μM Tamoxifen. There is marked reduction in cell viability compared to no treatment or treatment with electrical pulses only or drug only, illustrating the efficacy of the combination therapy using 5μM concentration of Tamoxifen and micro and millisecond pulses.

The viability of MCF-7 cancer cells treated with 40ms electroporation and 5μM Tamoxifen is around 38% and has the least cells alive of all samples.

Table 1. Parameters of electroporation for Tamoxifen delivery

Sample	Electric field intensity (V/cm)	Pulse Duration	Pulse number	Pulse interval (s)
EP-100μs	1200	100μs	8	1
EP-200μs	1200	200μs	8	1
EP-30ms	200	30ms	8	1
EP-40ms	200	40ms	8	1

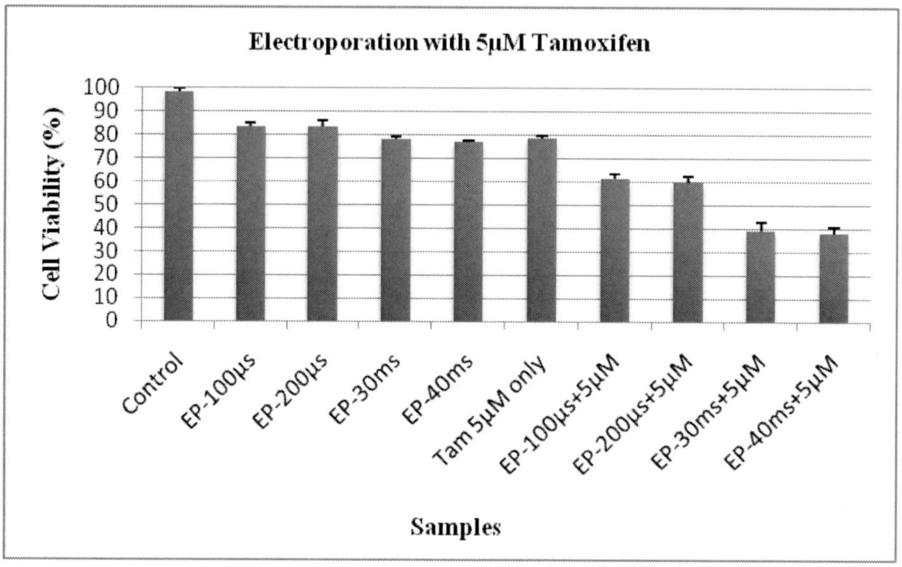

Figure 6. Viability of MCF-7 cancer cells treated with nothing, electrical pulses only, Tamoxifen only, and with electroporation+Tamoxifen.

The viability of cells treated with 30ms electroporation and 5μM Tamoxifen is 39%, almost the same as the 40ms sample with 5μM Tamoxifen. The viabilities of both samples have more than 50% reduction compared with control, almost 40% reduction compared with electroporation only and Tamoxifen only, and 20% compared with these samples treated with the 10 and 20millisecond electrical pulses and 5μM Tamoxifen.

Figure 7 shows yet another set of pulse conditions and Table 2 shows the details of the various pulses applied, ranging from high voltage to medium to low voltage pulses at micro and millisecond durations [27]. These pulse parameters were selected to see the efficacy of various pulse settings. Tamoxifen at one and five μM were studied under these pulse parameters.

The 1200V/cm, 100μs, 8 pulses seem to be the most lethal compared to other pulses in this group. The efficacy of 5μM is more severe than 1μM, causing more cell death for the all of the pulse parameters. This illustrates the dominance of the drug at higher doses for a given set of pulse conditions.

Using Nanosecond Pulses

Figure 8 shows the viability for various doses using 200, 500, and 1200V/cm, 20ns pulses for 10, 5 and 5 minutes, respectively, at 1 and 5μM concentration of Tamoxifen, along with control (no treatment) and Tamoxifen only (1μM). Each value is the average of three different sets of experiments (n=3, with very low standard deviation). There is a drastic reduction in the viability of the electroporated samples at 1 and 5μM compared to the control and drug alone for all of the three voltages. The viability of the control is around 89% in all three cases and it is 37.5%, 26.6% and 33,1% at 1μM for the 200V/cm, 1200V/cm, and 500V/cm pulses. The reductions were 36%, 57.5%, and 72.5%, respectively, for no drug, 1 and 5μM drug doses compared to the control when 200V/cm pulses were applied for10 minutes, indicating the excellent efficacy of these pulses at that dose.

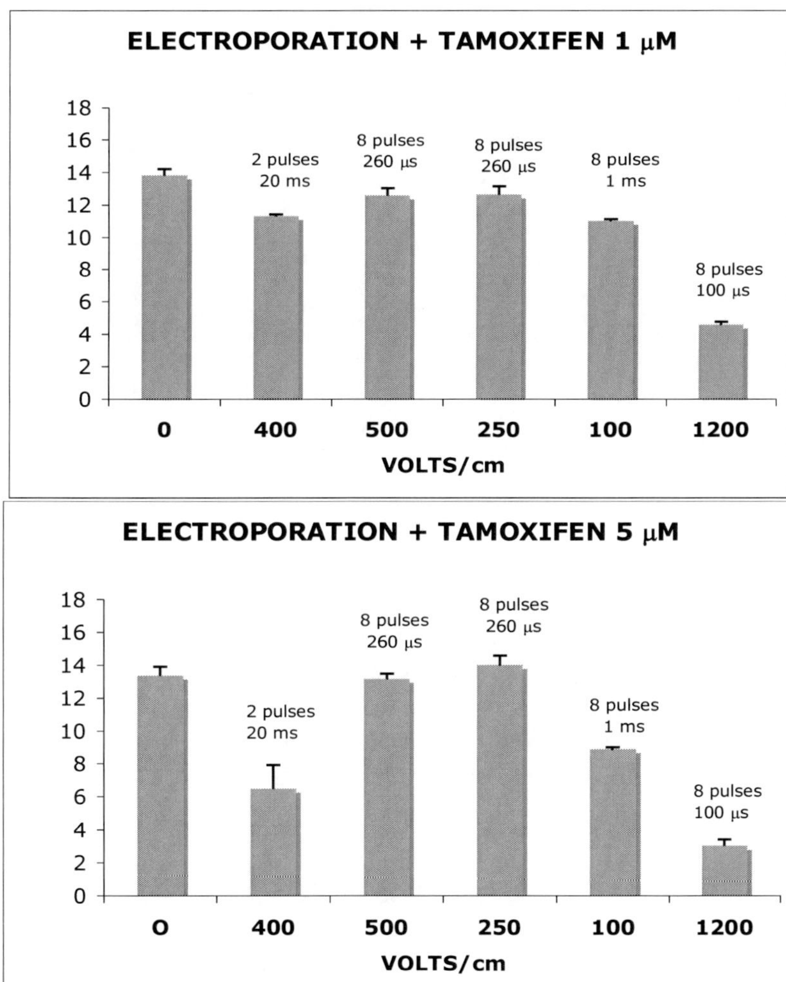

Figure 7. Effects of Tamoxifen and EP combination on MCF-7 cell growth using micro where the threshold p value < 0.05.) and millisecond pulses [27]. (Results are mean ± SEM from three experiments. Mean values significantly different from EP controls are indicated by an *. Statistical significance was determined by ANOVA and Tukey's tests, Y axis indicates number of cells).

Table 2. Parameters of electroporation for Tamoxifen delivery

Sample	Electric field intensity (V/cm)	Pulse Duration	Pulse number	Pulse interval (s)
1	-	-	-	-
2	100	1ms	8	1
3	250	260 μs	8	1
4	400	20ms	2	1
5	500	260 μs	8	1
6	1200	100μs	8	1

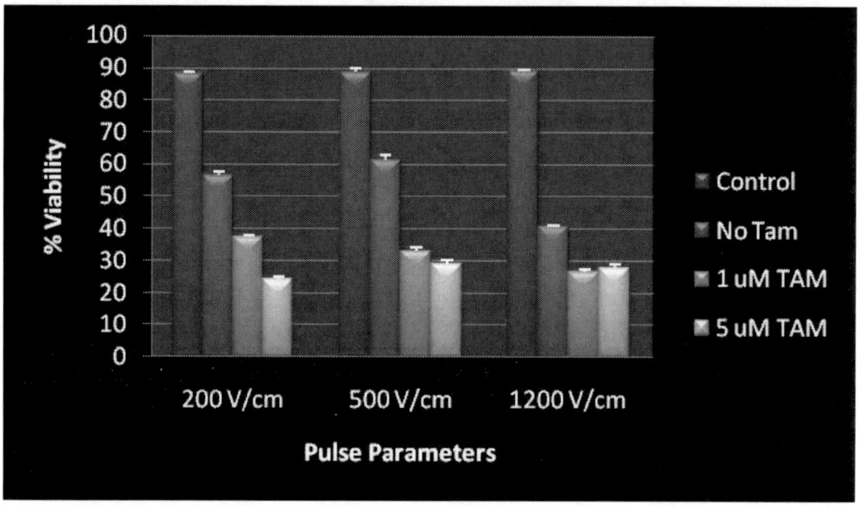

Figure 8. Comparison of percent viabilities at various voltages at various conditions – control (no treatment), Tamoxifen only, 1 and 5μM dose Tamoxifen.

It can be seen that the 200V/cm, 20ns pulses for 10 minutes has the highest viability at 1μM, compared to the other two pulses for 5 minutes each. This could be due to the lower intensity of electric field used despite twice the duration of application of pulses. A similar look at 5μM indicates that the percent viabilities are almost comparable at all the voltages. This could be due to the dominance of the higher dose at 5μM. The pulse parameters, the duration for a given voltage or the voltage for a given duration of pulses could be tailored to obtain the desired viability for a given type of cells. The energy levels of these pulses are extremely low and hence no heat or any other adverse effects are expected using these pulses.

Conclusion

Our pioneering study assessed the prospects of using low voltage, long duration pulses vs high voltage, short duration electrical voltage pulses, currently used in clinical trials to enhance the effect of minute doses of Tamoxifen, the anti-estrogen drug for breast cancer cells. The various milli- and microsecond pulses studied include 200V/cm, 10-40ms, 400V/cm, 20ms, 500V/cm, 260μs pulses, and 1200V/cm, 100 and 200μs, at reduced doses of 1 and 5μM. It proved that both high intensity, short duration and low intensity, long duration electrical pulse parameters, 1200V/cm with 200μs duration and 200V/cm with 40ms duration, eight pulses at 1Hz were equally effective to deliver these drugs.

Our study also demonstrated the use of low electrical voltage, nanosecond pulses of the orders of 200V/cm, 500V/cm, and 1200V/cm, for 10, 5 and 5 minutes to enhance the effect of minute doses of chemotherapeutics. Our results indicate that the MCF-7 cell line is receptive to low voltage, ns electroporation. Considering that the previous studies utilized 10s of kV/cm, these result indicate that lower voltages, but longer durations could be used. Reduced voltages are always safer and more economical than higher voltages.

For the first time, it is shown that the MCF-7 cells are receptive to electroporation at low as well as high voltages and using milli, micro and nano second pulses. It is also demonstrated that the combination therapy, electroporating cells in addition to a low dose of cytostatic drug, Tamoxifen administrations are more effective than treatment with the drug alone. This supports the hypothesis that electroporation and drug combination therapy will increase the cell's response to hormone drugs similar to chemo drugs, such as Bleomycin, the most commonly used for electrochemotherapy clinical trials for various cancers. Overall, the viable cell count has decreased in the electroporated sample, indicating that the proliferation control has been achieved in these cells due to apoptosis. The experiments also provide evidences that low voltage pulses with longer duration are effective towards permeabilization in MCF-7 breast cancer cells and may be used in clinics.

This will particularly be beneficial to drug-resistant patients as not all of the patients are responsive to conventional breast cancer treatments, and since this treatment allows targeted delivery of the therapeutic agents in a minute quantity, it would be less expensive and less toxic than the traditional treatments.

Acknowledgments

Authors, GV and RS acknowledge the assistance of Ms. R. Mathangi in preparation of Figure 1. Author GV acknowledges the financial support under the Fast Track scheme for young Scientists of the Department of Science and Technology, Government of India.

References

[1] Kingsbury,K. The changing face of breast cancer. *Time Magazine*. Oct 15 (2007).

[2] Gonzalez-Augulo, A.M., Morales-Vasquez, F. and Hortobagyi, G.N. "Overview of resistance to systemic therapy in patients with breast cancer", Ch 1, pp. 1-22, in *Breast Cancer Chemosensitivity,* D. Yu and M-C Hung (Eds), Springer Sciencc + Business Media, LLC, Landes Bioscience, New York, USA. (2007).

[3] Gehl, J. and Geertsen P.F. Efficient palliation of hemorrhaging malignant melanoma skin metastases by electrochemotherapy. *Melanoma Research.* 10, 1-5 (2000).

[4] Heller, R., Jaroszeski M., Grass L., Messina J., Rapaport D., Deconti R., Fenske, N., Gilbert, R., Mir, L., and Reintgen, D. Phase I/II trial for the treatment of cutaneous and subcutaneous tumors using electrochemotherapy. *Cancer.* 77, 964-971 (1996).

[5] Mir, L.M., *et al.* High efficiency gene transfer into skeletal muscle mediated by electric pulses. *Proc. Natl. Acad. Sci. US* 96, 4262-4267 (1999).
[6] Dev, S.B., Rabussay D.P., Widera, G., and Hofmann, G.A. Medical applications of Electroporation. *IEEE Trans. Plasma Sci. 28,* 206-223 (2000).
[7] Heller, R., Gilbert, R., and Jaroszeski, M. J. Clinical trials for solid tumors using electrochemotherapy, in *Electrochemotherapy, Electrogenetherapy, and Transdermal Delivery,* ed. Mark Jaroszeski, Richard Heller, and Richrd Gilbert, Humana Press, New Jersey, pp. 137-156 (2000).
[8] Gothelf, A., Mir, L., and Gehl, J. Electrochemotherapy: results of cancer treatment using enhanced delivery of bleomycin by electroporation. *Cancer Treatment Reviews* 29, 371-387 (2003).
[9] Campana, L., *et al.* Bleomycin-based electrochemotherapy: clinical outcome from a single institution's experience with 52 patients. *Annals of Surgical Oncology* 16, 191-99 (2009).
[10] Larkin, J.O., *et al.* Electrochemotherapy: aspects of practical development and early clinical experience. *Annals of Surgery.* 245 (2007).
[11] Nuccitelli, R., *et al.* Optimized nanosecond pulsed electric field theory can cause murine malignant melanomas to self-destruct with a single treatment. *Intl. J. of Cancer.* (2009).
[12] Nuccitelli, R., *et al.* Nanoseoncd pulsed electric fields cause melanomas to self-destruct. *Biochem Biophys Res Commun.* 343, 351-360 (2006).
[13] Schoenbach, K.H., Beebe, S.J, and Buescher, E.S. Intracellular effect of ultrashort electrical pulses. *Bioelectromagnetics.* 22, 440-448 (2001).
[14] Beebee, S.J., Fox, P.M., Rec, L.J. Willis, E.L., and Schoenbach, K.H. Nanosecond, high-intensity pulsed electric fields induce apoptosis in human cells. *FASEB J* 17, 1493-5 (2003).
[15] Desta, Z., Ward, B.A., Soukhova, N.V., Flockhart, D.A. Comprehensive evaluation of Tamoxifen sequential biotransformation by the human cytochrome P450 system in vitro: prominent roles for CYP3A and CYP2D6. *J. Pharmacol. Exp. Ther.* 310 (3): 1062–75 (2004).
[16] Wang, D.Y., Fulthorpe, R., Liss, S.N., Edwards, E.A. Identification of estrogen-responsive genes by complementary deoxyribonucleic acid microarray and characterization of a novel early estrogen-induced gene: EEIG1. *Mol. Endocrinol.* 18 (2): 402–11 (2004).
[17] Osborne, C.K., Bardou, V., Hopp, T.A., Chamness, G.C., Hilsenbeck, S.G., Fuqua, S.A., Wong, J., Allred, D.C., Clark, G.M., Schiff, R. Role of the estrogen receptor co-activator AIB1 (SRC-3) and HER-2/neu in Tamoxifen resistance in breast cancer. *J. Natl. Cancer Inst.* 95 (5): 353–61 (2003).
[18] Baum, M., Brinkley, D.M., Dossett, J.A., et al. Improved survival among patients treated with adjuvant Tamoxifen after mastectomy for early breast cancer. *Lancet.* 2(8347):450 (1983).
[19] Jordan, V.C. Fourteenth Gaddum Memorial Lecture. A current view of Tamoxifen for the treatment and prevention of breast cancer. *Br J Pharmacol.* 110(2):507-517 (1993).
[20] *UK C.* Breast cancer in men. *Cancer Research UK (*2007).
[21] Research CfDEa. Tamoxifen Information: reducing the incidence of breast cancer in women at high risk. (2005).

[22] Cuzick, J., Allen, D., Baum, M., et al. Long-term effects of Tamoxifen: Biological Effects of Tamoxifen Working Party. *European Journal of Cancer.* 29(1):15-21 (1993).

[23] Ring, A., Dowsett, M. Mechanisms of Tamoxifen resistance. *Endocrine-Related Cancer.* 11: 643-658 (2004).

[24] Drug Bank: a knowledge base for drugs, drug actions and drug targets. Wishart, D.S., Knox, C., Guo, A.C., Cheng, D., Shrivastava, S., Tzur, D., Gautam, B., Hassanali, M. Nucleic *Acids Res.* 36(Database issue):D901-6. PMID: 18048412 (2008).

[25] Osborne, C.K., Zhao, H., Fuqua, S.A.W. Selective Estrogen Receptor Modulators: Structure, Function and Clinical Use. *J. Clin. Oncol.* 18:3172-3186 (2000).

[26] Love, S.M., Dr. Susan Love's Breast Book. Capo Press, 3rd ed. New York (2000).

[27] Camarilo, I.G., Nichols, M.,Zhang, M., Sonnenburg, D. and Sundararajan, R. "Electro-Endocrine Combination Therapy for Aggressive Breast Tumors", *J. of Electrostatics.* 66, Issues 1-2, pp. 99-106 (2008).

In: Tamoxifen Concepts and Cancer: New Paradigms
Editor: Ramon Andrade de Mello
ISBN: 978-1-62081-520-5

Chapter XIII

Tamoxifen and Melanoma

Julieta Ruiz Beguerie
School of Public Health. The University of Sydney,
Sydney, Australia

Abstract

Throughout the years, multiple studies showed the benefits of tamoxifen (Tam) for cancers, other than breast and ovarian cancers, such as advanced melanoma, mesothelioma tumors, glioblastomas, colon cancer, lung cancer and urological cancer. Although tamoxifen is widely used in conjunction with cytotoxic agents for advanced melanoma and may modify the disease response to such drugs in a positive manner, there is still some controversy as to whether strong evidence exists to support this practice. Moreover, debate continues on which is the main mechanism of action of Tam in melanoma, the most life threatening form of skin cancer. Melanoma is one of the most common forms of cancers in the U.S., with approximately 63,130 new cases of diagnosed in 2010, according to the figures from the National Cancer Institute.

Recent data indicate that the estrogen receptor (ER) blocker, tamoxifen, can induce cell death in malignant melanoma cells through a variety of mechanisms. It can even enhance the synergy with other drugs used in melanoma treatments such as cisplatin (DDP). The specific biochemical interaction through which tamoxifen produces its pharmacological effect in this cancer, has been shown to be through a calcium channel blocking property, delaying the resistance to DDP, and consequently, sensitizing melanoma cancer cells to chemotherapeutic agents. Tam also works by stimulating the immune system, increasing the level of natural killers, along with other important modifications, which in turn, helps constraining the growth control of the most deadly skin cancer of all. Moreover, it has been found that induction of apoptosis and inhibition of angiogenesis are alternative ways in which tamoxifen suppresses tumor cell growth. At the same time, it has the potential of acting through endocrine and paracrine mechanism inhibiting the anchorage- dependent growth of melanoma. Additionally, tamoxifen has been found to increase the secretion of the transforming growth factor- beta (TGF β), which inhibits the growth of several estrogen-receptor-negative cancers.

Even though the tamoxifen is still used in the therapy of advanced melanoma (Stages III-IV), debate continues among scientists on which is the explanation of its mechanism of action. This chapter presents the updated knowledge regarding the biochemical interactions, particularly on melanoma response and resistance; through which tamoxifen produce its pharmacological effect.

Introduction

Melanoma, the most aggressive skin cancer of all, is of increasing concern as its incidence has continued to increase by 7% each year since 1985 (LaVecchia, Lucchini and Negri, 1999). However, the overall mortality rate has only slightly increased over the last years probably due to the earlier diagnosis of the lesion, yielding a better prognosis. According to recent data from the Skin Cancer Foundation, it kills an estimated of 8,700 people in the US annually.

Despite the fact that melanoma is not the most common skin cancer, it is the leading cause of death among skin diseases. Melanomas develop due to changes in the melanocytes that produce melanin pigment and they can spread very rapidly. This cancer can be found not only in the skin, but also in the uveal tract of the eyes, the upper digestive tract, anal canal, rectum and vagina (Gupta, Malpica and Deaverst, 2002; McLean 1995; Stringa, Valdez and Ruiz Beguerie, 2006). Rarely, melanomas appear in the mouth, iris of the eye, or retina at the back of the eye and they may be found during dental or eye examinations. Melanoma can appear on normal skin, or it may begin as a mole or other lesion that has changed in appearance. Even certain moles that are present at birth may develop later in life into melanomas (Goodson and Grossman, 2009).

There are four major types of melanoma:

- Superficial spreading melanoma is the most common type of melanoma. It is usually flat and irregular in shape and color, with different shades of black and brown in color. It may occur at any age or body site, and is most common in Caucasians.
- Nodular melanoma usually starts as a raised area that is dark blackish-blue or bluish-red. However, some do not have any particular color.
- Lentigo maligna melanoma usually occurs in the elderly. It is most common in sun-damaged skin on the face, neck, and arms. The abnormal skin areas are usually large, flat, and tan with areas of brown.
- Acral lentiginous melanoma is the least common form of melanoma. It usually occurs on the palms, soles, or under the nails and is more common in African Americans.

The risk of developing melanoma increases with age. However, the disease also frequently affects young, otherwise healthy people. The development of melanoma is related to sun exposure or ultraviolet radiation, particularly among people with fair skin, blue or green eyes, and red or blond hair. The risks for melanoma include the following: living in sunny climates or at high altitudes, long-term exposure to high levels of strong sunlight, one or more blistering sunburns during childhood, frequent use of tanning devices, first degree relatives with a history of melanoma or own personal history of this cancer, basal cell carcinoma or squamous cell carcinoma, exposure to chemicals that can cause cancer, such as arsenic, coal tar, and creosote, presence of atypical dysplastic moles and a weakened immune system due to HIV/AIDS, leukemias/ lymphomas, organ transplant or certain immunosuppressant medications (Markovick, Erickson and Rao, 2007, 2007).

A team of prestigious photobiologists from Ireland reported in the Irish Journal of Medical Science a connection between breast cancer and melanoma, establishing that having either one raises the odds of developing the other. While earlier studies have noted this association between the two malignancies, this is the first time researchers have explicitly advised doctors to monitor breast cancer patients for signs of melanoma, and vice versa. They also recommend that melanoma patients with a family history of breast cancer have regular mammographies or breast magnetic resonance imaging (MRI). Between 1994 and 2007, The Beaumont Hospital in Dublin and the Skin Cancer Foundation, examined 6,788 cases of melanoma and 27,597 cases of breast carcinoma documented in Ireland's National Cancer Registry. They mathematically determined that if there was no statistically significant relationship between the two, 30–35 patients could be expected to have both malignancies. Instead, there were 127 cases. This is a fourfold increase, which raises the possibility of a genetic predisposition linking these two cancers. Earlier findings published in the Annals of Oncology and Breast Cancer Research and Treatment, reported that breast cancer patients have between 1.4 and 2.7 times the risk of developing melanoma. And the danger is reciprocal: The International Journal of Cancer noted that female melanoma patients have a 1.4 times greater chance of developing breast cancer. In most countries, female melanoma patients are now advice to have routine breast exams (Ho, Comber and Murphy, 2009).

It is yet unclear just how great a role genes play in the development of breast cancer and melanoma. Researchers suggest that mutations in the gene CDKN2A, which indicate high risk of developing melanoma, also put carriers at up to 3.8 times greater risk of breast cancer. Similarly, mutations in the gene BRCA2 for breast cancer susceptibility increase carriers' risk of melanoma by as much as 2.58 times. However, only a minority of melanoma cases has identifiable genetic mutations. We must not forget that still there is a lot of unknown in genetic or not well understood. Just 5 to 10 percent of melanomas occur in families with multiple cases of the disease, and in only 20-40 percent of these families is there a mutation in CDKN2A (Monnerat, Chompret and Kannengiesser, 2007; Buecher, Gauthiers-Millars and Desjardins, 2010).

Metastatic spread involves several different stages and, in escaping from the primary tumor and in forming distal metastatic deposits, neoplastic cells need to attach to and subsequently invade through stromal extracellular matrix (ECM). Metastatic melanoma cells express a greater range of adhesion molecules than their non-transformed precursor, the melanocytes. Initial attachment of cells to ECM proteins then leads to the organization of the cell cytoskeleton to form focal adhesions (Dewhurst, Gee and Rennie, 1997).

Treatment success depends on many factors, including the patient's general health and whether the cancer has spread to the lymph nodes or other organs. The outcome for patients with stage IV melanomas, which are those tumors with distant metastasis, is poor and the resistance to systemic therapy is high. This classification in stages is based on the American Joint Committee on cancer criteria. Surgery remains the cornerstone of curative treatment in earlier stages but for advanced stages the use of a systemic therapy is usually applied. However, it remains highly resistant to systemic therapies. The median survival for this advance stage is only six to nine months, with an estimated five-year survival of 5-10% depending on the prognostic factors, the site of metastasis, the number of metastatic sites and the elevated serum lactate dehydrogenase levels (LDH) (Australian cancer network/ Ministry of Health, New Zealand, 2008). Building upon recent laboratory discoveries on the resistance of melanoma cells to therapies, The Cancer Institute of New Jersey is conducting a clinical trial that further explores how to prevent that action. The goal is to determine if hydroxychloroquine, an anti-malaria drug used to treat malaria and certain types of arthritis, is able to interfere with the cellular process that acts as a survival method for human melanoma. Hydroxychloroquine has been shown to block autophagy, the process by which cells eat themselves in order to survive through times of stress. This mechanism of survival apparently allows cells to become resistant to cancer therapies. The scientists believe this particular drug may help melanoma treatments work more effectively by providing an easier path for the cancer drugs to enter the cell. They would like to further examine the process of autophagy and learn if the mentioned drug is able to interrupt this process in human blood and tumor samples of adults with stage III or stage IV melanoma

Even though many attempts have been made in the last years in finding a satisfactory new therapy for advanced stages of melanoma, the treatment response of patients remains unsatisfactory. Hence, the prognosis is still poor. According to the American Cancer Society, melanoma accounted for about 59,940 cases of skin cancer in 2007 and most (about 8,110 of the 10,850) of the deaths due to skin cancer each year. Consequently, an effective and safe treatment is of critical importance for the survival of these patients.

Overall results have changed only marginally over the last 25 years with five-year survival improving from 88% in 1980 to 90 % in 2004 in Australasia. However, in the rest of the world the outcomes are slightly better with the USA reporting 92% five-year survival and the UK 82% (Australian cancer network/ Ministry of Health, New Zealand, 2008).

Tamoxifen is a nonsteroidal, triphenylethylene antiestrogen molecule, which was first synthesized as a contraceptive pill in 1960 in the United Kingdom. Tamoxifen mimics the effects of the estrogens and has a complex mechanism of action, with anticancer and carcinogenic effects. Interestingly, these divergent effects are shown in the same tissue, where Tam induces progesterone receptors in an agonist way and inhibits cancer proliferation in an antagonist effect. Tam is one of the selective estrogen receptor modulators with tissue-specific activities, acting as an anti-estrogen (inhibiting agent) in the mammary tissue, but as an estrogen agonist (stimulating agent) in cholesterol metabolism, bone density, and cell proliferation in the endometrium. It is well known that patients expressing estradiol receptors in melanoma cells have been reported to have a better prognosis suggesting a putative inhibitory action of estradiol on the growth of this tumor. Estrogen receptor -alpha (ER-α) belongs to a superfamily of transcription activators involved in many physiologic processes, including melanoma progression as reported in 2006 (Mori, Martinez and O'Day, 2006). In addition to acting on reproductive functions, estrogens are known to affect growth and differentiation of a variety of cell types. It has been reported that estrogens and progestins may elicit hyperpigmentary responses by the stimulation of melanogenesis within skin melanocytes. It was reported in 2004, the presence of type II estrogen binding sites in human cancer cell lysates and extracts; SK-Mel 23 cells, which, once activated by estradiol, induce phosphorylation of 16- and 46-dalton (kDa) proteins. These events lead to differentiation of melanoma cells, as there is a decrease of proliferation and an increase in melanogenesis (Sarti MS and Castrucci, 2004). Tamoxifen offers additional health benefits other than in cancer treatment. By activating estrogen's action in bone and liver cells, it improves the blood cholesterol profile by lowering LDL levels and it helps maintain bone density. Therefore, it lowers the risk of osteoporosis and bone fractures. It is also used for the treatment of gynecomastia in men with prostate cancer, in multiple sclerosis, Parkinson's disease, Alzheimer's disease and systemic lupus erythematosus (Ernst, Chang and Cooray, 2002; Rohlff, Blagosklonny and Kyle, 1998; Sthoeger Z, Zinger H, Mozes, 2003).

The Food and Drug Administration has approved Tamoxifen in 1977 for the treatment of breast cancer. Current scientific literature suggests that Tam reduces the incidence of breast cancer in healthy women at high risk of breast cancer as it blocks the tumor's ability to use estrogen. The actual mechanism of action is explained by its ability to bind to the estrogen receptors, inducing a conformational change in the receptor. The anti-estrogen effects of tamoxifen are mediated through the ERs, which are present in the cytosol but also within the cell membranes. The prolonged binding, results in reduced deoxyribonucleic acid (DNA) polymerase activity, impaired thymidine utilization, blockade of estradiol uptake, and decreased estrogen response. It is likely that it interacts with other co-activators or co-repressors in the tissues where melanocytic cells are present. Moreover, it exerts a variety of activities including the regulation of cytokines such as transforming growth factor- β1which stimulates stromal cells and angiogenesis.

During the last two decades numerous trials evidenced the benefits (Gelmann, 1997). One of the explanations for the mentioned positive result is that this drug works by increasing the level of natural killers helping control the growth of tumors and by sensitizing cancer cells to chemotherapeutic agents. Furthermore, many experimental studies have shown that induction of apoptosis and angiogenesis inhibitions are alternative ways in which this drug suppresses tumor cell growth, independent of the expression of ERs. It is well known now that Tam as a single agent has little activity in patients with melanoma, but it is of additional benefit in combination therapy. As the combined therapy of tamoxifen and dacarbazine has shown to be superior to dacarbazine alone, now they are prescribed together (Cocconi, Bella and Calabresi, 1992). Most published studies started reporting response rates of less than 10% when this combination therapy began. It was in 1984, that prestigious trialists reported the results of the first clinical trial combining cytotoxic chemotherapy with tamoxifen in patients with metastatic melanoma (Del Petre, Maurer and O'Donell, 1984). The role of Tam in combination therapy to treat advanced melanoma is still controversial. Overall response rates reported from nonrandomized clinical trials of tamoxifen added to chemotherapeutic agents to treat metastatic melanoma (with or without historical controls) ranged from 8% to 60% (Gelmann, 1997; Eigentler, Caroli and Radny, 2003). Several randomized controlled trials have evaluated the role of tamoxifen in the treatment of metastatic melanoma, with inconsistent results.

Despite the side effects reported in the literature, the benefit of tamoxifen in pre- and post- menopausal women diagnosed with breast cancer in controlling the tumor and preventing relapse is without debate. Many women and men who take tamoxifen have no side effects at all while others experience some. The most common side effects reported are flushes and sweats, weight gain, change in periods, nausea and indigestion. It is nowadays indicated in both women and men for the treatment of invasive and metastatic breast cancer, in women at high risk of breast cancer and in ovarian cancer. It is also one of the most used regimens for treatment of advanced melanoma along dacarbazine, cisplatin and carmustine. This regimen is known as the Dartmouth regimen. Many institutions have confirmed high response rates of 40 to 50% when the Dartmouth regimen was given for melanomas. In 1984, a publication showed a response rate of 55% in 20 patients with confirmed melanoma treated with this same systemic plan (Del Petre, 1984).

Previous primary studies looking on the efficacy of Tam in melanoma have been inconclusive. They were often underpowered and produced conflicting conclusions. Furthermore, previous systematic reviews were poorly done and sometimes mixed Tam's results with other treatments results. Therefore, controversies remain regarding the real benefit of using tamoxifen in advanced melanoma. An additional concern is the potential toxicity and quality of life generated by its use. The purpose of the 2010 meta- analysis on tamoxifen and advanced melanoma was to quantitatively assess whether the inclusion of Tam to the systemic therapies is more effective and safe compared to non- tamoxifen regimens in terms of clinical response, mortality, quality of life, haematological and non -haematological toxicity and treatment- related mortality, in patients with advanced melanoma (Stage III/IV). The conclusion of this meta-analysis was that Tamoxifen is more effective than non-tamoxifen regimens in overall and partial response for patients with advanced melanomas. The treatment effect was consistent irrespective of funding source, Tam dose or gender of participants, although a greater benefit in response towards tamoxifen was seen in trials with female predominance. However, the improvement in response was not associated with a reduction in 1 and 2-year-mortality, which shows a non-statistically significant increase in the Tam group (RR 1.03, 95% CI 0.95 to 1.12, P-value 0.47 and RR 1.03, CI95% 0.94 to 1.12, P-value 0.55 respectively) (Ruiz Beguerie, Xingzhong and Valdez, 2010).

Conclusions regarding toxicity are difficult to make as the chemotherapy regimen and the follow-up periods of some trials differ from the others. The stage-appropriate surveillance strategy is not detailed in some of the studies done in the past and some differ from current recommendation (Garbe, Paul and Kohler-Spath, 2003; Weiss, Loprinzi and Creagan, 1995). Before 2003, there were no standardized agreed guidelines in existence for the follow-up of patients with melanoma. The results of this review suggest that the recommendation of incorporating Tam into chemotherapy regimens for advanced melanoma to introduce a better response are still narrow and more information should be obtained regarding the harm of the treatment to be able to assess its applicability. Patients exposed to this drug have 1.39 times more chances of overall response than those not exposed, increasing the absolute risk of this benefit by seven events per 100. On the other hand, imprecise results on mortality suggest the opposite; a slightly higher risk of mortality at 2 years with those regimens using Tam (90 vs. 87%). A beneficial effect from tamoxifen was seen in studies with a higher female/male ratio. This tendency could be further explored in studies comparing females and males' responses to Tamoxifen, linking its anti estrogen effect with this outcome.

As commented previously in the chapter, tamoxifen has been used in chemotherapy and bio-chemotherapy regimens for over a decade. The pharmacological targets of tamoxifen are multiple, including estrogen receptor, multi-drug resistance gene product, permeability-glycoprotein (P-glycoprotein), and recently discovered 7-transmembrane G protein-coupled receptor. Most probably in the near future, more targets will be discovered which are unknown at the present time and they could help us better understand the mechanism of action of this multifaceted drug (Behjati and Frank, 2009).

Dr.Mori and colleagues carried out the first study, which reported a potential explanation for the failure of tamoxifen in improving the reduction of mortality in the treatment of melanoma. They have shown that the variable down-regulation of ER in melanoma is due to epigenetic control of its expression though hypermethylation via a gene promoter region. Tamoxifen, a member of the selective ER modulator family, is still used in the bio-chemotherapy regimen for melanoma patients as we explained before. Patients without serum methylated ER-α, who therefore expresses ER-α, may be more likely to respond to the antitumor effects of tamoxifen. Conversely, the deficiency of patients to respond to bio chemotherapy may be partially explained by the faultiness of tamoxifen to exert its antitumor effects when ER-α expression is silenced due to the hypermethylation of a promoter region. This is akin to the clinical situation seen in breast cancer in which tumors not expressing ER-α do not respond to hormone therapy, therefore, carrying a poorer prognosis. ER-α methylation could also reflect a pathophysiologic event that involves a more global hypermethylation of tumor-related genes, thereby supplying tumor cells with a growth advantage (Mori, 2006).

Several in vitro studies have reported the presence of ERs on melanoma cells derived from metastatic tumors (Fisher, Neifeld and Lippman, 1976; Walker, Beattie and Patel, 1987). Although biochemical assays have shown that estrogen-binding proteins are present in malignant melanoma, later studies using a sensitive and more specific immunohistochemical technique have not found ERs in melanoma. Many experimental studies have shown that induction of apoptosis and inhibition of angiogenesis are alternative ways in which tamoxifen suppresses tumor cell growth, independent of the expression of ERs. These studies provided the rationale for the clinical investigation of therapy regimens that include tamoxifen.

Mechanism of Action of Tamoxifen in Melanoma

The modulatory actions of Tam on melanoma cells and its mechanism of action are still poorly understood, but many investigators have been postulating their hypothesis in several trials to explain this intriguing action. Hence, there are a considerable number of studies published in the literature trying to find the best rationale to explain the response of the melanocytic cells to the drug: tamoxifen.

Mechanism of synergy with cisplatin. Multidrug resistance mechanisms underlying the intractability of malignant melanomas remain largely unknown. I read with great interest a study published in 2006, concerning the synergy of Tam with cisplatin, which suggests that the development of multidrug resistance in melanomas involves subcellular sequestration of intracellular cytotoxic drugs such as cisplatin (CDDP) (Chen, Valencia and Lai, 2006). CDDP is initially sequestered in subcellular organelles such as melanosomes, which significantly reduces its nuclear localization when compared with non-melanoma□epidermoid carcinoma cells, which produce the squamous cell carcinoma in skin (SCC). The melanosomal accumulation of cisplatin modulates melanogenesis through a marked increase in tyrosinase activity. The altered melanogenesis manifests a □8- fold increase in both intracellular pigmentation and extracellular transport of melanosomes containing CDDP. Hence, this trial provides evidence that melanosomes contribute to the refractory properties of melanoma cells by sequestering cytotoxic drugs and by increasing melanosome-mediated drug exports. Preventing melanosomal sequestration of cytotoxic drugs by inhibiting the functions of melanosomes may have great potential as an approach to improving the chemosensitivity of melanoma cells. This action could be done through the addition of tam to cisplatin in the systemic therapy. According to some experts in the field, tamoxifen enhances the synergy with other drugs used in melanoma treatments at the cellular level (Agarwala, Ferri and

Gooding, 1999). This mechanism of action reported in 1998, was previously observed in several studies of melanoma cell lines conducted by different authors (McClay, Albright and Jones, 1992, 1993). Likewise, it has been previously demonstrated that cisplatin and tamoxifen act synergistically to kill human melanoma cells. They have identified the intracellular antiestrogen-binding sites (AEBSs), defined by their ability to bind antiestrogen while having no affinity for estrogen, as a possible mediator of this synergy. This implicates AEBSs as a critical component of the mechanism that mediates the synergistic interaction of DDP and Tam in human melanoma cells (Jones, Aibright and Christen, 1997).

Mechanism of calcium channel blocking. Tam has been shown to work through a calcium channel blocking property, delaying the resistance to DDP, and consequently sensitizing melanoma cancer cells to chemotherapeutic agents. The attachment of melanoma cells to ECM proteins appears to involve intracellular signaling systems, in particular calcium and calmodulin (Cocconi, 1992). It was demonstrated that tamoxifen and two of its major metabolites could inhibit cell attachment to ECM (stromal extracellular matrix) proteins. Their data suggest that the action of Tam and its metabolites in this respect is a result of their ability to inhibit calmodulin activity even at micromolar concentrations.

Invasion through ECM is part of the complex, multistep process of tumour cell invasion and metastasis. It was previously emphasized the importance of calcium and calmodulin in the main steps of the metastatic cascade, which includes the attachment of cancer cells to the ECM. One of the main objectives of this study was test whether tamoxifen might reduce melanoma cell invasion, possibly by acting as a calmodulin antagonist rather than through its ability to compete with estrogen binding to estrogen receptors (Dewhurst, 1997). As reviewed in 1984, calmodulin itself mediates many different actions of calcium in cells such as cell proliferation, microtubule disassembly and secretion of agents from the cell (Tomlinson, MacNeil and Walker, 1984; Walker, MacNeil and H Senior, 1984). Interestingly, tamoxifen, which also has calmodulin antagonist activity, is used in the treatment of various cancers including metastatic cutaneous melanoma, and is able to inhibit the attachment of normal and neoplastic cells to stromal extracellular matrix. In 1997 these same scientists investigated whether tam and its metabolites (N-desmethyltamoxifen and 4-hydroxytamoxifen), could also reduce tumor invasion through a layer of human fibronectin using uveal melanoma cells. They found that submicromolar concentrations of tamoxifen reduced the invasiveness of melanoma cells. All cells used in this study were found to be negative for nuclear oestrogen receptors, reinforcing the possibility that tamoxifen and estradiol can act via mechanisms unrelated to binding to classical estrogen receptors to inhibit tumour cell invasion (Dewhurst, 1997). In 1984, reports were published regarding the mechanism of metastasis of melanoma through adhesion receptors. It is known that melanoma often develops from clinically and histologically well-defined precursor lesions. Throughout the progression of normal melanocytes to cancerous cells, dramatic changes in the expression of adhesion receptors are observed, most notably loss of E-cadherin, which mediates adhesion of melanocytes to keratinocytes in the skin. This gains at the same time the melanoma cell adhesion molecule (MEL -CAM), which mainly mediates heterotypic adhesion between cells. The integrin subunit beta 3 is up- regulated, whereas other integrins such as alpha 6 beta 1 and alpha V beta 1 are down- regulated. Moreover, the review published in Invasion Metastasis in 1994 highlights the major changes in adhesion receptor expression on melanocytes at multiple stages of melanoma progression in accordance with that commented above (Nesbit and Herlyn, 1994).

Mechanism of the immune system. Tamoxifen impacts the immune system as well by increasing the level of natural killers and by helping regulate the growth control of human tumors. In 1993, investigators found an increase of natural killer cells in a study that was carried out on 48 postmenopausal breast cancer patients receiving an adjuvant therapy with 30 mg tamoxifen for an average of 22 months. The effect of hormonal therapy on different immunologic parameters was examined and compared with an age-matched control group of breast cancer patients without hormonal therapy. Previous to the start of the trial and at the end of the tamoxifen treatment, several examinations were performed such as Leucocyte Migrations-Inhibition-Test (LMI-Test) against autologous and homologous tumor and recall antigens, serum levels of tumor necrosis factor alpha, interleukin 2 and interferon alpha, as well as lymphocyte subsets (total T-, T-helper-, T-Suppressor- and natural killer cells) in the peripheral blood. Compared to the control group under a tamoxifen therapy, the percentage of patients with a migration inhibition in the LMI-test increased, whereas the percentage of patients with an enhancement decreased (Mallmann and Krebs, 1991). There is a growing body of evidence, which demonstrates immunomodulatory effects of tamoxifen, including several *in vitro* and *in vivo* studies. Taken together these various clinical studies, it is suggested that tamoxifen is capable of inducing a shift from cellular (T-helper 1) to humoral (T-helper 2) immunity. Interestingly, the immunomodulatory effects of Tam appear to be independent of the estrogen-receptor and may be mediated through the multi-drug resistance gene product known as the Permeability-Glycoprotein (P-Glycoprotein). An interesting role of Tam in immunity has recently emerged in a recent study published in 2009 (Behjati, 2009). This P-Glycoprotein is a well-characterized ABC-transporter of the MDR/TAP subfamily distributed and expressed in intestinal cells, renal cells, hepatocytes and endothelial cells. ABC proteins transport various molecules across extra-and intra- cellular membranes. ABC genes are divided into seven families, and one of them is the MDR/TAP (antigen peptide transporter), which is involved, in multidrug resistance.

Proinflammatory cytokines IL-1α and IL-1β promote tumor angiogenesis, an action that might be counteracted by the IL-1 receptor antagonist (IL-1Ra): anakinra. The mentioned antagonist, blocks the biologic activity of naturally occurring IL-1, including inflammation and cartilage degradation by competitively inhibiting the binding of IL-1 to the Interleukin-1 type receptor, which is expressed in many tissues and organs. IL-1 is produced in response to inflammatory stimuli and mediates various physiologic responses, including inflammatory and immunologic reactions. Tamoxifen increases IL-1Ra levels significantly. The tumor stroma contains macrophages, which express the estrogen receptors. In vitro, estradiol decreases IL-1Ra release from breast cancer cells and from cultured macrophages. IL-1Ra decreases endothelial cell proliferation significantly. Finally, IL-1Ra therapy of tumor-bearing mice opposes estrogen-dependent breast cancer growth and decreases angiogenesis. The study concluded that the release of IL-1s both by cancer cells and by the stroma, where macrophages are a key component, might offer feasible targets for tamoxifen (Lindahl, Saarinen and Abrahansom, 2011). Tamoxifen, which has once failed as a contraceptive and then revolutionized the treatment of breast cancer, could re-emerge as a novel modulator of the immune system. The blood lymphocyte population was studied in 23-breast cancer patients treated with adjuvant tamoxifen for 1.5-2 years, and in an equal number of control patients. The size and cellular composition of the blood lymphocyte population, as assessed by monoclonal antibodies directed against various subsets, did not differ between the two patient groups. However, lymphocytes of the tamoxifen-treated patients exhibited a significantly lower natural killer (NK) activity against K562 cells. K562 cells were the first human immortalized myelogenous leukemia line to be established. K562 cells are of the erythroleukamia type, and the line is derived from a 53-year-old patient diagnosed with chronic myelogenous (or myeloid) leukemia in blast crisis. The results from this study indicate that tamoxifen may modulate the immune system (Agarwala, 1999). Moreover, in 1993 it was reported the effects of Tam in patients with two of the non-melanomas skin cancer (NMSCs) which are Squamous Cell Carcinoma (SCC) and the most common form of skin cancer: the Basal Cell Carcinoma (BCC). The NMSCs include 82 types of tumors with wide variability in prognosis, ranging from those with generally good prognosis such as BCC and SCC to those that generally portend a worst prognosis such as Merkel cell carcinoma. Patients with BCC, who received tamoxifen, also show a reduction in the proportion of CD4+ T cells and in AMLR (Autologous Mixed Lymphocyte Reaction) proliferative responses, compared to the levels in normal controls. Taken together, these results indicate that long-term tamoxifen treatment modulates immune responses in BBC patients as well (Robinson, Rubin and Mekori, 1993).

Tamoxifen is found to increase the secretion of TGF Beta, which inhibits the growth of several estrogen-receptor-negative cells such as melanoma cells (Behl, Weilbach and Apfel, 1990; Cocconi, 1992). Activated T lymphocytes and malignant melanocytic cells are known to induce TGF Beta. The most investigated endogenous anti-tumor hormone is the pineal hormone, melatonin (MLT), whose immunomodulation and oncostatic properties have been well demonstrated in experimental conditions. MLT has improved the clinical status of untreatable metastatic solid tumors mainly by efficiently affecting a macrophage-mediated immunosuppression and through inhibition of the release of tumor necrosis factor alpha (TNF- α), especially in several tumor histotypes (Beutler and Cerami, 1987). Alternatively, MLT might amplify Tam efficacy, as suggested by the evidence of disease stabilization in patients previously with a progressing disease on Tam alone, perhaps by stimulating endocrine receptor expression on cancer cells. Since MLT alone is generally unable to induce objective tumor regressions, this phase I study suggests that the concomitant administration of Tam may amplify the oncostatic activity of MLT, perhaps through a stimulation of TGF- α release (Lissoni, Paolorossi and Tancini, 1996).

The immune system is the target of a variety of studies searching new drugs for melanoma. On March 25, the Food and Drug Administration (FDA) approved a new medication, Yervoy, which has been found to prolong the lives of patients with late-stage melanoma by an average of four months. It is administered intravenously and stimulates the body's immune system to fight cancer by blocking a molecule connected to the development of melanoma. The molecule prevents the activity of white blood cells. After the molecule is blocked, cells can function properly and attack the cancer.

Mechanism of apoptosis and anti-angiogenesis. Moreover, it has been found that induction of apoptosis and angiogenesis inhibition are alternative ways through which tamoxifen suppresses tumor cell growth. Tam induced apoptosis in 289-melanoma cells in the trial conducted in 1996. In contrast, the drug did not induce apoptosis 289 cells of Tam-resistant variant. To my knowledge, these are the first data connecting Tam resistance with the inhibition of apoptosis (McClay, Jones and Winski, 1996). Tamoxifen treatment leads to a rapid decrease in the number of S-phase cells, an accumulation of cells in the G1-fraction, and the induction of apoptosis *in vivo* and in *vitro*. It was reported for the first time in 2010, that claudin-1, a membrane protein of tight junctions which is associated with the development of various cancers, has anti-apoptotic effects in tamoxifen-treated MCF-7 cells involving the regulation of apoptosis-related factors and subcellular localization of adherents junctions (Akasaka, Sato and Morohashi, 2010). MCF-7 is a breast cancer cell line and the acronym for Michigan Cancer Foundation - 7, referring to the institute in Detroit where Herbert Soule established the cell line in 1973. In 2005, it was established that tamoxifen and estradiol exert dual effects on the angiogenic environment in breast cancer by regulating extracellular levels of important angiogenic factors secreted by cancer cells as well as by exerting effects on receptor expression of endothelial cells. Their results suggest an estrogen-driven angiogenic switch, explained by the inhibition of sVEGFR-1 (Vascular endothelial growth factor receptor 1) and stimulation of VEGF (Vascular endothelial growth factor) and VEGFR-2 (Vascular endothelial growth factor receptor 2), tipping the angiogenic scale to promote angiogenesis, and possibly encouraging breast carcinoma progression. Tamoxifen, on the other hand, tips the balance to favor angiogenic inhibition (Garvin, Nilsson and Dabrosin, 2005).

Another spectrum of the apoptosis mechanism in tumors has been related to hyperthermia, which has been shown to produce regression of human cancer. Because hyperthermia has produced only limited results, attention has focused on searching for chemicals that are able to sensitize cancer cells to the effects of hyperthermia. The flavonoid quercetin has been reported to be a hyperthermic sensitizer in ovarian and uterine cervical tumors, as well as in leukemia. Tamoxifen and quercetin can both inhibit melanoma cell growth. Therefore, in a recent study it was investigated whether these substances are able to sensitize M10, M14 and MNT1 human melanoma cells to hyperthermia. It was observed that quercetin and tamoxifen synergize with hyperthermia (42.5°C) in inducing apoptotic cell death in all three-cell lines and in reducing the clonogenic activity of M14 and MNT1. Using flow cytometries and Northern blot analyses, quercetin and tamoxifen reduced heat shock protein-70 expression at mRNA and protein levels. The trialists suggest that quercetin and tamoxifen can be usefully combined with hyperthermia in the therapy of recurrent and/or metastatic melanoma (Piantelli, Tatone and Castrilli, 2011).

Mechanism of Insulin –like growth factor pathway. According to some scientists, tamoxifen induces cell death in malignant melanoma cells through the insulin-like growth factor-1 (IGF-1) pathway. However, melanoma cells usually do not express classical ERs, as it is shown in this mentioned study. It was investigated whether the cytotoxic effect of Tam on melanoma cells could depend on interference with the expression or function of the insulin-like growth factor-1 receptor (IGF-1R), a plasma membrane receptor important for cell survival in this tumor cell type. Several melanoma cell lines were included in the analysis. Administration of Tam at a concentration of 15 μm or more resulted in cell death of the melanoma cells within 48 hours. Tam treatment was correlated to a slight to moderate inhibition of IGF-1 (Insulin-like growth factor 1) binding to IGF-1R (Insulin-like growth factor 1 receptor). Since it has been reported that Tam can increase the release of IGF binding proteins (IGFBPs) they then investigated whether this mechanism could underlay the decreased IGF-1 binding. However, they were not able to demonstrate that the amount of released IGFBPs was unchanged or decreased in Tam-treated cells. Whereas Tam did not have any strong effect on IGF-1 binding and the expression of IGF-1R at the cell surface, it was found to efficiently block tyrosine phosphorylation of IGF-1R β-subunit. Taken together, the evidence suggests that the induction of cytotoxicity done by Tam on malignant melanoma cells can be due to the inactivation of IGF-1R (Kanter-Lewensohn, Girnita and Girnita, 2000).

Mechanism of hypermethylation. DNA methylation is a modification of DNA in which methyl groups are added to certain positions on the nitrogen bases. In bacteria, adenine and cytosine are commonly methylated, while in eukaryotic cells, cytosine is most commonly methylated. In eukaryotic cells, methylation is a method of inhibiting gene expression.

Hypermethylation of gene promoter CpG islands plays a significant role in the development and progression of various cancers, including melanoma. In genetics, CpG islands are genomic regions that contain a high frequency of Cytosine-phosphate-guanine sites and typically occur at or near the transcription start site of genes. The identification of hypermethylated genes in cancer has become an accepted approach to assess tumor-related gene inactivation. It was previously reported tumor-related gene hypermethylation in primary and metastatic melanomas (Kanter-Lewensohn, Girnita and Girnita, 2006). Thereafter, investigators showed the hypermethylation of multiple tumor-related and tumor suppressor genes during the progression phase from primary to metastatic lesions. Several genes methylated in primary and metastatic melanomas could also be detected in serum as methylated circulating DNA.

Estrogen receptor α (ER-α) belongs to a superfamily of transcription activators involved in many physiologic processes, including tumor progression. In breast cancer, the loss of ER-α expression has been associated with aberrant CpG island hypermethylation, showing to regulate its progression. Several studies have demonstrated the presence of ER in melanoma cell lines but analysis of human melanomas has shown variable ER-α expression. Unfortunately, mechanisms regulating the expression of ER-α in melanoma are still poorly defined. There is still no mutation or other gross structural alteration of the *ER-α* gene, which has been reported in melanoma. It is hypothesized that *ER-α* gene is silenced via a gene promoter of hypermethylation in primary and metastatic melanoma which plays an important role in melanoma progression and may be extremely important in the future as a prognostic molecular biomarker. Several *in vitro* trials established that tamoxifen is an effective growth inhibitor of melanoma cells. Based on the inconsistent presence of ER-α in melanoma cells, multiple trials with patients diagnosed with melanoma looking at clinical responses to antiestrogen therapy were coordinated finding various results. For this reason, colleagues from the University of Sydney based in Australia, and The Austral Hospital based in Argentina, designed the 2010 meta-analysis of published and unpublished randomized controlled studies, without language restriction, to assess the benefits of tamoxifen in the treatment regimens for advanced melanoma. The conclusion of this meta-analysis was that the results do not confirm the findings from previous reviews (Lens, Reiman and Husain, 2003). In this systematic review, the use of tamoxifen in the chemotherapy regimens has been shown to be beneficial in overall and partial response as well as in mortality-related to the treatment but has not been shown to be beneficial looking at mortality or toxicity. These relevant findings are strengthened by the fact that all eligible trials reported both major outcomes of interest, excluding the possibility of "outcome reporting bias".

The reported expression level of ER-α in melanoma has been variable, with several studies failing to show the presence of ER-α using monoclonal antibodies. Tamoxifen has been used in chemotherapy and biochemotherapy regimens for over a decade. Although improved response rates have been reported with its use, it has not been shown to significantly improve overall survival in advanced melanoma according to several trialists. It has been reported that the variable down-regulation of ER in melanoma is due to epigenetic control of its expression via a gene promoter region of hypermethylation.

Additionally, methylated ER-α can be detected in paraffin-embedded primary and metastatic melanoma tumors, showing its value as a biomarker of tumor progression (Mori, O'Day and Umetani, 2005). Methylated ER-α DNA was detected in the serum of melanoma patients with The American Joint Committee on Cancer (AJCC) stage IV disease and was a biomarker of disease progression. Furthermore, serum-circulating hypermethylated ER-α in AJCC stage IV melanoma patients predicted response to biochemotherapy, progression-free survival, and overall survival.

This suggests that *in vitro* culturing may promote the epigenetic silencing of ER-α or select for a subpopulation of cells with methylated ER-α. Similar epigenetic regulation in other cancers such as breast cancer, ovarian cancer, prostate cancer, and hepatocellular cancer has been reported. The frequency of ER-α methylation served as a marker of progression from primary to metastatic disease and from regional nodal metastasis to distant visceral metastasis. As with breast cancer, the expression of ER-α mRNA as regulated by ER-α methylation is directly or indirectly related to the development of metastasis.

In the current study, methylated ER-α was detected in the serum of stage IV melanoma patients in a pattern related to disease progression. In a subset of matched melanoma tumor and serum sample pairs, all participants with methylated DNA detected in serum had either primary or metastatic tumors with methylated ER-α as well (Mori, 2006).

The trialists attempted to predict the response to treatment based on the methylation status of ER-α in serum. The use of chemotherapy in conjunction with immune modulators (biochemotherapy) has produced better response rates in the past but outcomes differ greatly between responders and nonresponders. Before or in the early stages of biochemotherapy, it has been challenging to predict melanoma response. Identifying molecular predictors of therapeutic response may permit physicians to treat those patients most likely to respond to therapy while sparing nonresponsive patients unnecessary treatment, which usually carries side effects and pocket money. Methylated ER-α was more commonly detected in the serum of patients who failed to respond to the combine therapy mentioned above. Serum methylated ER-α was the only independent predictor of progression-free and overall survival in a multivariate analysis, surpassing even known clinical prognostic factors.

There are several plausible explanations for these findings. First, tamoxifen, a member of the selective ER modulator family, was used in the biochemotherapy regimen of 44 of 50 patients. Patients without serum methylated ER-α, who therefore expresses ER-α, may be more likely to respond to the antitumor effects of tamoxifen. On the other hand, the lack of response to biochemotherapy may be partially explained by the inability of Tam to exert its antitumor effects when ER-α expression is silenced due to promoter region hypermethylation. This fact is akin to the clinical outcome seen in patients diagnosed with breast cancer in which tumors not expressing ER-α do not respond well to hormone therapy and, hence, carrying a worst prognosis.

In this particular trial, however, the ER-α was not detected in the serum from normal healthy participants. Non-tumor cells containing methylated ER-α would be expected to release DNA into the bloodstream. The investigators believe that methylated ER-α from tumors is less efficiently than methylated ER-α from normal cells. The destruction of normal cells is primarily through an apoptosis-related mechanism, finishing in the release of small-degraded fragments of DNA, which is rapidly cleared and not easily detected in blood. On the other hand, those tumor cells that are disrupted by physical trauma or cell necrosis, release large and intact fragments of DNA. Patients diagnosed with melanoma release both cancer cells and free DNA into the blood stream. Circulating cancer cells release large fragments of DNA as a result of non-apoptotic mechanisms. The detection of methylated ER-α in melanoma patients strongly suggests that the circulating DNA is cancer - related. There was no age difference in the ER-α methylation in this trial. Among the 40 healthy patients included in the trial, methylated ER-α was detected only in one senior participant, which may be due to factors unrelated to aging (Mori, 2006; Koyanagi, Mori and O'Day, 2005).

These findings indicate that detection of methylated ER-α in serum may be an extremely useful tool to identify the population of patients with poor melanoma outcome and poor response to systemic therapy in whom alternative treatment management should be considered.

Because it is difficult to predict which primary tumors will progress to regional or distant metastases, cutaneous melanoma remains a challenging disease to manage. New strategies for the identification of epigenetic biomarkers may improve the clinical management of melanoma by facilitating earlier disease diagnosis and providing more accurate prognostic information. No major study has examined the epigenetic alterations of hormone receptors in the progression from primary to metastatic melanoma in a large series of patients before the study done by the Department of Molecular Oncology of Santa Monica, California, in 2006 (Mori, 2006).

Even though there is a variety of the mechanism of action of Tam in melanoma contented in the literature, still the adjuvant treatment of high-risk malignant melanoma remains problematic. Previously, investigators from the University of California reported moderate success in the treatment of metastatic disease using tamoxifen, cisplatin, dacarbazine and carmustine. Based upon data that suggested tamoxifen and cisplatin were the active agents in this regimen, they initiated a phase II trial of this combination of drugs for melanoma. They treated 153 patients with 4 cycles of tamoxifen (160 mg day) and cisplatin (100 mg day) for 28-day intervals. During the first 2 years of follow-up, patients were evaluated every 2 months with a history, physical exam, and laboratory work and computed tomography scans of the chest, abdomen and pelvis every 4 months. Thereafter, patients were evaluated every 3 months and radiographic studies were performed if necessary. They used a median follow-up of 36 months where they found a disease-free survival (DFS) of 68.4% and an overall survival (OS) of 84.5%. Kaplan-Meier analysis predicts a 5-year DFS of 62% with an OS of 79%. Relapses after 20 months have been rare. No effect of gender or number of positive lymph nodes was noted, however, stage of disease prior treatment was an important factor. The major toxicity proved to be gastrointestinal with nausea the most prevalent symptom. These preliminary results suggested that there is a positive impact of tamoxifen and cisplatin on both the DFS and OS of high-risk malignant melanoma patients (McClay, McClay and Monroe, 2000).

Conclusion

The most updated data with the least bias results comparing chemotherapies with and without tamoxifen shows that those systemic therapies including tamoxifen improve overall and partial response. But, on the other hand, they do not improve survival in patients with advanced melanoma. The biological reason to explain these results is still not clear, as the drug's mechanism of action in melanoma is complex and still debatable among investigators worldwide. Therefore, the most accepted theories of its role in the deadliest skin cancer of all, are the synergy role that it plays with other drugs included in the chemotherapy for advanced melanoma, the apoptosis and the anti-angiogenesis mechanism, and the interaction it exercises with the immune system.

These results suggest that there must be more than one effective process by which the tamoxifen interacts with the melanoma cells and better quality randomized clinical trials are needed to prove this.

References

Agarwala S.S., Ferri W. and Gooding W. (1999). A phase III randomized trial of dacarbazine and carboplatin with and without tamoxifen in the treatment of patients with metastatic melanoma. *Cancer, 85*, 1979–1984.

Akasaka H., Sato F. and Morohashi S. (2010). Anti-apoptotic effect of claudin-1 in tamoxifen-treated human breast cancer MCF-7 cells. *BMC Cancer, 10, 548.*

Behjati S. and Frank M.H. (2009). The Effects of Tamoxifen on Immunity. *Current Medicinal Chemistry,16*, 3076-3080.

Behl C., Weilbach F.and Apfel R. (1990). Melanoma inhibiting activity 9 MIA) –biological characterization of a neuroectodermal derived tumor growth inhibitor. *Proceedings American Association Cancer Research,* 31, 59.

Beutler B. and Cerami A. (1987). Cachectin: more than a tumor necrosis factor. *New England Journal of Medicine, 316,* 379-385.

Buecher B., Gauthiers-Millars M. and Desjardins L. (2010). Contribution of CDKN2A/P16 (INK4A), P14 (ARF), CDK4 and BRCA1/2 germline mutations in individuals with suspected genetic predisposition to uveal melanoma. *Familial Cancer, 9,* 663-667.

Chen K.G., Valencia J.C. and Lai B. (2006). Melanosomal sequestration of cytotoxic drugs contributes to the intractability of malignant melanomas. *Proceedings of the national academy of science; PNAS.*

Clinical Practice Guideline for Melanoma: *NCCN Medical Practice Guidelines and Oncology*: V.2. (2009).

Cocconi G., Bella M. and Calabresi F. (1992). Treatment of metastatic malignant melanoma with dacarbazine plus Tamoxifen. *New England Journal of Medicine, 327,* 516-523.

Del Petre S.A., Maurer L.H. and O'Donell J. (1984). Combination chemotherapy with cisplatin, carmustine, dacarbazine, and tamoxifen in metastatic melanoma. *Cancer Treatment Reports, 68,* 1403-1405.

Dewhurst L.O., Gee J.W. and Rennie I.G. (1997). Tamoxifen, 17-oestradiolandthecalmodulin antagonists J8 inhibit human melanoma cell invasion through fibronectin. *British Journal of Cancer, 75,* 860-868.

Eigentler T.K., Caroli U.M. and Radny P. (2003). Palliative therapy of disseminated malignant melanoma: a systematic review of 41 randomized clinical trials. *Lancet Oncology, 4,* 748–759.

Ernst T., Chang L. and Cooray D. (2002). The effects of tamoxifen and estrogen on brain metabolism in elderly women. *Journal of the National Cancer Institute, 94,* 592–597.

Fisher R.I., Neifeld J.P. and Lippman M.E. (1976). Estrogen receptors in human malignant melanoma. *Lancet, 2,* 337-338.

Garbe C., Paul A. and Kohler-Spath H. (2003). Prospective evaluation of a follow-up schedule in cutaneous melanoma patients: recommendations for an effective follow-up strategy. *Journal of Clinical Oncology, 21*, 520–529.

Garvin S., Nilsson U.W.and Dabrosin C. (2005) Effects of estradiol and tamoxifen on VEGF, soluble VEGFR-1, and VEGFR-2 in breast cancer and endothelial cells. *British Journal of Cancer, 93,* 1005-1010.

Gelmann E.P. (1997). Tamoxifen for the treatment of malignancies other than breast and endometrial carcinoma. *Seminars of Oncology, 24,* (Suppl 1): S1-65–S1-70.

Goodson A.G. and Grossman D. (2009). Strategies for early melanoma detection: Approaches to the patient with nevi. *Journal of the American Academy of Dermatology, 60*, 719-735.

Gupta D., Malpica A. and Deaverst M.T. (2002). Vaginal melanoma: a clinicopathologic and immunohistochemical study of 26 cases. *American Journal of Surgery and Pathology, 26*, 1450-1457.

Ho W.L., Comber H. and Murphy G.M. (2009). Malignant melanoma and breast carcinoma: a bidirectional correlation. *Irish Journal of Medical Science, 4*, DOI: 10.1007/s11845-009-0297-5.

Jones J.A., Aibright K.D.and Christen R.D. (1997) Synergy between Tamoxifen and Cisplatin in Human Melanoma Cells Is Dependent on the presence of antiestrogen – binding sites. *Cancer Research, 68,* 1403-1405.

Kanter-Lewensohn L., Girnita L. and Girnita A. (2000). Tamoxifen-induced cell death in malignant melanoma cells: possible involvement of the insulin-like growth factor-1 (IGF-1) pathway. *Molecular Cell Endocrinology, 165,* 131-137.

Koyanagi K., Mori T. and O'Day S.J. (2006). Association of circulating tumor cells with serum tumor-related methylated DNA in peripheral blood of melanoma patients. *Cancer Research, 66,* 6111-6117.

La Vecchia C., Lucchini F. and Negri E. (1999). Recent declines in worldwide mortality from cutaneous melanoma in youth and middle age. *International Journal of Cancer, 81*(1), 62-66.

Lens MB, Reiman T, Husain AF. (2003). Use of Tamoxifen in the Treatment of Malignant Melanoma. *Cancer, 98,* 1355-1361.

Lindahl G, Saarinen N, Abrahamsson A. (2011). Tamoxifen, flaxseed, and the lignan enterolactone increase stroma- and cancer cell-derived IL-1Ra and decrease tumor angiogenesis in estrogen-dependent breast cancer. *Cancer Research, 71,* 51-60.

Lissoni P., Paolorossi F. and Tancini G. (1996). A phase II study of tamoxifen plus melatonin in metastatic solid tumour patients. *British Journal of Cancer, 74,* 1466–1468.

Mallmann P. and Krebs D. (1991). Effect of tamoxifen on parameters of cell-mediated immunity in postmenopausal patients with breast carcinoma. *Zentralbl Gynakol, 113,* 689-696.

Markovick S.N., Erickson L.A. and Rao R.D. (2007). Malignant melanoma in the 21st century, part 1: epidemiology, risk factors, screening, prevention, and diagnosis. *Mayo Clinical Proceedings, 82*,364-380.

Markovick S.N., Erickson L.A.and Rao R.D. (2007). Malignant melanoma in the 21st century, part 2: staging, prognosis, and treatment. *Mayo Clinical Proceedings, 82*,490-513.

McClay E.F., Albright K.D. and Jones J.A. (1992). Modulation of cisplatin resistance in human malignant melanoma cells. *Cancer Research, 52*, 6790-6796.

McClay E.F., Albright K.D. and Jones J.A. (1993). Tamoxifen modulation of cisplatin sensitivity in human malignant melanoma cells. *Cancer Research, 53*, 1571-1576.

McClay E.F., Jones J.A. and Winski P.J. (1996). Determinants of tamoxifen sensitivity control the nature of the synergistic interaction between tamoxifen and cisplatin. *Cancer Research, 56,* 3993-3997.

McClay E.F., McClay M.E. and Monroe L., (2000). The effect of Tamoxifen and cisplatin on the disease-free and overall survival of patients with high-risk malignant melanoma. *British Journal of Cancer, 83,* 16-21.

McLean I.W. (1995). Prognostic features of uveal melanoma. *Ophthalmology Clinics of North America, 1*, 143-153.

Monnerat C., Chompret A. and Kannengiesser G. (2007). BRCA1, BRCA2, TP53, and CDKN2A germline mutations in patients with breast cancer and cutaneous melanoma. *Familial Cancer, 6*, 453-461.

Mori T., Martinez S.R. and O'Day S. J. (2006). Estrogen Receptor-alpha methylation predicts melanoma progression. *Cancer Research, 66,* 6692-6698.

Mori T., O'Day S.J. and Umetani N. (2005). Predictive utility of circulating methylated DNA in serum of melanoma patients receiving biochemotherapy. *Journal of Clinical Oncology, 23,* 9351-9358.

Nesbit M. and Herlyn M. (1994). Adhesion receptors in human melanoma progression. *Invasion Metastasis, 14,* 131-146.

Piantelli M., Tatone D. and Castrilli G. (2011). Quercetin and tamoxifen sensitize human melanoma cells to hyperthermia. *Cancer Research Resources: Hyperthermia, Melanoma, Quercetin.*

Robinson E., Rubin D. and Mekori T. (1993). In vivo modulation of natural killer cell activity by Tamoxifen in patients with bilateral primary breast cancer. *Cancer Immunology Immunotherapy, 37,* 209-212.

Rohlff C., Blagosklonny M.V. and Kyle E. (1998). Prostate cancer cell growth inhibition by tamoxifen is associated with inhibition of protein kinase C and induction of p21 (waf1/cip1). *Prostate, 37,* 51-59.

Rotstein S., Blomgren H. and Petrini B. (1988). Influence of adjuvant tamoxifen on blood lymphocytes. *Breast Cancer Research Treatment, 12,* 75-79.

Ruiz Beguerie J., Xingzhong J. and Valdez R.P. (2010). Tamoxifen vs. non-tamoxifen treatment for advanced melanoma: a meta-analysis. *International Journal of Dermatology, 49,* 1194–1202.

Sarti M.S. and Castrucci A.M.L. (2004). Biological activity and binding of estradiol to SK-Mel 23 human melanoma cells. *Brazilian Journal of the Medical and Biological Research, 37,*901-905

Sthoeger Z., Zinger H. and Mozes E. (2003). Beneficial effects of the anti-oestrogen tamoxifen on systemic lupus erythematosus of F1 female mice are associated with specific reduction of IgG3 autoantibodies. *Annals of the Rheumatic Diseases, 62,* 341–346.

Stringa O., Valdez R. and Ruiz Beguerie J. (2006). Primary amelanotic melanoma of the esophagus. *International Journal of Dermatology, 45*, 1207-1210.

The Clinical Practice Guidelines for the Management of Melanoma in Australia and New Zealand. (2008). The cancer council Australia/ *Australian cancer network/ Ministry of Health, New Zealand.*

Tomlinson S., MacNeil S. and Walker S.W. (1984). Calmodulin and cell function. *Clinical Science, 66,* 497–507.

Walker M.J., Beattie C.W. and Patel M.K. (1987). Estrogen receptor in malignant melanoma. *Journal of Clinical Oncology, 5,* 1256-1261.

Walker S.W., Mac Neil S. and Senior HJ. (1984). Calmodulin activation of cyclic AMP phosphodiesterase in the B16 mouse melanoma. *Biochemical Journal, 219,* 941–946.

Weiss M., Loprinzi C.L. and Creagan E.T. (1995). Utility of follow-up tests for detecting recurrent disease in patients with malignant melanomas. *JAMA, 274,* 1703–1705.

Index

#

A

D

E

F

G

H

M

N

O

P

T

U

V

W

X

Y

Z